NEWBORN FAMILY and NURSE

Second Edition

MARY LOU MOORE, R.N., M.A., F. A. A. N.

Nursing Coordinator and Instructor
North Carolina Perinatal-Neonatal Nursing Program
Bowman Gray School of Medicine
Winston-Salem, North Carolina

Certified Childbirth Educator (ASPO)

Nursing Staff, Intensive Care Nursery
North Carolina Baptist Hospital
Winston-Salem, North Carolina

With a contribution by

KAREN G. GALLOWAY, R.N., M.S.N.

Formerly Assistant Professor, Graduate Program
College of Nursing
University of Arkansas for Medical Sciences
Little Rock, Arkansas

1981
W.B. SAUNDERS COMPANY
Philadelphia London Toronto Sydney

W. B. Saunders Company: West Washington Square
Philadelphia, PA   19105

1 St. Anne's Road
Eastbourne, East Sussex BN 21   3UN, England

1 Goldthorne Avenue
Toronto, Ontario   M8Z   5T9, Canada

9 Waltham Street
Artarmon, N.S.W.   2064, Australia

Library of Congress Cataloging in Publication Data

Moore, Mary Lou.

Newborn family and nurse.

Earlier ed. published in 1972 under title: The newborn
and the nurse.

1. Infants (Newborn)—Care and hygiene.   2. Pediatric
   nursing.   3. Infants (Newborn)—Diseases—Nursing.
   I. Title [DNLM: 1. Pediatric nursing.   2. Infant,
   Newborn. WY159 M823n]

RJ253.M66 1981   618.92'01   80–52773

ISBN 0–7216–6491–1

Listed here is the latest translated edition of this book together with the language of the translation and the publisher.

Spanish (1st Edition)—NEISA, Mexico City, Mexico

Cover photograph courtesy of **Suzanne Szasz**

Newborn, Family and Nurse   ISBN   0-7216-6491-1

Last digit is the print number: 9   8   7   6   5   4   3   2   1

To our children:

Richard Dudley Moore, Jr.
William Eric Moore
John Christopher Moore
Virginia Anne Moore

PREFACE TO SECOND EDITION

Few experiences highlight the changes in our care of newborns in such a dramatic fashion as the revision of a textbook. Nine years have elapsed between the publication of the first edition of *Newborn and the Nurse* and this second edition. During those years, newborn care has changed in many respects.

More attention has been given to the fetus. Increased awareness of factors in the fetal environment, assessment of fetal growth, and early recognition of potential problems has resulted in improved neonatal outcome.

Family-centered care at childbirth is much more widespread than in 1972, although many families, particularly from lower income groups, are still denied this opportunity. The recognition of the importance of the family is reflected in the change in the title of this volume as well as in its content.

The care of the high risk newborn has changed markedly. Fortunately, technological change in this area has been accomplished, in most instances, with an increasing sensitivity to the needs of the baby's family. As technology continues to advance, questions of ethical values and of the infant's long-range development must be raised and addressed.

Our belief that many nurses must be knowledgeable about the newborn, expressed in the first edition, is stronger than ever. Nurses who guide mothers through pregnancy, who care for adolescents and prepare them for possible future pregnancies, who work to improve the quality of psychological and physical health for future mothers who are children today, all contribute to the well-being of newborns.

Parents and parents-to-be seek information from a large and growing group of nurses in community and hospital practice. Nurses who are knowledgeable about newborn issues can be strong advocates for change in their local community, their state, the nation, and the world.

ACKNOWLEDGMENTS

Many colleagues, friends, nurses, other professionals, and childbearing families have contributed to this volume by sharing specific information, ideas, and concerns through day-by-day conversations and through their continuing support.

In particular I want to acknowledge Dr. Keith Moore for permission to use many excellent illustrations from his book *The Developing Human,* second edition; Dr. Lewis Nelson for the ultrasound photographs; Dr. Elsie Broussard for permission to use the Broussard assessment; Drs. Ralph Traylor, Richard Trippie, and Rosita Pildes for photographs and charts; Barbara Laughinghouse, who typed the manuscript; Cathy Shaffner, who helped with many, many details; Dr. Richard Weaver, who read and commented on Chapter 8; and Bill Moore, our son, for photographs. Special recognition is due Karen Galloway, both for the chapter she contributed and for her useful suggestions in other aspects of the revision. The nursing editors at W. B. Saunders, Kathy Pitcoff and Elizabeth Cobbs, provided valuable advice.

My husband and our children, through their love and support, made it possible for me to grow and learn and write.

CONTENTS

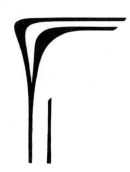

THE UNSEEN INFANT

For nine months the infant-to-be grows unseen. The chromosomes, with their genes, which are inherited from the parents, interact constantly with the environment surrounding the fetus and determine what he will be at birth and to a certain extent what he will be in the months and years that follow. By understanding what happens to the fetus during the first nine months, we are better able to understand why a newly born infant behaves as he does, and we are in a better position to answer the many questions posed by his parents. This knowledge also helps to reduce the number of ill and malformed newborns and enables us to plan for the improved health of all infants.

Embryonic Age versus Menstrual Age

Embryonic age is calculated from the time of fertilization. Menstrual age, used to describe the length of the pregnancy, is calculated for convenience from the first day of the last menstrual period. Thus, 14 days are subtracted from the menstrual age to determine the embryonic age. Embryologists describe the fetus in terms of embryonic age; obstetricians speak of weeks of pregnancy in terms of menstrual age. Thus, a woman who is "six weeks pregnant" is carrying a four-week-old em-

bryo. The descriptions in this chapter refer to embryonic age.

FERTILIZATION

Fertilization is the fusion of a sperm and an ovum. Within the head of a sperm are the nucleus, which contains the sperm's chromosomes (Chapter 2), and the acrosome, which contains the enzymes that enable the sperm to penetrate the *corona radiata* and the *zona pellucida*, which surround the ovum (Fig. 1–1). When one sperm head attaches itself to the ovum, changes in the zona pellucida and the cell membrane of the ovum inhibit the entry of additional sperm.

It has not yet been determined precisely when fertilization occurs in humans, but research indicates that it is within 12 to 24 hours after ovulation and coitus. Sperm are believed to remain alive for 24 to 48 hours in the reproductive tract, although they may survive for a longer period. Semen, which contains sperm, may be kept for as long as 10 years at temperatures between −79 and −196°C.

Between 24 and 60 hours after fertilization the fertilized egg begins to divide, first into two cells, then four, then eight, and so on. Each division is called a *cleavage*. At the same time, the fertilized egg or *zygote* passes from the fallopian tube to

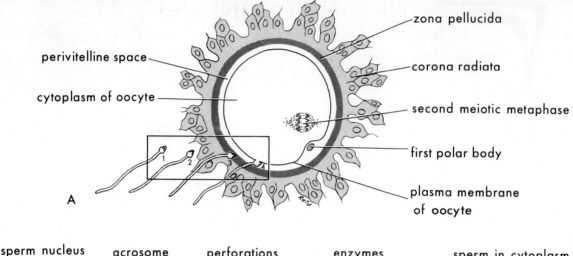

perivitelline space

cytoplasm of oocyte

zona pellucida

corona radiata

second meiotic metaphase

first polar body

plasma membrane
of oocyte

A

sperm nucleus
containing
chromosomes

acrosome
containing
enzymes

perforations
in acrosome
wall

enzymes
breaking down
zona pellucida

sperm in cytoplasm
of oocyte without its
plasma membrane

plasma membrane
of sperm

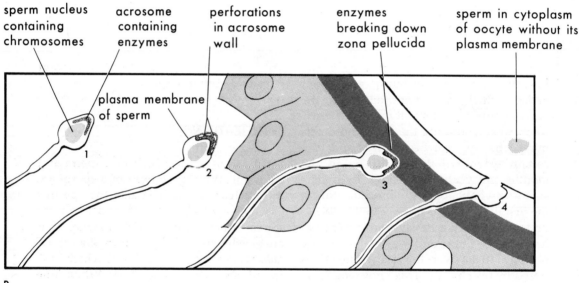

B

Figure 1–1. Diagrams illustrating the acrosome reaction and sperm penetration of an ovum. The detail of the area outlined in *A* is given in *B*. *1*, sperm during capacitation. *2*, sperm undergoing the acrosome reaction. *3*, sperm digesting a path for itself by the action of enzymes released from the acrosome. *4*, sperm head fusing with ovum. (From Moore: The Developing Human. 2nd Edition. W. B. Saunders, 1977.)

the uterus. The *morula*, a solid ball of cells, has been found in the uterus approximately three days after ovulation (Fig. 1–2).

Toward the end of the third day or early in the fourth day the morula begins to change from a solid mass of cells into a ball with a central cavity called the *blastocyst*. The cells from which the embryo will develop (*embryoblast* or inner cell mass) remain at one end of the blastocyst, while those cells that along with uterine tissue will form the placenta (*trophoblast*) gather around the periphery (Figs. 1–3, 1–4).

During the time in which the blastocyst has been dividing and traveling to the uterus (Fig. 1–5), the secretory phase of the menstrual cycle has been preparing the uterine endometrium for the ovum, as it does during every menstrual cycle. By the beginning of the second week after fertilization the trophoblast has begun to attach itself to the endometrium. The attachment of the blastocyst to the uterine wall is called *implantation*. Attachment is usually in the midposterior or midanterior segment of the fundus. In the process of implantation the blastocyst penetrates the

Figure 1–2. The morula, a solid ball of cells, about 3 days after ovulation. (Courtesy of the Carnegie Institution of Washington.)

Figure 1–3. A 58-cell blastocyst, 4 days after ovulation. (Courtesy of the Carnegie Institution of Washington.)

Figure 1–4. A 107-cell blastocyst, 4.5 days after ovulation. (Courtesy of the Carnegie Institution of Washington.)

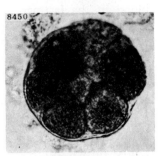

Figure 1–2.

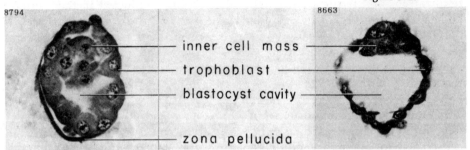

inner cell mass
trophoblast
blastocyst cavity

zona pellucida

Figure 1–3. Figure 1–4.

uterine wall, destroying the epithelium at the implantation site and sinking into the underlying connective tissue. By the ninth day after fertilization the uterine wall closes over the implanted blastocyst.

At the time of implantation the blastocyst is approximately 0.2 mm in diameter; it disappears within the uterine wall without a marked distortion of the endometrium. Thus, in humans, the embryo does not actually develop within the uterine cavity, but within a cavity of its own deep within the lining of the uterus.

The trophoblast begins a profuse proliferation by which its outgrowths further penetrate the uterine wall. At the same time it develops cavities called *lacunae*. Maternal blood flowing into the lacunae provides nutrition to the fetal tissues. Strands of trophoblast bathed by maternal

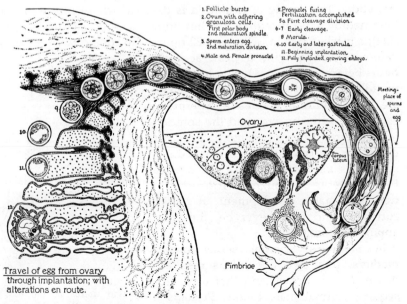

Figure 1–5. As the fertilized ovum divides to form the morula, the blastocyst, and finally the trophoblast, it travels through the fallopian tube to the uterus. (From Dickinson In Arey: Developmental Anatomy. 7th Edition revised. W. B. Saunders, 1974.)

blood in the lacunae develop into *villi*. Through progressive stages, the placenta develops at the site of interface between the uterine wall and the embryonic villi.

IN VITRO FERTILIZATION

With the birth of an infant girl named Louise Brown in England in 1978, in vitro fertilization, i.e., fertilization outside the body of a living organism, resulted in a normal human infant. Nearly 90 years of research, beginning with embryo transplants in rabbits in the 1890s, preceded this infant's birth. Human ova were first harvested from the ovaries in the 1920s.

Steptoe, the English obstetrician who cared for Louise Brown's mother, has specific criteria for potential candidates for in vitro fertilization. The mother must be less than 35 years of age, have a normal ovary and uterus, and be free of infection. Initially a diagnostic laparoscopy is performed to make sure the ovary is accessible. Any adhesions surrounding the ovary are lysed and the uterine tubes, which are scarred (the basis of the woman's infertility), are cauterized to prevent a tubal ectopic pregnancy.

The egg itself is retrieved during a subsequent laparoscopy at the time of natural ovulation. The timing of ovulation is determined by a rise in leutenizing hormone (LH); a marked rise in LH occurs 22 hours before ovulation with a peak at eight hours before ovulation. During laparoscopy, follicular fluid and the developing egg are aspirated through a needle. Sperm are combined with the egg, and the solution is transferred to a culture media until the eight- or 16-cell stage is reached. A syringe is used to introduce the morula into the uterus. Although in vitro fertilization is a major development, it is not currently, and may never be, the chief approach to infertility.

In Steptoe's original series of 79 mothers, only two live births resulted, that of Louise Brown and that of a subsequent normal male infant. Perhaps a more important result of the in vitro research has been a better understanding of normal fertilization and the early stages in the development of the embryo.

In the United States, federal funding of in vitro fertilization experiments was suspended in 1975. Such research has now been declared "ethically acceptable" by an advisory board of the Department of Health, Education and Welfare; a decision on federal funding is pending. Some research, funded through private sources, is being conducted in the United States. In late 1979 the first United States clinic offering in vitro fertilization was established in Norfolk, Virginia.

PLACENTA

The embryo is embedded within the uterine wall by nine days following conception. The layer of endometrium lying beneath the embryo at the site of implantation is the *decidua basalis*. That portion of endometrium above the embryo is the *decidua capsularis*. The remainder of the endometrium is the *decidua parietalis* (Fig. 1–6).

Until the fourth week, chorionic villi cover all of the chorionic sac, but as the sac enlarges, those portions that come in contact with the decidua capsularis begin to degenerate because of compression, which results in reduction of the blood supply. At the same time, the villi that are in contact with the decidua basalis enlarge

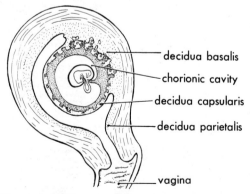

decidua basalis
chorionic cavity
decidua capsularis
decidua parietalis
vagina

Figure 1–6. Drawing of a sagittal section of the gravid uterus at the fourth week, showing the relation of the fetal membranes to the decidua. (From Moore: The Developing Human. 2nd Edition. W. B. Saunders, 1977.)

and proliferate to form the *chorion frondosum* (leafy chorion). The chorion frondosum forms the fetal component of the placenta, and the decidua basalis forms the maternal component. As the villi continue to invade the decidua basalis, wedge-shaped areas called *septa*, remain, which divide the fetal placenta into 15 to 30 *cotyledons*. Cotyledons are clearly visible on the maternal surface of the placenta at birth. Grooves are present at the locations of the septa. Fetal blood circulates within the villus, whereas maternal blood circulates outside the villus within the intervillous space (Fig. 1–7). Thus, fetal blood circulates in close proximity to maternal blood, but under normal circumstances there is no intermingling of maternal and fetal blood.

Maternal blood enters the intervillous space through the spiral endometrial arteries and flows over the villi, permitting the exchange of gases, metabolic products, and other substances, and then out through the endometrial veins (Fig. 1–7). Fetal blood flows from the fetus through the umbilical arteries (which are carrying deoxygenated blood) into the villi; following the exchange of substances, fetal blood returns to the umbilical vein and the fetus. The umbilical vein carries oxygenated blood.

Amnion and Chorion

The amniotic cavity, which will eventually surround the embryo/fetus and which contains the amniotic fluid, is present by the eighth day after fertilization when the embryo itself is a two-layer disc. The *amnion*, the inner of the two fetal membranes, begins to develop from cells in the roof of the cavity. The *chorion*, the outer

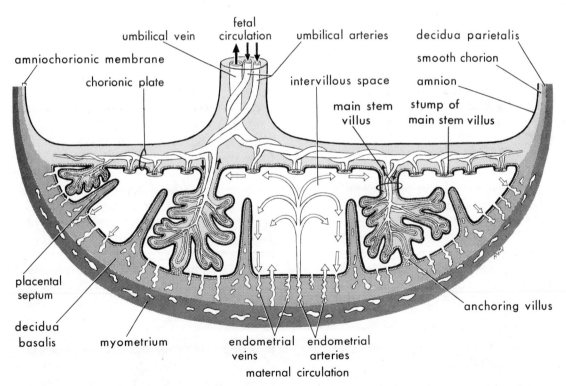

Figure 1–7. Schematic drawing of a section through a mature placenta, showing (1) the relation of the villous chorion (fetal placenta) to the decidua basalis (maternal placenta), (2) the fetal placental circulation, and (3) the maternal placental circulation. Maternal blood is driven into the intervillous space in funnel-shaped spurts, and exchanges occur with the fetal blood as the maternal blood flows around the villi. The inflowing arterial blood pushes venous blood out into the endometrial veins, which are scattered over the entire surface of the decidua basalis. Note that the umbilical arteries carry deoxygenated fetal blood to the placenta and that the umbilical vein carries oxygenated blood to the fetus. (Based on Ramsey, 1965. *In* Moore: The Developing Human. 2nd Edition. W. B. Saunders, 1977.)

fetal membrane that forms a sac in which the embryo, amnion, and yolk sac are suspended by a "stalk," forms by the end of the second week.

AMNIOTIC FLUID

Maternal blood is the principal source of amniotic fluid early in pregnancy. By seven to eight weeks the fetus begins to excrete urine into the amniotic fluid; in the late weeks of pregnancy almost half of the amniotic fluid volume (approximately 1000 ml) is fetal urine. The fetus also swallows amniotic fluid, as much as 400 ml a day, as term approaches. Thus, a fetus with nonfunctioning or absent kidneys or with a urinary tract obstruction may have decreased amounts of amniotic fluid (*oligohydramnios*), whereas a fetus with an obstruction of the gastrointestinal tract or central nervous system may have increased amniotic fluid (*polyhydramnios*) because of a decreased ability to swallow or to absorb the fluid in the intestine.

The volume of amniotic fluid is approximately 1 oz (29.6 ml) at 10 weeks, increasing to approximately 350 ml at 20 weeks and 1000 ml at term.

Umbilical Cord

The beginnings of the umbilical cord date to the fourth week, during the period in which the flat, three-layer embryo folds and becomes cylindrical. The cord contains two arteries and one vein surrounded by connective tissue called *Wharton's jelly*.

GESTATION

The First Month

While the blastocyst is becoming implanted in the uterine wall, changes are also taking place in the inner cell mass. The amniotic cavity forms, splitting the inner cell mass into an outer layer of cells, which will become the amniotic sac, and

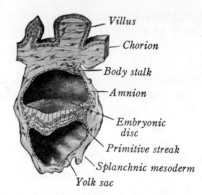

Figure 1–8. Right half of the human embryo (Brewer) of 14 days (× 85). The chorionic villi have partially penetrated the mucosa of the uterus. (From Arey: Developmental Anatomy. 7th Edition revised. W. B. Saunders, 1974.)

an inner layer, the embryonic disc. The amniotic sac forms above the embryonic disc; the yolk sac forms below it (Fig. 1–8). The human yolk sac does not contain yolk; it is so named only because it resembles the yolk sac in birds and reptiles. Thus, of all the cells that have resulted from the cleavage of the original egg, only those that form the embryonic disc will be part of the developing embryo. All the rest — amniotic sac, placenta, and cord — form its environment.

The embryonic disc begins to differentiate into two layers during the second week. By the third week there will be three layers — ectoderm, mesoderm, and entoderm. Specific types of tissue arise from each of these layers (Table 1–1). These germ layers are, in a sense, assembly grounds. During the early stages of development each germ layer had the potential for a variety of types of development. Cells first differentiate chemically and later physically. Although the master controller of this process is the genetic code, cell differentiation is more immediately influenced by *induction*, the process by which one tissue transmits a chemical stimulus that leads to the development of another tissue. For example, the nervous system begins with a median cord of cells, the notochord, which forms from the embryonic plate. The notochord then induces the cells above it to form first the neural plate and subsequently the neural tube by the end of the fourth week. When

Table 1–1 The Germ Layer Origin of Human Tissues*

Ectoderm	Mesoderm (including mesenchyme)	Entoderm
Epidermis, including cutaneous glands, hair, nails, lens	Muscle (all types)	Epithelium of pharynx, includ-ing root of tongue, auditory
Epithelium of sense organs, nasal cavity, sinuses, mouth, (including oral glands, enamel), anal canal	Connective tissue, cartilage, bone, notochord	tube, tonsils, thyroid, parathyroids, thymus
	Blood, bone marrow	Larynx, trachea, lungs
	Lymphoid tissue	Digestive tube, including associated glands
Nervous tissue, including hypophysis, chromaffin tissue	Epithelium of blood vessels, lymphatics	Bladder
	Body cavities	Vagina (all?), vestibule
	Kidney, ureter	Urethra, including associated glands
	Gonads, genital ducts	
	Suprarenal cortex	
	Joint cavities, etc.	

*From Arey: Developmental Anatomy. 7th Edition revised. W. B. Saunders, 1974, p. 83.

contact between the notochord and the cells above it is prevented experimentally, the neural plate does not develop. Moreover, if the notochord tissue is implanted under ectodermal tissue elsewhere in the body, a neural plate will develop there.

If induction fails either because of inadequate inductive stimulus or because the tissue does not react, an organ may fail to appear (agenesis), may be smaller than normal (hypoplasia), or may be incompletely differentiated. Irregularities in induction can also lead to organ duplication, such as a double kidney and ureter, or to abnormal positioning of an organ.

During the third and fourth weeks of embryonic life, a time when the mother is scarcely aware that she is pregnant, several major systems undergo remarkable development. The rudimentary nervous system has already been mentioned. The neural tube is open at first, but by the end of the fourth week the anterior end has closed to form brain tissue, and the posterior portion has closed to form the spinal cord. If for some reason the neural tube fails to close, anencephalus will occur at the anterior end; if the posterior neural tube fails to close, myelomeningocele results. For whatever reasons these defects happen, they occur very early in pregnancy.

Heart formation also begins early, at about the sixteenth day. In just eight days the circulatory system progresses from young blood cells clustered in the walls of the yolk sac, to a fine network of blood vessels, to two symmetrical tubes, to a single heart tube that is present on the twenty-second day and begins to beat about the twenty-fourth day (Fig. 1–9). Fetal heart movement may be observed by ultrasound examination in the tenth week; fetal heart sounds can be heard by Doppler ultrasound at 10 to 12 weeks and by stethoscope at 18 to 20 weeks. Further heart and circulatory development will take place over the next several weeks so that by the end of six weeks the exterior heart form is essentially what it will be at

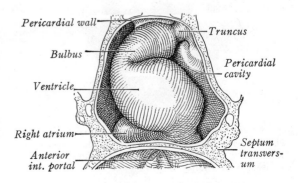

Figure 1–9. The heart at approximately three weeks. Even before the anatomical structure of the heart reaches its final form, the heart has started to beat to maintain circulation within the embryo and to provide a placental circuit. (After Davis In Arey: Developmental Anatomy. 7th Edition revised. W. B. Saunders, 1974.)

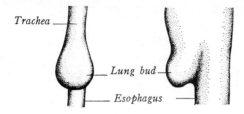

Figure 1–10. Both trachea and esophagus develop from a single entodermal tube. (After Grosser and Heiss *In* Arey: Developmental Anatomy. 7th Edition revised. W. B. Saunders, 1974.)

birth. By the seventh week the heart valves are present.

In the third week the rudimentary respiratory and digestive tracts exist as a single tube (Fig. 1–10); the potential for tracheoesophageal fistula is not difficult to imagine. By the end of the fourth week the esophagotracheal septum has begun the initial division of the two systems, and lung buds have appeared on the trachea.

Embryonic skin, a bud which will become the liver, arm and leg buds, and rudimentary kidneys are also present by the end of four weeks, only two weeks after the mother has missed a menstrual period (Fig. 1–11). Yet the embryo is no larger than a fingernail (Fig. 1–12).

The Second Month

Equally crucial to the embryo is the second four-week period. At the start of

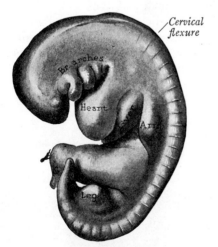

Figure 1–11. A human embryo at four weeks. (From Arey: Developmental Anatomy. 7th Edition revised. W. B. Saunders, 1974.)

this period, the embryo looks something less than human; before the four weeks are completed he is not recognizable, but he has begun to develop every system to some degree, several of them to a very high level. It is hardly surprising that disturbances in normal development during this period can lead to serious malformations.

NERVOUS SYSTEM AND MUSCLE TISSUE

During the second month, the brain becomes the largest and most complex of the embryo's developing organs. Both motor nerves, which innervate muscle tissue, and sensory nerves, which carry messages from receptors to the central nervous system, have begun to form and, in some instances, to function. Meanwhile, the muscle tissue is also developing; if for some reason innervation fails to occur, the muscle will subsequently atrophy.

HEART AND CIRCULATORY SYSTEM

The major development of the heart and great vessels occurs during the second month. In the fifth week the *endocardial cushions*, which have been developing in the dorsal and ventral walls of the heart, fuse to divide the right and left atrioventricular canals (Fig. 1–13).

The *septum primum* and *septum secundum* are developing during the same period to separate the right atrium from the left (Fig. 1–14). Because the upper part of the septum primum gradually disappears and the septum secundum forms an incomplete partition, an oval opening, the *foramen ovale*, remains. The foramen ovale is one of two fetal structures (the other being the ductus arteriosus) that shunts most blood away from the lungs during fetal life but functionally closes at birth when the lungs begin to function. The foramen ovale may not close anatomically. Abnormalities in the development of the endocardial cushions, the septum primum, or the septum secundum lead to various types of atrial septal defects.

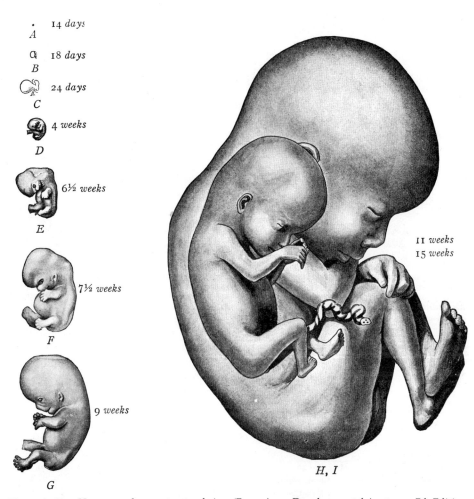

Figure 1–12.   Human embryos at natural size. (From Arey: Developmental Anatomy. 7th Edition revised. W. B. Saunders, 1974.)

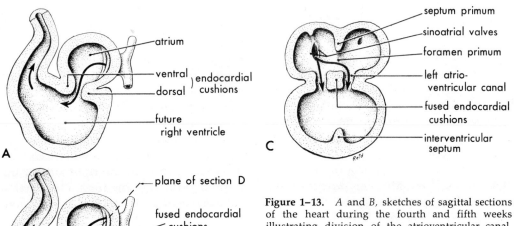

Figure 1–13.   *A* and *B*, sketches of sagittal sections of the heart during the fourth and fifth weeks illustrating division of the atrioventricular canal. *C*, frontal section of the heart at the plane shown in *B*. The interatrial and interventricular septa have also started to develop. (From Moore: The Developing Human. 2nd Edition. W. B. Saunders, 1977.)

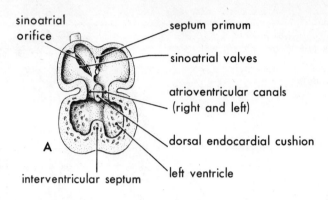

sinoatrial orifice

septum primum

sinoatrial valves

atrioventricular canals (right and left)

dorsal endocardial cushion

A

left ventricle

interventricular septum

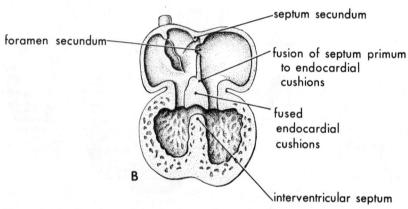

septum secundum

foramen secundum

fusion of septum primum to endocardial cushions

fused endocardial cushions

B

interventricular septum

Figure 1–14. Drawings of the developing heart showing partitioning of the atrioventricular canal, the atrium, and the ventricle. *A,* about 28 days, showing the early appearance of the septum primum, the interventricular septum, and the dorsal endocardial cushion. *B,* about 35 days, showing the foramen secundum. (Adapted from various sources, especially Patten, 1968. *In* Moore: The Developing Human. 2nd Edition. W. B. Saunders, 1977.)

The *interventricular septum* develops to close the *interventricular foramen* by the end of the seventh week. A ventricular septal defect, the result of a failure of the interventricular septum to close completely, is the most common of all congenital cardiac defects.

At five weeks, blood leaving the heart flows through a continuous structure consisting of the *bulbus cordis* and the *truncus arteriosus* (Fig. 1–15A). Truncal and bulbar ridges develop into the spinal *aorticopulmonary septum*, separating the aorta from the pulmonary trunk (Fig. 1–15B, C, D). Figure 1–15E shows the spiral form of the aorticopulmonary septum that causes the great arteries to twist around each other as

they leave the heart. Failure of the aorticopulmonary septum to develop results in persistent truncus arteriosus. Transposition of the great arteries occurs when the aorticopulmonary septum is straight rather than spiral, so that blood from the left ventricle enters the pulmonary circulation and blood from the right side of the heart flows through the aorta. Oxygenated and deoxygenated blood mix only through defects in the atrial and ventricular septa.

Unequal partitioning of the truncus arteriosus can lead to a small pulmonary trunk (pulmonary stenosis) and a large aorta that overrides both ventricles (Fig. 1–16). The small pulmonary artery causes

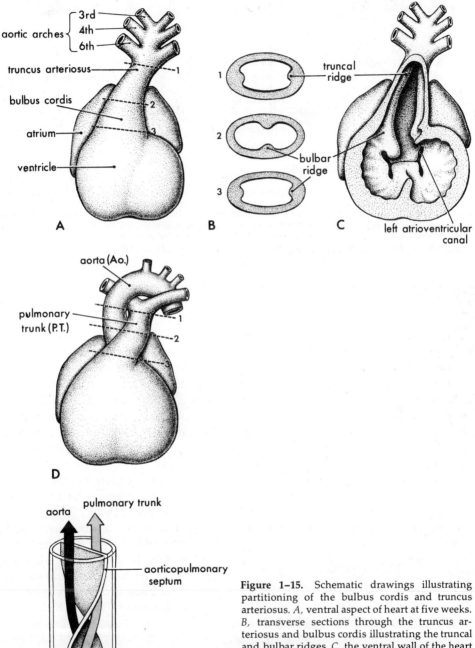

Figure 1–15. Schematic drawings illustrating partitioning of the bulbus cordis and truncus arteriosus. *A,* ventral aspect of heart at five weeks. *B,* transverse sections through the truncus arteriosus and bulbus cordis illustrating the truncal and bulbar ridges. *C,* the ventral wall of the heart has been removed to demonstrate the ridges. *D,* ventral aspect of heart after partitioning of the truncus arteriosus. *E,* diagram illustrating the spiral form of the aorticopulmonary septum. (From Moore: The Developing Human. 2nd Edition. W. B. Saunders, 1977.)

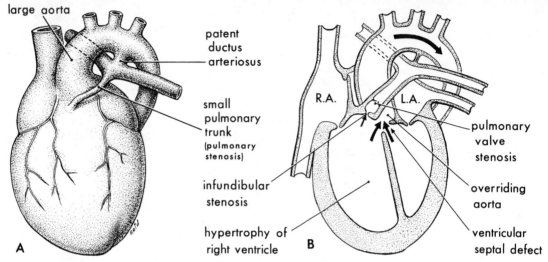

large aorta

patent
ductus
arteriosus

small
pulmonary
trunk
(pulmonary
stenosis)

infundibular
stenosis

hypertrophy of
right ventricle

R.A.   L.A.

pulmonary
valve
stenosis

overriding
aorta

ventricular
septal defect

A   B

Figure 1–16. *A,* drawing of an infant's heart showing a small pulmonary trunk (pulmonary stenosis) and a large aorta resulting from unequal partitioning of the truncus arteriosus. There is also hypertrophy of the right ventricle and a patent ductus arteriosus. *B,* frontal section of a heart illustrating the tetralogy of Fallot. (From Moore: The Developing Human. 2nd Edition. W. B. Saunders, 1977.)

right ventricular hypertrophy. These three anomalies (pulmonary stenosis, overriding aorta, right ventricular hypertrophy), in combination with a ventricular septal defect, comprise the defect called *tetralogy of Fallot.*

During the sixth to eighth weeks, aortic arch arteries, which arise from the truncus arteriosus, are transformed into their adult forms. Anomalies of the aortic arch include coarctation of the aorta, which may occur just above or below the ductus arteriosus (Fig. 1–17) and patent ductus arteriosus (Fig. 1–18). Fetal circulation is described in Chapter 5 in relation to the changes that take place at the time of birth.

RESPIRATORY SYSTEM

Respiratory development proceeds during the second month as the respiratory tract becomes separated from the digestive system and begins to subdivide into the main bronchi (Fig. 1–19). Unlike some systems, the respiratory system is not completed until after birth, with significant changes occurring at virtually the moment of delivery. This is one reason, perhaps, that the respiratory system is so vulnerable in the newborn (Chapter 8).

Until the seventh week, the diaphragm does not completely separate the thoracic cavity from the abdomen. Large openings on either side of the *septum transversum,* the major component of the diaphragm, are known as the *pleural canals.* During the sixth week, fast-growing lung buds extend down into these canals, but further longitudinal growth of the chest enables the lungs to reenter the thorax and the diaphragm to be completed in the seventh week. Failure of the canals to close results in a diaphragmatic hernia, which in the majority of instances is on the left side. The stomach, spleen, liver, or intestines may then enter the thoracic cavity, compressing the lungs and displacing the heart (Fig. 1–20). Babies with diaphragmatic hernia have severe respiratory difficulty at birth and require immediate surgical treatment (Chapter 8).

DIGESTIVE SYSTEM

The intestinal tract grows so rapidly during the second month that the abdominal cavity temporarily becomes too small to contain it. During the sixth week a portion of the intestinal loop enters the coelom (i.e., cavity) in the umbilical cord, where it will remain until the 10-week

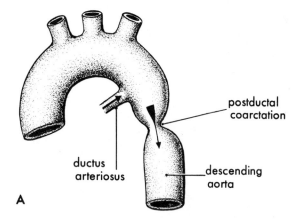

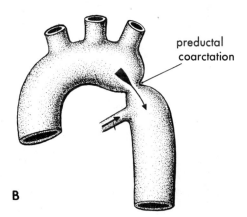

Figure 1–17. *A,* postductal coarctation of the aorta, the commonest type. *B,* preductal coarctation. (From Moore: The Developing Human. 2nd Edition. W. B. Saunders, 1977.)

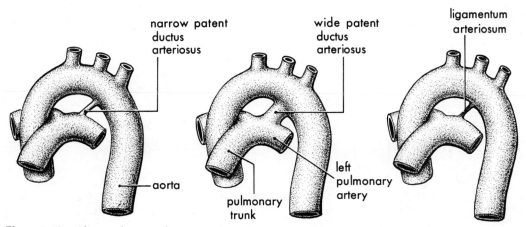

Figure 1–18. Abnormal patent ductus arteriosus in a six-month-old infant. The ductus is nearly the same size as the left pulmonary artery. (From Moore: The Developing Human. 2nd Edition. W. B. Saunders, 1977.)

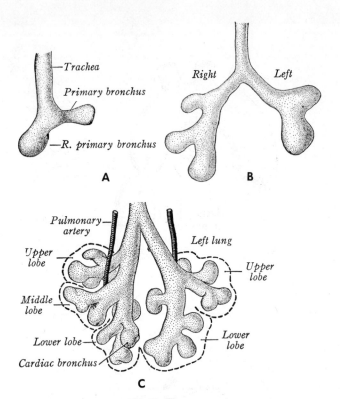

Trachea

Primary bronchus

R. primary bronchus

A

Right   Left

B

Pulmonary artery

Upper lobe

Left lung

Upper lobe

Middle lobe

Lower lobe

Lower lobe

Cardiac bronchus

C

Figure 1–19. Anatomical development of the respiratory tract. A, at 4 weeks. B, at 5 weeks. (After Heiss and Merkel.) C, at 6½ weeks. (After Ask.) (From Arey: Developmental Anatomy. 7th Edition revised. W. B. Saunders, 1974.)

gestation period, by which time the expanded length of the fetal torso along with the reduced growth of the liver and the degeneration of the *mesonephroi,* one set of rudimentary kidneys, allows sufficient room in the abdomen. Occasionally this withdrawal from the umbilical cord fails to occur and some of the intestinal loops remain outside the abdominal wall in a defect known as *omphalocele.* Or, rather than protruding through the umbilicus, intestines and sometimes all of the ab-

dominal viscera may protrude through a circular defect in the central part of the abdominal wall. Viscera are covered by peritoneum and amnion but not by skin. The thin covering sac often ruptures at the time of birth or shortly afterward.

Between the fourth and sixth weeks the *cloaca,* a common tube at the caudal end of the digestive tract, is divided laterally by the urorectal septum into the anorectal canal and the beginnings of the urogenital sinus. Urorectal and rectovaginal fistulas

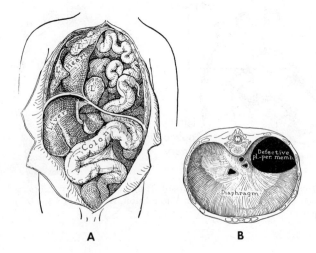

A

B

Figure 1–20. *A,* herniation of intestines into the left pleural cavity. *B,* the actual defect in the diaphragm. (From Arey: Developmental Anatomy. 7th Edition revised. W. B. Saunders, 1974.)

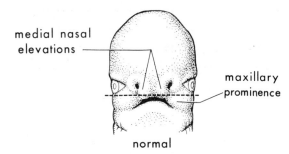

medial nasal
elevations

maxillary
prominence

normal

Figure 1–21. Drawing illustrates the embryological basis of complete unilateral cleft lip in a five-week-old embryo. (From Moore: The Developing Human. 2nd Edition. W. B. Saunders, 1977.)

are anomalies related to this part of development.

At five weeks, a labial groove is normal in embryos (Fig. 1–21). By six weeks the maxillary process should merge with the medial nasal elevation, "filling in" the groove. When this fails to occur, either unilaterally or bilaterally, a cleft lip results. A cleft palate results from a failure in the fusion of the lateral palatine processes after the eighth week of development (Fig. 1–22).

SKELETAL SYSTEM

Although there is no bony skeleton in the second month, cartilage prototypes in the shape and position of future bone already support the embryo to some extent. Ossification, the replacing of this cartilage with bone tissue, begins in the second month and continues not only throughout fetal life but until adulthood, some 18 to 20 years later. Once the cartilaginous vertebral column has formed, the embryo begins to straighten. A distinct difference in curvature can be seen in comparing the embryo at 6½ and 7½ weeks (Fig. 1–12). The embryonic period concludes at the end of the seventh week, when bone marrow formation begins in the humerus. Figure 1–23 depicts the events of the first two months of gestation.

And so the embryo reaches two months, still only an inch long, with his head

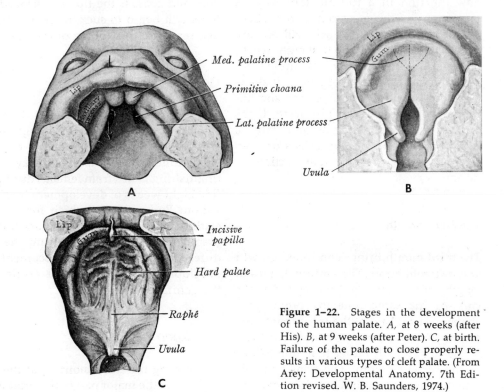

Med. palatine process

Primitive choana

Lat. palatine process

Uvula

A

B

Incisive papilla

Hard palate

Raphé

Uvula

C

Figure 1–22. Stages in the development of the human palate. *A,* at 8 weeks (after His). *B,* at 9 weeks (after Peter). *C,* at birth. Failure of the palate to close properly results in various types of cleft palate. (From Arey: Developmental Anatomy. 7th Edition revised. W. B. Saunders, 1974.)

Last Normal Menstrual Period ⟶						
Fertiliza-tion	2	3	4	Blasto-cyst	Implanta-tion begins	7
8	9	10	11	Implantation Completed		14
First Missed Menstrual Period				19	20	21
22	23	Heart beat	25	26	27	28
29	Lateral Separation: trachea & foregut	31	32	33	34	35
Fusion: lat & medial nasal processes	37	38	39	40	41	42
Second Missed Menstrual Period						

Figure 1–23.   Menstrual and embryonic timetable.

accounting for approximately half of that length. Yet many of his organ systems now function in a rudimentary way. A great many of the most common congenital defects present at birth will already have occurred during the first eight weeks of gestation. The mother has missed her second menstrual period by now; if she is a middle- or upper-class patient she has probably been seen by a physician. If she is poor, though she may be quite sure of her pregnancy, it may be weeks or even months before she will visit a clinic or doctor.

The Third Month

The third month brings continued growth and differentiation. The embryo triples in length, from 1 inch to 3 inches (2.5 to 7.5 cm). At the same time the proportions change. At the end of the third month the embryo's head accounts for only one third of the total length rather than one half as in the second month. The arms and legs also increase in length. Thin skin develops

in the third month; eyelids develop and fuse, and nails begin to grow on the fingers and toes. If the lips are stroked, the fetus will begin to suck; there is also a reflex response to stroking of the eyelids.

GENITAL SYSTEMS

Sexual differentiation is one of the major changes in this period. Although sex is determined at conception by chromosomal inheritance, there is no way of distinguishing males from females during the first eight weeks of development by observation. Both gonads, which form in the sixth week, and genital ducts are initially identical for both sexes during the "indifferent stage." Table 1–2 documents the development of some major portions of the genital systems.

RED BLOOD CELLS

It is during the third month that the liver takes over the major part of the production

Table 1–2 Homologues in the Male and Female Genital Systems*

Male	Indifferent Stage	Female
Testis	Gonad	Ovary
Seminiferous tubules	Germinal cords	Pflüger's tubules
Bladder; prostatic urethra	Primitive urogenital sinus	Bladder; greater part of urethra
Appendix testis	Paramesonephric duct (Müllerian duct)	Uterine tubes
		Uterus
		Vagina
Glans penis	Glans of phallus	Glans clitoris
Floor of penile urethra	Urethral folds	Labia minora
Scrotum	Genital swelling	Labia majora

*Adapted from Hamilton, Boyd, and Mossman: Human Embryology. Williams and Wilkins, 1962.

of red blood cells, with some blood formation also beginning in the bone marrow. Prior to this, red blood cells are produced in the yolk sac in the third and fourth weeks and by numerous blood islands scattered throughout the embryo in the ensuing four weeks.

The Second Trimester

At 12 weeks the fetus weighs 14 g (approximately one-half ounce) and is 7 cm (2.75 inches) long. During the next four weeks body growth is particularly rapid. Ossification of the skeleton is also rapid during this period, so that the fetal skeleton may be seen on x ray by 16 weeks, although only in very rare instances would x rays be taken at this stage of development. Bone marrow begins to play an increasingly important role in blood formation after the fourth month.

The rate of growth is slower in the fifth month, but this period is especially significant for the mother becuase it is the time during which *quickening,* the perception of fetal movements by the mother, occurs. Quickening is usually reported at about 20 weeks gestation (18 weeks embryonic age) by primiparous mothers and about two weeks earlier by multiparous mothers, because the latter are quicker to recognize the meaning of the faint internal flutters they are experiencing. Fetal heart tones can be heard by auscultation during this same period. The experiences of quickening and hearing the fetal heart tones make the presence of the fetus much more real to the mother.

Vernix caseosa, the white cheeselike material that covers the fetus and protects fetal skin from amniotic fluid, and *lanugo,* a fine downy hair covering the skin, are present by the twentieth week. The fetus has eyebrows and head hair. *Brown fat,* important in heat production in the newborn infant, develops in the fifth month between the shoulder blades, beneath the sternum, and around the kidneys.

By the end of the sixth month most fetal systems are mature, but a fetus born at this time will almost never survive because of respiratory tract immaturity. At the end of the second trimester the fetus weighs roughly 2 lbs (approximately 900 g), 10 times his weight at the end of the first trimester. In the fetal position, the fetus is the approximate size of an adult's hand span — 36 to 37 cm or 14 to 15 inches (Fig. 1–24).

The Third Trimester

In the third trimester, unlike the first and second, extrauterine survival is possible, although the mortality associated with birth early in the trimester is high. In the seventh month the formation of subcutaneous fat smooths out many of the wrinkles in the fetal skin. The eyes open.

During the twenty-eighth week the testes descend from the dorsal abdominal wall to the inguinal rings because of the

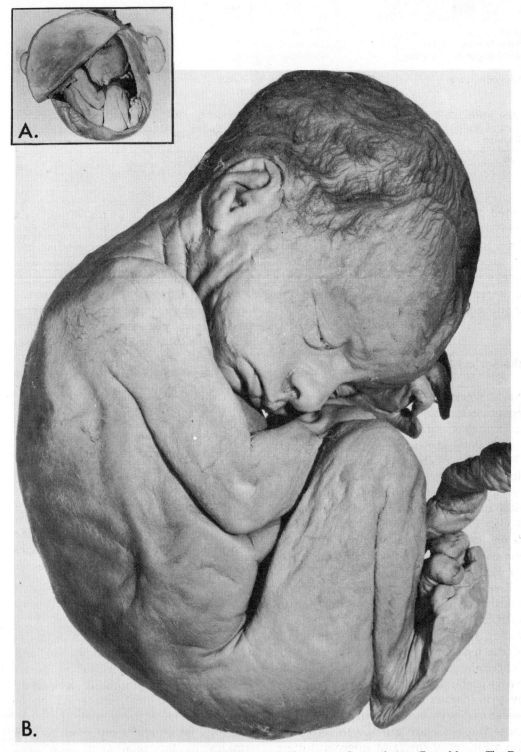

Figure 1–24.   Photographs of a 25-week-old fetus. *A,* in the uterus. *B,* actual size. (From Moore: The Developing Human. 2nd Edition. W. B. Saunders, 1977.)

elongation of the fetal trunk. Subsequently, the testes pass through the inguinal canals, entering the scrotum at about 32 weeks.

By 32 weeks the fingernails reach the tips of the fingers; toenails reach the tips of the toes by 36 weeks. Lanugo has virtually disappeared by 36 weeks. The mammary glands are prominent by 38 weeks. Many of these characteristics form the basis for the assessment of the gestational age of the newborn infant (Chapter 5).

RESPIRATORY TRACT

Between 24 and 26 weeks fertilization age (26 to 28 weeks menstrual age), thin-walled terminal air sacs, the primitive alveoli, are developing. At the same time capillaries develop in the surrounding tissue. By 26 to 28 weeks (fertilization age) gas exchange and, therefore, extrauterine life, is possible. However, even at full term, the newborn infant has only 12 to 15 per cent of the alveoli that are present at eight years of age, when the respiratory tract is fully mature. Lining the alveoli are two types of cells, Type I and Type II.

Production of pulmonary surfactant, a phospholipid substance produced by Type II cells, begins at approximately 24 weeks. By lowering surface tension within the alveoli, surfactant prevents collapse of the alveoli on expiration. Inadequate surfactant results in respiratory distress syndrome (RDS), also called hyaline membrane disease —HMD (Chapter 8). The measurement of surfactant in amniotic fluid, a test of fetal maturity, is described in Chapter 4.

EYES

Until the fourth month of gestation the retina of the eye has no blood vessels. During the fourth to eighth months vessels grow anteriorly toward the retina. Much of the anterior retina in a baby born at seven months still lacks these vessels and is consequently highly susceptible to damage by oxygen. Once vascularization is complete, the retinal vessels are no longer in danger. Unfortunately, it is the young premature baby who is most susceptible and most likely to be in need of oxygen because of other problems.

KIDNEYS

The structure of the kidney continues to change as glomeruli form throughout the third trimester. In spite of this there is not much difference in kidney function in surviving premature infants and term infants. However, the kidneys of both preterm and term infants do not tolerate stress well.

BIRTH DAY

Approximately 266 days after fertilization or 280 days from the first day of the last menstrual period (LMP) birth is expected. The majority of births occur within one to two weeks of this date. The expected date of confinement (EDC) is commonly calculated by using Nagele's rule: subtract three months from the first day of the LMP and add seven days. Thus, if the LMP began on February 25, one would count back three months to November 25 and add seven days to calculate the EDC as December 2.

SIGNIFICANCE OF EARLY DEVELOPMENT

In the review of embryological and fetal development, the important developments of the early weeks of pregnancy are obvious. During these weeks, all the major systems begin to develop. Yet during the first two weeks following conception, prior to the time of the first missed menstrual period, few women realize they are pregnant. In the weeks that follow, while many women may begin to suspect the possibility and some seek actual confirmation, most will not be active participants in the health care system until a minimum of six to eight weeks following fertilization. For many women, particularly those who are young or poor, who have limited formal education, or who have limited access to health care, entry into the system will come much later. Thus, the need for educating not only women who are pregnant but men and women about the facts of embryo/fetal development and the potential hazards to that development described in the chapters that follow, are of paramount importance in assuring the health of the unseen infant.

Bibliography

Arey, L.: Developmental Anatomy. 7th Edition revised. Philadelphia: W. B. Saunders, 1980.

Moore, K.: The Developing Human: Clinically Oriented Embryology. 2nd Edition. Philadelphia: W. B. Saunders, 1977.

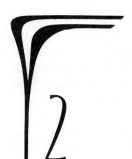

THE GENETIC BASIS OF DEVELOPMENT

The development of a single fertilized egg into a marvelously complex human infant is governed continually by hereditary factors, by the infant's own internal environment, by the environment of his mother's body, and by the environment surrounding his mother. After several decades of debate it now seems evident that both the genetic potential of the *gametes* (the single sperm cell and the single ovum that it penetrates) and the environment interact continually from the time of conception until death.

How does a gene determine development? Genes are chemical complexes of information that govern the specific traits an individual will develop. A specific gene governs a specific trait (e.g., eye color), although a trait may be affected by more than one gene (see polygenic traits). It has been estimated that human genes govern approximately 50,000 traits.

The chemical complex of which genes are composed is deoxyribonucleic acid or DNA. The DNA molecule consists of two sugar phosphate strands arranged in a double helix. Attached to these strands are four chemical substances: adenine, guanine, cystosine, and thymine (Fig. 2–1). As the two strands of the molecule unwind, two new identical molecules are formed. In this way the genetic material in the cells duplicates itself to pass an exact copy of its biological information to the next generation of cells.

A single segment of the helical strand, involving one sugar portion to which one phosphate group and one purine or pyrimidine are attached, is termed a *nucleotide*. Each gene is estimated to be made up of a chain of from 200 to 2000 nucleotides.

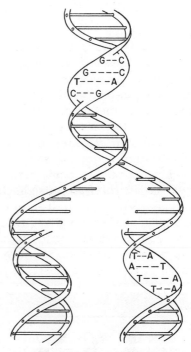

Figure 2–1. Replication of DNA. Note that the original molecule (top) unwinds, and the halves separate. The new half molecules of DNA are formed on the old halves by adenine (*A*) pairing with thymine (*T*) and by guanine (*G*) pairing with cytosine (*C*). (From Moore: Realities in Childbearing. W. B. Saunders, 1978.)

21

As many as 3000 genes, in turn, make up a single chromosome.

Chromosomes are threadlike strands of genetic material. Unlike the number of genes, which can only be approximated, the number of chromosomes for a given species is known and is specific to that species. For example, there are 20 chromosomes in corn, 48 in the chimpanzee, and 46 in the human. Since chromosomes exist in pairs, except in the gametes, man has 23 pairs of chromosomes.

The genes associated with each chromosome are transmitted as a group called a *linkage group*, rather than independently. If chromosomes (or linkage groups) always remained intact, and humans always inherited 23 groups of genes, possible trait combinations would be somewhat more limited than they are. However, because of a process termed *crossing over*, in which two chromosomes of a pair may interchange sections and thus genes, linkage groups do not remain constant (Fig. 2–2).

Each gene is located at a particular spot on a particular chromosome called the *locus*. For example, the gene for color-blindness will always be found at the same locus on the same chromosome. The function of the genes at any specific point on each chromosome is the same for all chromosomes of that type. Thus, not only chromosomes but also genes exist in pairs. In any pair of genes there may be two contrasting forms or states of the gene, known as *alleles*. Some genes have multiple alleles; there are three alleles for blood type — A, B, and O. If an individual has similar alleles for a given trait, he is said to be homozygous for the particular gene. He may, for example, have two alleles for A type blood, designated AA.

When alleles differ, the individual is heterozygous, such as the man with AB blood. In heterozygous combinations, one allele, the *dominant* allele, may manifest itself in the *phenotype* (visible characteristic), whereas the other allele, which is *recessive,* is not apparent. Only when the zygote receives two recessive alleles will recessive traits be expressed. Examples of the inheritance of dominant and recessive traits are found on page 27.

Twenty-two of man's 23 pairs of chromosomes are *autosomes*, i.e., they are alike in both sexes. The *sex chromosomes,* designated XX in the female and XY in the male, are the remaining pair. In egg cells the sex chromosome is always X. Half of the sperm cells carry the X chromosome, the other half the Y chromosome. The sperm cell as it unites with the egg to form the zygote determines the sex of the new organism, a sperm cell with an X chromosome producing a female (XX) and a sperm cell with a Y chromosome producing a male (XY). The X chromosome is much larger than the Y chromosome and carries genes for a number of traits as well as determines sex. These traits are called X-linked traits; hemophilia and red-green colorblindness are two examples. There is currently disagreement among geneticists as to whether the Y chromosome in humans contains genetic information other than maleness; one trait, the hairy pinna, is specifically known to be carried by the Y chromosome (Thompson and Thompson 1980).

Human chromosomes have been classified on the basis of size and the position of the *centromere* (the point at which the *chromatids* or strands of the chromosome are joined). Since it is often difficult to identify all 23 pairs of chromosomes in an individual sample, it has become an accepted practice to organize them into seven groups, identified by the letters A through G in order of decreasing length. A systematically arranged set of chromosomes is called a *karyotype* (Fig. 2–3). Cells for karyotyping may be white blood cells (red blood cells have no nucleus so they have no chromosomes) or tissue cells obtained in biopsy.

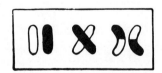

Figure 2–2. Crossing over: the exchange of material between paired chromosomes. (From Arey: Developmental Anatomy. 7th Edition revised. W. B. Saunders, 1974.)

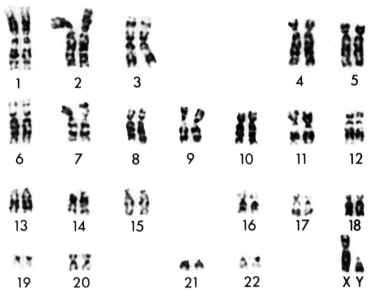

Figure 2–3. A karyotype of human chromosomes. (Courtesy of R. G. Worton *In* Thompson and Thompson: Genetics in Medicine. 2nd Edition. W. B. Saunders, 1975.)

Cells from amniotic fluid, obtained through amniocentesis (Chapter 4), are used to study fetal chromosomes. These cells are fetal in origin and some of them will grow in culture. The most successful results have been with 10 to 20 ml of amniotic fluid obtained between 14 and 16 weeks of gestation. It takes approximately four weeks to culture the cells for karyotyping, a fact parents must understand. Cell growth is successful in about 85 to 90 per cent of cultures; when fetal cell growth is poor a second amniocentesis is necessary.

Following culture, the cells are chemically treated to arrest mitosis at metaphase (Fig. 2–4). The chromosomes are spread out and flattened. Slides can then be made for examination and photography. Individual chromosomes are cut from the photograph, matched in pairs, and mounted according to the standard classification, usually called the Denver classification because of its adoption at a meeting in Denver, Colorado, in 1960.

CELL DIVISION

Two different processes of cell division keep the number of chromosomes in both gametes and other cells constant. *Mitosis* is the process by which all cells, other than those that produce the gametes, divide. Just prior to division each chromosome duplicates to form two identical chromosomes. The two daughter cells are identical to each other and to the parent cell (Fig. 2–4).

Gametes are produced by *meiosis* rather than mitosis so that the number of chromosomes will always be halved in these germ cells. The zygote, formed when sperm and egg unite, will then contain the correct number of chromosomes for each species. Unlike the daughter cells produced by mitosis, the daughter cells of meiosis are not identical to each other or the parent cell, each containing only half the genetic material of the mother cell. For instance, if the mother cell contained one allele for blue eye color and one allele for brown eye color, each gamete would contain only one of these alleles.

In meiosis, chromosomes join in pairs, one chromosome of each pair coming from each parent cell. Each chromosome then duplicates, forming four similar strands called *tetrads*. The mother cell divides into two daughter cells, each of which divides again, so that each of the resulting four

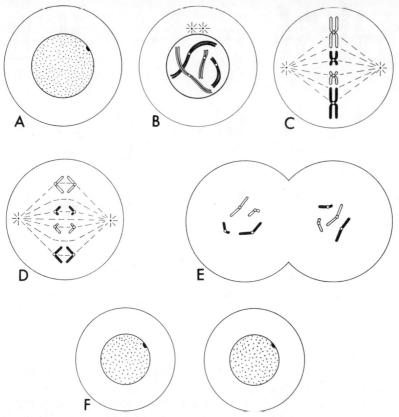

Figure 2–4. The stages of mitosis showing two of the 23 pairs of chromosomes. *A,* before mitosis (interphase). *B,* chromosomes have duplicated and become visible (prophase). *C,* chromosomes line up at the equatorial plane of the cell (metaphase). *D,* division (anaphase). *E,* chromosomes arrive at the poles of the cells; the division of cytoplasm begins (telophase). Eventually a complete membrane is formed across the cell, producing two new daughter cells. *F,* two daughter cells, identical with the former single cell. (From Thompson and Thompson: Genetics in Medicine. 3rd Edition. W. B. Saunders, 1980.)

daughter cells contains one strand from the tetrad (Fig. 2–5).

Since each gene contributes 23 chromosomes to the zygote, inheritances from the parent cells are equal. Moreover, of the 46 available chromosomes possessed by each parent, only 23 will actually be available to the new individual. Genetically there is no "chip off the old block" in the sense that no child can be just like either parent. Two children of the same parents may resemble each other closely in genotype (total gene content) or in phenotype, or they may be very different, depending on the genes they have received (and discounting the fact that the environment of each will also vary). The real surprise is not that some children fail to resemble either parent very closely, considering the tremendous number of potential combinations between two people, but that strong similarities can be seen rather frequently in even more distant relatives.

Twins may or may not have the same genotype. Dizygotic (fraternal) twins result when two separate ova are fertilized by two separate sperm. Their genotype, including their sex, is no more likely to be alike than is the genotype of any other brother and sister. Monozygotic (identical) twins result when one egg and one sperm unite to form a single zygote and then split at an early stage of zygote development. These twins have the same genotype and must, of course, be of the same sex.

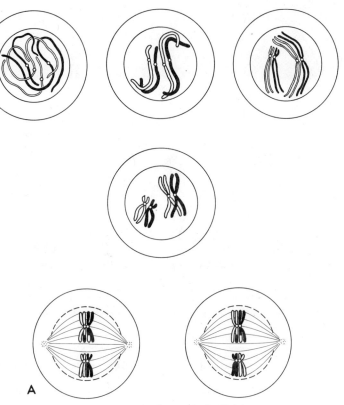

A, the first meiotic division.

Figure 2–5. *A,* the first meiotic division.

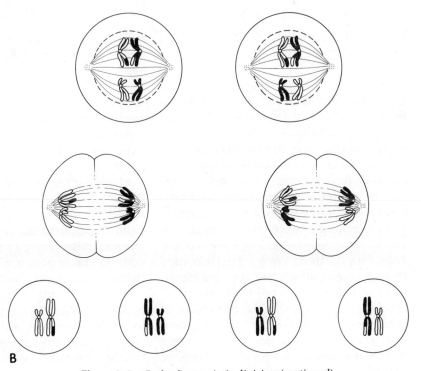

Figure 2–5. *B,* the first meiotic division (continued).

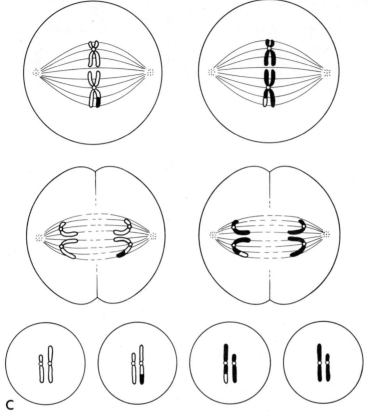

C

Figure 2–5. *C,* the second meiotic division. (From Thompson and Thompson: Genetics in Medicine. 3rd Edition. W. B. Saunders, 1980.)

THE GENETIC INHERITANCE OF CHARACTERISTICS

As genetic counseling becomes increasingly prevalent, it is important that nurses be aware of some of the basic principles governing inheritance. Many of these principles can be applied in very practical ways to help answer some of the questions about unborn and newborn infants and about future pregnancies that are of great concern to parents. Often questions revolve around characteristics that are debilitating or deforming. Both normal and pathological traits may be inherited through alleles of a gene that are dominant, recessive, X-linked, or polygenic.

Before considering the various modes of inheritance, it is essential to understand that when there is a one in four chance that a particular genetically controlled condition will be inherited by the child of a specific man and woman, those same odds prevail for every pregnancy involving those two individuals because of the way genes segregate during meiosis und recombine at fertilization. It does not mean that if they have one child with a particular disorder (e.g., cystic fibrosis) in which there is a one in four risk that the next three children will not have cystic fibrosis.

Moreover, no matter how many children of whatever genotype have been produced by the parents, each succeeding child has exactly the same probability as the first child. The possibilities are analogous to the toss of a coin. If the coin is tossed a large number of times, one expects an approximately equal number of heads and tails. But if a person happens to throw 50 heads in a row, the odds are still even on the fifty-first toss. So too does chance determine which alleles will be present in a particular zygote.

It is equally important to recognize that

every individual carries from four to eight deleterious genes, i.e., genes for some genetic disorder. Most of these genes will never be expressed in our phenotype because of the principles that govern inheritance, but the genes exist nevertheless.

Dominant Inheritance

Hyperphalangy (an extra phalanx) of the thumb and one type of achondroplasia, a disorder of cartilage that leads to a specific type of dwarfism (Fig. 2–6), are examples of hereditary malformations caused by dominant alleles.

If "A" is used to represent the allele for achondroplasia and "a" the nonachondroplastic form of the gene, the possible situations in which achondroplasia is inherited can be demonstrated. Since the dominant allele will be expressed in the phenotype, any combination of alleles that includes "A" will result in an achondroplastic dwarf:

1. If one parent is of normal stature (genotype aa) and the other parent has achondroplasia (genotype Aa) there are four possible combinations of alleles. (Remember that because of meiosis the egg cell and the sperm cell will each contain only one of the parent's two alleles.) The children who inherit the genotype aa will be normal with respect to achondroplasia; the children who inherit the genotype Aa will be achondroplastic dwarfs.

Parents	*A*	*a*
a	*Aa*	*aa*
a	*Aa*	*aa*

2. If neither parent has achondroplasia, the child cannot inherit the condition from his parents. However, achondroplastic dwarfs are born to normal parents. Mørch, reviewing 94,075 births in a Danish hospital, found 10 achondroplastic dwarfs. Two of these children had one parent who was achondroplastic and thus inherited the condition from the parent. The other eight, however, were born into families in which neither parent was achondroplastic. In these cases the gene may have been a new mutant, or the child may have been homozygous for a recessive gene carried by each parent for Ellis van Creveld syndrome, which includes achondroplasia as well as other symptoms.

Recessive Inheritance

Cystic fibrosis and phenylketonuria (PKU) are examples of traits inherited through recessive genes. Unlike dominant alleles, which may appear in every generation in the phenotype, recessive alleles may be carried for many generations without being manifest; this is the mode of transmission for most of our own deleterious

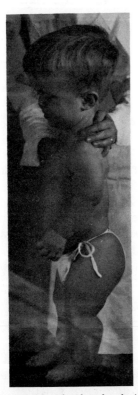

Figure 2–6. A child with achondroplasia, a cartilage disorder that leads to a specific kind of dwarfism. Because the long bones are most severely affected, body disproportion becomes increasingly obvious with growth. One type of achondroplasia is governed by a dominant gene. Another syndrome, Ellis van Creveld, which is autosomal recessive, leads to congenital achondroplasia plus other symptoms. (From Speck *In* Vaughan, McKay, and Behrman (eds.): Nelson Textbook of Pediatrics. 11th Edition. W. B. Saunders, 1979.)

genes mentioned previously. It is only when two recessive alleles for the same trait are present in a single genotype that the trait is expressed.

PKU will be used to illustrate the inheritance of recessive alleles. The allele for PKU, since it is recessive, is designated "p"; the normal, dominant allele as "P." To have PKU, the infant must have the genotype "pp", i.e., two recessive alleles.

1. If neither parent carries an allele for PKU, neither the condition nor any allele for the condition can be transferred to the infant.

2. One parent may carry the recessive allele for PKU. Since the allele is recessive and will not appear in any outward characteristic, the individual will probably be unaware of its presence. He will differ in genotype but not in phenotype. If the other parent does not carry the recessive allele "p" none of the children will have PKU, but the odds are that half the children will carry the recessive allele. It is in this manner that a recessive allele may be carried for many generations before finding expression in the phenotype.

Parents	P	P
P	PP	PP
p	Pp	Pp

3. If both parents carry the recessive allele for PKU, although they will display no outward evidence of the condition, the possibility now exists for a child to be born with PKU, i.e., a child with the genotype "pp."

Parents	P	p
P	PP	Pp
p	Pp	pp

4. If one parent has the genotype "pp" and the other carries no allele for PKU, every child will be a carrier of the recessive allele but no child will have PKU.

Parents	p	p
P	Pp	Pp
P	Pp	Pp

5. However, if a person with PKU mates with a person carrying the recessive allele, the odds are now two in four that they could have a child with PKU; any child who did not have PKU would be a carrier.

Parents	p	p
P	Pp	Pp
p	pp	pp

6. If both parents have PKU, all the children will have the condition.

Parents	p	p
p	pp	pp
p	pp	pp

Once a child with PKU is born to phenotypically normal parents, the genotypes of the parents in relation to PKU are known; both must carry the recessive allele. All future children should be observed carefully from the time of their birth and appropriate treatment instituted when necessary.

Until recently, few infants with PKU became reproducing adults. However, with early identification and treatment, adults with the genotype "pp" may become parents.

X-linked Characteristics

The majority of genes are carried by the 22 pairs of autosomal chromosomes, and it makes no difference whether the alleles causing a specific condition are inherited from the mother or the father. It has already been mentioned, however, that X chromosomes, in addition to determining sex, carry other genes as well. Hemophilia is one of the best known of the X-linked characteristics. If the symbol "h" represents the X gene that transmits hemophilia and "H" represents the X gene that does not, we have the following possible combinations of genes:

hY: hemophiliac male
HY: normal male
hh: hemophiliac female
Hh: carrier female
HH: normal female

Consider the possible combinations:

1. If the mother carries no gene for hemophilia (HH) but the father is a hemophiliac (hY), all the daughters will be carriers but the sons will neither have the disease nor be carriers. The daughters are carriers rather than hemophiliacs because one X chromosome, the one inherited from their mother, has the normal gene that is dominant over the allele for hemophilia inherited from their father.

Father	Mother	
	H	H
h	Hh	Hh
Y	HY	HY

2. If the mother carries the hemophiliac allele (Hh) but the father is not a hemophiliac (HY), the chance at each pregnancy is 50 per cent that a daughter will be a carrier and 50 per cent that a son will have hemophilia.

Father	Mother	
	H	h
H	HH	Hh
Y	HY	hY

3. If a woman who carries the recessive allele (Hh) marries a man with hemophilia (hY), their daughters will all be either carriers or hemophiliacs, but there is a 50 per cent probability that a son will have hemophilia.

Father	Mother	
	H	h
h	Hh	hh
Y	HY	hY

Polygenic Inheritance

Unfortunately, at least from the standpoint of unraveling genetic puzzles, not all traits are inherited in as straightforward a manner as the three modes described. Polygenic or multifactorial inheritance is due to the combined action of two or more genes. Variations in height, fingerprint ridges, and arterial blood pressure are examples of traits in which there is a polygenic component (Roberts and Pembrey 1978). Neural tube defects, such as spina bifida and anencephaly (Chapter 4) are examples of polygenic disorders in the newborn. Other conditions believed to be transmitted by polygenes include clubfoot, congenital dislocation of the hip, cleft lip and palate, and pyloric stenosis.

It is not possible to calculate potential risks for polygenic traits in the same way as they are calculated for single gene traits. Instead, risk factors are based on actual birth records. For example, when parents have one child with cleft lip, there is a four in 100 chance of recurrence. When one child has spina bifida or anencephaly, the chances of recurrence are five in 100. Notice that the risks in these polygenic conditions are much lower than the risks in single gene disorders. In general, the risks for polygenic traits are approximately 5 per cent (five in 100).

Genetic Penetrance

Penetrance refers to the fact that at times a gene may produce an effect that is easily recognized and at other times it may produce no effect at all. When an effect is produced or expressed, penetrance is said to be complete. When the effect is not produced, penetrance is partial or incomplete. Incomplete penetrance may be due to the action of other genes or to environmental factors. For example, environmental factors such as maternal nutrition and maternal illness may affect the fetus's genetic potential for growth and thus modify birth weight. The possibility of incomplete penetrance makes interpreting genetic probabilities more difficult.

Summary

Genes, which direct the growth and differentiation of the infant-to-be, can cause abnormal development if they themselves are abnormal. Mutant (abnormal) genes may be passed from generation to generation through decades and even centuries, or they may be newly developed in the infant's parents. Dobzhansky (1962) has estimated that perhaps as much as 20 per cent of the population carries mutant genes that arose for the first time in the immediately preceding generation. Some mutants arise because of environmental influence; others seem to occur spontaneously for reasons that are not clear at this time, though it is known that radiation and certain drugs increase the probability of mutation. In the case of x ray, the probability of mutation increase may be double the natural rate (Papazian 1967).

CHROMOSOMAL ABNORMALITIES

Abnormalities can occur in chromosomes as well as in genes, with consequent abnormalities in the infant. Because of the large number of genes located on each chromosome, chromosomal changes produce not just one but a constellation of irregularities.

Several types of chromosomal abnormalities can occur, involving either the autosomes or the sex chromosomes. The most common is *nondisjunction*. If, during the meiotic process, a chromosome pair fails to separate as it should, one gamete will contain not one but two of a given chromosome (Fig. 2–7). If the two-chromosome gamete then unites with a normal gamete to form a zygote, the zygote will then have three of that particular chromosome; hence the term *trisomy* (Fig. 2–8). During the same meiotic division, one gamete will recieve no chromosome, but gametes lacking an autosome do not seem to form a viable zygote. Nondisjunction can also occur during mitosis after the zygote has been formed.

Down's syndrome, which most often results from trisomy of the twenty-first chromosome (Figs. 2–9, 2–10), is usually a result of nondisjunction. Occasionally Down's syndrome is due to a second type of abnormality called *translocation*. During meiosis, translocation occurs when chromosomes of two different pairs exchange segments. When Down's syndrome is due to translocation, the exchange is usually, but not always, between a chromosome of the D group, frequently number 14, and a number 21 chromosome. In this instance the child with Down's syndrome will have only two number 21 chromosomes (not three, as in trisomy 21). However, there is a chromosome that is a composite of number 14 and number 21 chromosomes and contains the genetic material of each; thus, the total amount of genetic material for the number 21 chromosome is equivalent to that of three chromosomes. The effect on the child is the same; the child has Down's syndrome.

When translocation occurs at the first meiotic division, four types of gametes are possible: (1) normal chromosomes and a

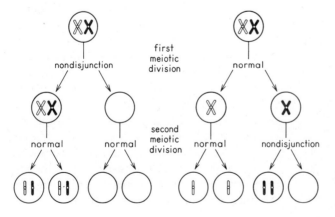

Figure 2–7. Nondisjunction can occur during either the first or second meiotic division. (The term "normal" in this diagram refers to the process of cell division, not to the cells themselves.) (From Thompson and Thompson: Genetics in Medicine. 3rd Edition. W. B. Saunders, 1980.)

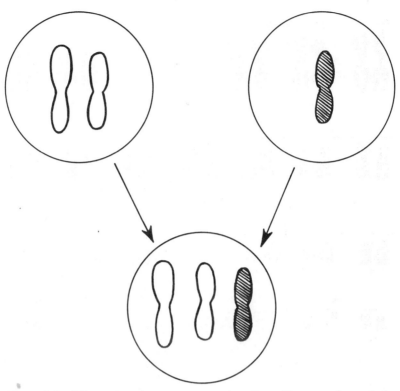

Figure 2–8. When a two-chromosome gamete unites with a normal gamete the zygote exhibits trisomy.

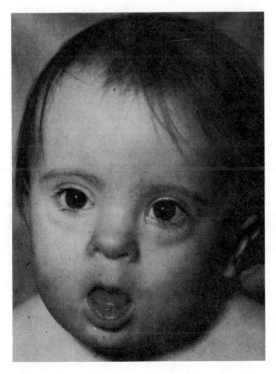

Figure 2–9. A child with trisomy 21 (Down's syndrome). (From Smith: Recognizable Patterns of Human Malformation. 2nd Edition. W. B. Saunders, 1976.)

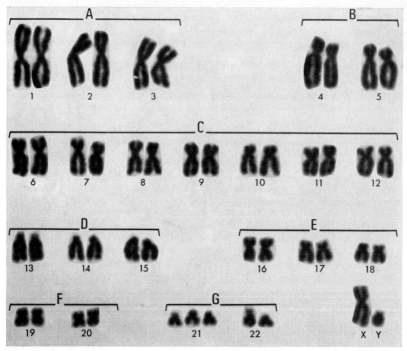

Figure 2–10. Trisomy 21 karyotype. Note that in the G group there are three 21 chromosomes. Compare this karyotype with Figure 2–3. (From Walker, Carr, Sergovich, Barr, and Soltan: J Ment Defic Res 7:150–163, 1963.)

normal gamete; (2) a normal number 14 chromosome and a fragment but no number 21 chromosome, so that if fertilized the zygote would not be viable; (3) a composite of number 14 and number 21 chromosomes and a normal number 21 chromosome, which would result in a child with Down's syndrome although there are 46 chromosomes; (4) a composite of number 14 and number 21 chromosomes and a fragment; following fertilization the individual would have only 45 chromosomes but would have the normal amount of genetic material and would be a translocation carrier.

Of children with Down's syndrome born to mothers younger than 30, 8 to 10 per cent of the cases are due to translocation. Of these translocation Down's children, approximately two thirds of the parent pairs have a normal karyotype, and the translocation occurred with the cell division at this pregnancy. In the remaining third one parent is a translocation carrier. For some reason that is not now apparent, the likelihood of a child with Down's syndrome is 10 per cent when the

mother is the translocation carrier and only 2 per cent when the father is the translocation carrier.

One might well wonder whether these seemingly highly technical differences are merely medical curiosities. It should be stressed that they do have some value in genetic counseling. When the basis of Down's syndrome in an individual child is determined (by obtaining family history related to Down's syndrome, by karyotyping the infant, and sometimes by karyotyping parents as well), the likelihood that the syndrome may be repeated in future children can be evaluated more accurately. In the case of trisomy 21, the risk of having another affected child is considered to be two to three times the risk for the normal mother in the same age group, the risk rising with the age of the mother. The prenatal detection of Down's syndrome is discussed in Chapter 4.

In addition to trisomy 21, trisomy 18 —E syndrome (Fig. 2–11) — and trisomy D also result from nondisjunction, the letters in both instances referring to the groups of chromosomes involved. Affect-

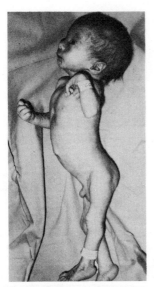

Figure 2–11. A 4-day-old male with trisomy 18 (E syndrome). Note the prominent occiput, micrognathia, low set ears, short sternum, narrow pelvis. (Courtesy of Robert E. Carrel from Uchida and Summitt *In* Vaughan, McKay, and Behrman (eds.): Nelson Textbook of Pediatrics. 11th Edition. W. B. Saunders, 1979.)

Mosaicism is difficult to detect when tissue is taken from a single site for examination.

The Sex Chromosomes and Abnormalities

Several anomalies are a result of abnormalities of the sex chromosomes with the individual possessing a number of possible combinations of X and Y chromosomes other than the normal female XX or the normal male XY. The XXY (Klinefelter's syndrome), occurring once in 400 male births (Fig. 2–12) and XO (Turner's syndrome), occurring once in 3000 live births (Fig. 2–13), are two of the more common abnormal combinations.

In general, those persons with unusual

ed infants are born with severe multiple deformities and usually die in the first months after birth. Sufficient data on which to base risk figures for recurrence are not currently available.

Other chromosomal aberrations include *deletion,* in which a piece of chromosome breaks off and is lost; *duplication,* with an extra piece of chromosome either in the chromosome itself, attached to another chromosome (translocation), or existing as a separate unit; the development of *isochromosomes* because of an abnormal splitting; and *chromosomal mosaicism,* in which an individual has at least two different cell lines with different chromosome compliments. Mosaicism always occurs after fertilization during mitosis, leaving cells with two different types of chromosomes to develop. It may involve the sex chromosomes or, less commonly, the autosomes. In rare instances, children with Down's syndrome may have mosaicism, with some cells having 46 chromosomes and others 47 chromosomes. Some of these children will have only a few symptoms of the syndrome, whereas others will have a full range of symptoms.

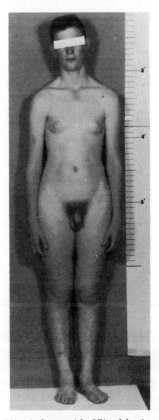

Figure 2–12. A boy with Klinefelter's syndrome, showing small testes and gynecomastia (female development of the breasts), the latter not always being present. Many affected males are mentally retarded. (Courtesy of M. L. Barr *In* Thompson and Thompson: Genetics in Medicine. 3rd Edition. W. B. Saunders, 1980.)

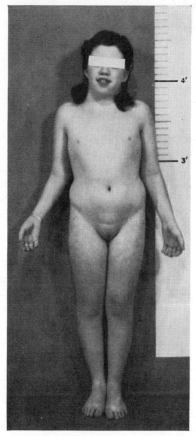

Figure 2–13. A girl with Turner's syndrome. Note the short stature, low-set ears, mature facial appearance, wide chest with broadly spaced nipples, poorly developed breasts, and juvenile external genitalia. The ovary is usually only a streak of connective tissue. (From Barr: Am J Hum Genet 12:118–127, 1960.)

Nondisjunction can occur at either the first or the second meiotic division. For the sake of example, assume that it occurs at the first:

XX
First meiotic divison
XX   O
Second meiotic division
XX   XX   O   O

The potential combinations following fertilization with a normal sperm (XY) would then be:

| | Mother | |
Father	XX	O
X	XXX	XO
Y	XXY	YO

XO represents Turner's syndrome and XXY represents Klinefelter's syndrome. YO would not be viable. Females with the XXX pattern have been frequently found in surveys of hospitals for the retarded and among women in infertility clinics. They may be relatively common in the general population as well.

Causes of Chromosomal Breakage

What causes chromosomal breakage, with resultant deletions, translocations, and other abnormalities? Like genetic mutations some appear to arise spontaneously. Radiation is a factor in certain deletions and translocations. Maternal age correlates with nondisjunction. Since viruses can produce fragmentation of chromosomes, they may play a role in resultant abnormalities. LSD has been suspect in relation to chromosomal breakage, but a final verdict awaits further research.

genotypes will be phenotypically male if they have a Y chromosome (e.g., XXY) and phenotypically female if they do not (e.g., XO). The higher the number of extra chromosomes, the greater the likelihood of abnormality in the phenotype.

One example of nondisjunction in a single ovum illustrates how some unusual combinations can arise. Nondisjunction can take place in the sperm as well.

In the normal process of meiosis the XX chromosomes of the normal female would be divided:

XX
First meiotic division
X   X
Second meiotic division
X   X   X   X

GENETIC COUNSELING

Before considering the process of genetic counseling for others, each of us must recognize that every individual carries from four to eight deleterious genes that, under specific circumstances of mating or environment, would become manifest in our phenotype. The idea that couples who produce infants with genetic defects are in some way different from the rest of us is fallacious. Anyone, rich or poor, of any racial or ethnic group, may have a child with a genetic defect.

Who, then, is a candidate for genetic counseling? Counseling is predominantly for three groups of couples: (1) the couple with a relative who has a genetic disease or who have a genetic disease themselves (e.g., the woman's brother has hemophilia or cystic fibrosis or the man's cousin has sickle cell disease); (2) the couple who have borne a child with physical or mental abnormalities; and (3) the couple in which the mother is older than 35 or the father is older than 55. The availability of genetic counseling should be suggested to any couple or individual when the basic health history indicates the birth of a child with a possible abnormality of some type. Age is important because of the increased likelihood of Down's syndrome.

Nurses may meet these individuals in any area of practice where basic assessment is a part of care. It has been estimated that as many as 90 per cent of persons in the United States who could benefit from genetic counseling do not receive that counseling, often because either they are unaware of counseling per se or they do not recognize the need for counseling. Nurses who are aware of the values of genetic counseling to these people are important in the prevention of genetic disease.

The Process of Genetic Counseling

What happens when a couple comes for genetic counseling? First, a diagnosis is made or confirmed. Although the diagnosis may appear obvious, as in a cleft lip, the obvious problem may be part of a group of defects comprising a particular genetic entity.

A family history is carefully developed. Table 2–1 indicates who is included in the history. For each individual, sex and date

Table 2–1 Developing a Genetic Family History*

Man	Woman
pregnancies and outcomes	
brothers or sisters (living or dead)	
mother's stillbirths and miscarriages	
children of siblings	
father and mother	
aunts, uncles, cousins, cousins' children	
more distant relatives (grandparents, aunts and uncles of parents, etc.)	

*After Roberts and Pembry: An Introduction to Medical Genetics. 7th Edition. Oxford University Press, 1978.

of birth are noted as are abnormalities that the person can identify. The genetic history is not directed only toward the specific condition that brought the couple to counseling; other genetic conditions may become evident. One should always ascertain if the man and woman are related to each other other than by marriage.

After the history and appropriate literature are reviewed, risks are discussed with the couple at a subsequent interview. Risks may be described in mendelian terms, as in this chapter, for some specific dominant or recessive disorders. Often, however, although the disorder is genetic in origin, such clear-cut risk figures cannot be given. In these instances empirical risk figures, i.e., based on observation of the recurrence in actual practice, are given.

The couple must decide what use to make of the information they receive. It is not the role of the genetic counselor to decide a course of action for them. The counselor should, of course, make them aware of the availability of prenatal diagnosis (Chapter 4) if it is appropriate. But here again, the final decision is that of the parents.

Couples will react differently to risk figures. For example, for a couple who has had a child with a ventricular septal defect (VSD), the most common of all congenital heart defects, the chances at each subsequent pregnancy of having a second child with a VSD are about one in 20 or 5 per cent. One couple will focus on these figures as indicating there is a 95 per cent chance that a subsequent child will not have a VSD, and another couple will find the 5 per cent risk too high.

Differences in the acceptability of risk vary with the condition itself. Some couples would risk a condition that is fatal in the neonatal period, as difficult as that situation is at the time, but would be more hesitant to risk a condition that involves a long-term disease, such as Duchenne muscular dystrophy.

Bibliography

Bogdanovic, S.: Prenatal detection of Down's syndrome. JOGN Nurs 4(6):35, 1975.

Dobzhansky, T.: Mankind Evolving. New Haven: Yale University Press, 1962.

Lubs, H., de la Cruz, F. (eds.): Genetic Counseling: A Monograph of the National Institute of Child Health and Human Development. New York: Raven Press, 1977.

Hendin, D., Marks, J.: The Genetic Connection. New York: New American Library, 1979.

Milunsky, A., Atkins, L.: Prenatal diagnosis of genetic disorders. In The Prevention of Genetic Disease and Mental Retardation. Philadelphia: W. B. Saunders, 1975.

Mørch, E.: Chondrodystrophic dwarfs in Denmark. Opera ex Domo Biol Hered Hum Univ Hafniensis 3:1, 1941.

Murphy, E., Chase, G.: Principles of Genetic Counseling. Chicago: Year Book Medical Publishers, 1975.

Papazian, H.: Modern Genetics. New York: W. W. Norton, 1967.

Roberts, J., Pembrey, M.: An Introduction to Medical Genetics. 7th Edition. Oxford: Oxford University Press, 1978.

Sahin, S.: The multifaceted role of the nurse as genetic counselor. MCN 1(4):211, 1976.

Sorenson, J., Culbert, A.: Genetic counselors and counseling orientations — unexamined topics in evaluation. In Genetic Counseling. H. Lubs and F. de la Cruz (eds.). New York: Raven Press, 1977.

Steele, M., Breg, W.: Chromosome analysis of human amniotic fluid cells. Lancet 1:383, 1966.

Thompson, J. S., Thompson, M. W.: Genetics in Medicine, 3rd Edition. Philadelphia: W. B. Saunders, 1980.

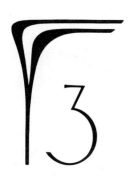

THE ROLE OF FETAL ENVIRONMENT

Chromosomes and genes constantly interact with the embryonic-fetal environment. Any part of that environment, chemical or physical, that affects the unborn infant adversely is known as a *teratogen*. The term *teratogen* is derived from a Greek word meaning monster. The word *monster* originates from the Latin *monstrum*, meaning a portent or omen. People of some ancient societies believed that the birth of an infant with a congenital anomaly was an omen for the future. Thus teratogen is used to describe a substance that can cause a congenital malformation. Human teratogens include certain drugs, alcohol, radiation, and certain microorganisms. Although smoking has not been linked with congenital anomalies, it is associated with the birth of infants who are small for gestational age.

Before considering the specific varieties of environmental teratogens, there are three general principles to recognize. First, either too much or too little of almost any physical or chemical agent can have a teratogenic effect on some species of mammals. However, not every agent that affects one species or even one subspecies will necessarily affect another species in the same way or even in a way that is harmful. The practical implication of this is that there are limits to what animal research can tell us about the way in which a specific agent will affect humans.

The experience with thalidomide, which did not show the characteristic effect in animal tests that it was to show in humans, is an example of this.

Second, the timing of the insult is of great importance. Prior to implantation, a teratogen will either (1) destroy the blastocyst or (2) have no effect because cells of the blastocyst are not yet differentiated and can be replaced by other undifferentiated cells (Hawkins 1976). A teratogen introduced between the third and sixth weeks of embryonic life (fifth and eighth weeks by menstrual age) when the principal body systems are being established is likely to do far more harm than one introduced in the eighth or ninth month of pregnancy, because the nutritional and energy requirements of differentiating tissue are so much greater than those of tissue either before or after differentiation. Metabolic and nutritional disturbances, which can be tolerated by tissues that are less active, may be disastrous for tissues actively undergoing differentiation. This does not mean that the fetus is free from environmental hazard after the first trimester; environmental agents can cause difficulty late in pregnancy. For example, syphilis and toxoplasmosis in the late months can cause malformations in organs that were originally normal.

In addition to timing, it seems that some teratogens have a predilection for a specific system or area within the embryo. With certain drugs this appears to be due to a higher concentration in these tissues, but in other instances the reason for a special predilection is unknown. Thalidomide, for example, affects the limbs. With other agents, however, a broad range of deformities is possible.

Fetal tissues may respond to teratogens in several ways. They may hypertrophy or they may atrophy. Structures may split where they should have remained one, or they may fuse where they should have remained separate. Or there may be a general inhibition of normal growth and development. Underlying these more obvious responses may be failure of induction, i.e., failure of the tissue or organ to transmit the appropriate stimulus that leads to the development of a neighboring tissue, or failure of competence, in which the inductive stimulus is normal but the adjacent tissue is unable to respond normally. In both instances these initial failures may lead to still more change.

Embryos of different species react in different ways to teratogens. This fact poses a real problem in the evaluation of the safety of drugs. For example, thalidomide showed no evidence in animal studies of the disastrous effects it was to cause in humans. Some drugs that have caused defects in animals have not been found to do so in humans. Withholding a needed medication from a mother can also present a problem. The possible teratogenic effects of the condition for which the drug is given rather than the drug itself is something that must be considered.

External environmental factors that have or are suspected of having the potential to affect the embryo or fetus include: (1) maternal infection, both viral and bacterial, (2) medication and drugs, including alcohol, (3) maternal nutrition, (4) smoking, (5) lead, (6) pica, and (7) radiation.

INFECTION: THE *TORCH* DISEASES

The first letters of the major infectious diseases that may seriously affect the embryo or fetus form the acronym TORCH: Toxoplasmosis, Other (Syphilis), Rubella, Cytomegalic inclusion disease, and Herpes genitalis.

Toxoplasmosis

It has been estimated that as many as four to six of every 1000 mothers in the United States may contract toxoplasmosis, a disease caused by a protozoan, during pregnancy and that as many as one of every 1000 infants may have congenital toxoplasmosis. In a small proportion of these babies, the result is severe mental retardation.

The incidence of toxoplasmosis varies from one population to another. In Paris, the maternal infection rate is as high as 50 of 1000 pregnancies. Principal routes of infection are the consumption of raw or undercooked meat (frequent in Paris) and direct or indirect contact with cat feces. Thus, cooking methods, exposure to cats, and warm, moist soil conditions that favor the survival of the protozoan oocytes are factors in the incidence of the disease and also suggest preventative measures.

Congenital infection appears to be a result of a primary infection of the mother during pregnancy. Frequently the mother has no symptoms; when symptoms are present infection of the lymph nodes is most common. Spread of the infection to the fetus varies with the stage of pregnancy; fetal infection was found to occur in 20 per cent of first trimester infections, 30 per cent of second trimester infections, and 66 per cent of third trimester infections. Thus, early education of mothers concerning prevention should be of value in reducing the incidence.

Even when the fetus is infected, only 10 per cent of infected infants will have symptoms in the newborn period. Signs and symptoms may occur in the central nervous system (abnormal cerebrospinal fluid, convulsions, hydrocephalus, microcephalus) or the eyes (chorioretinitis), or they may be more general (anemia, jaundice). In infants with CNS or eye disease, there is a strong possibility that the infant will be severely mentally retarded. When toxoplasmosis is identified, infants are treated for 30 days with oral sulfadiazine and pyrimethamine. Since pyrimethamine is an antifolate that affects cell growth, folic acid is also given to the baby.

The nurse's most important role, as suggested above, is the prevention of exposure of pregnant women to the protozoan. Specific suggestions to all pregnant women should include the following:

1. Eat no raw or undercooked meat during pregnancy.
2. Wear gloves and/or wash hands thoroughly when handling raw meat to ensure against inoculation through breaks in the skin.
3. Feed house cats only dry, cooked, or canned meat; do not allow them to hunt.
4. Let someone else handle the cat litter; clean cat litter pans daily.
5. Avoid soil potentially contaminated with cat feces.

Syphilis

Standards of prenatal care, and in many instances state laws, require that all pregnant women be screened for syphilis by blood tests that measure antibody response. The tests are either the VDRL (Venereal Disease Research Laboratory) or the newer, more sensitive RPR (rapid plasma reagin). Testing is usually performed on an initial prenatal visit and again in the eighth month of pregnancy. If the VDRL or RPR is positive, the diagnosis is confirmed by FTA-ABS (fluorescent treponemal antibody absorption test). This confirmation is important because occasional false-positive results occur (1:2000) with both the VDRL and RPR, particularly following acute infection, mononucleosis, systemic lupus erythematosus, immunization, and exposure to some drugs.

Yet not every instance of maternal syphilis is detected, and congenital syphilis continues to occur. Reasons include absence of prenatal care, failure to perform the screening test, failure to treat the mother after a positive test, and infection after the initial testing.

Serological tests for syphilis should be part of prenatal care for every woman. However, not all mothers receive prenatal care, and some women may contract syphilis following testing or recontract the disease after initial treatment. Moreover, because of the characteristics of the test, the results will not become positive until four to six weeks after the initial infection. The mean length of time between treatment and a negative serological reaction is 245 days, so the test may remain positive following delivery even though the mother has been treated and is no longer infected. Thus, important as serological testing is, it must be supplemented by education of mothers and their sexual partners about the significance of syphilis during pregnancy. The patient must come to trust the nurse so that she will tell the nurse if she suspects she may have become infected. If initial tests are negative, repeat testing during the third trimester is often recommended.

Regardless of when syphilis is discovered during pregnancy, it should be treated. Effective treatment with penicillin prior to the eighteenth week of pregnancy prevents fetal infection because the organism apparently does not cross the placenta until after that time. Treatment after 18 weeks is also highly effective, however, because penicillin crosses the placenta to reach the fetus quickly and in adequate amounts. Fortunately, penicillin has never been associated with teratogenicity, in spite of its common use during pregnancy for many years. For patients sensitive to penicillin, erythromycin or tetracycline is used. Failure to treat syphilis may lead to abortion, stillbirth, premature labor, and signs and symptoms in the infant.

The earliest sign of syphilis in the newborn may be a nasal discharge that is at first clear but later becomes purulent. The nose becomes obstructed by the discharge; these symptoms are called *snuffles*. Skin lesions may appear after two weeks; common sites are around the nose and mouth, in the diaper region, and on the palms and soles of the feet. Characteristic bone changes are seen on x ray. Treatment of the baby, as of the mother, is with penicillin. Untreated, syphilis may lead to death in 10 to 30 per cent of infants or to central nervous system damage.

Rubella

Rubella is certainly the best known of the teratogenic viral infections; it is the one that first alerted researchers to the idea that there could be an environmental source of congenital deformity. This discovery followed rubella epidemics in Australia in 1939 and 1940. Because there had been no major rubella outbreak in Australia in the previous 17 years, the vast majority of young, pregnant women had no immunity and contracted rubella in large numbers, with a subsequent high incidence of what are now recognized as the classic signs and symptoms in their newborn infants: cardiac defects (particularly patent ductus and pulmonary stenosis), cataracts, deafness, mental and motor retardation, dental and facial defects, retarded intrauterine growth, enlarged livers and spleens, encephalitis, thrombocytopenia, and thrombocytopenic purpura.

In the United States population it has been estimated that of those mothers exposed to rubella during the first trimester, 82.5 per cent will already be immune. About 3 per cent will actually contract rubella, but another 6 per cent will have subclinical infections that can also harm the fetus.

Through what mechanism the rubella virus affects development remains a mystery. It is known that the virus enters the fetus through the placenta where it may persist in the tissues of the embryo for as long as one to four years after birth. Thus, a newborn with evidence of congenital rubella may himself be a source of infection to susceptible hospital personnel and should be isolated.

RUBELLA TESTING AND IMMUNIZATION

Although rubella immunization for all children between one year of age and puberty has been recommended since the rubella vaccines were first licensed in 1969, only 60 to 70 per cent of infants and children in the United States receive rubella vaccines. This level of immunization has led to a continuous decline in the incidence of rubella, congenital rubella, and therapeutic abortion performed because of rubella during pregnancy. However, many unimmunized children now reach adolescence with no exposure to rubella, so that the disease occurs primarily in persons older than 15.

To prevent congenital rubella syndrome, several solutions are worthy of consideration.

1. If rubella immunization were required for admission to school, as DPT, polio, and measles immunizations are now, the unimmunized segment of the future childbearing population would be decreased.

2. The Advisory Committee on Immunization Practices of the U. S. Public Health Service recommends that educational and training institutions, such as colleges and military bases, require proof of rubella immunity from all women of childbearing age and vaccinate those who lack proof. Proof consists of a positive serological test or documentation of previous rubella vaccination (Rubella vaccine 1978).

3. Many health agencies and hospitals screen certain personnel for rubella immunity but not others (some states require that all female employees in hospitals be screened). For example, nurses who work on pediatric units may be routinely screened, a policy that protects the nurse herself but not nurses who work in other areas. Given the changing age range of rubella patients, such a policy may not protect the nurse most at risk. Pediatric patients may be the least in need of protection from a nurse who might have rubella.

4. Little consideration has been given to males who work in hospitals. In July 1978 a male house officer in New York contracted rubella; 170 staff members and 11 prenatal patients, three of whom were susceptible to rubella, were exposed to the disease. None of the prenatal patients

contracted rubella, but the potential seriousness of even a single infection suggests that men as well as women who work in hospitals and clinics should be screened and immunized (McLaughlin and Gold 1979).

Cytomegalovirus Infection

Cytomegalovirus (CMV) is the most common of the known infectious causes of mental retardation in childhood. From 3 to 6 per cent of pregnant women have a cytomegalovirus infection during pregnancy. Fetal infection rates are considerably lower; from 0.5 to 2.0 per cent of newborns excrete the virus. Approximately one infant in 3000 will develop cytomegalic inclusion disease. Signs in the newborn include hyperbilirubinemia, an enlarged spleen, petechiae, intrauterine growth retardation, and, in some instances, microcephaly. The baby may have seizures or other signs of central nervous system disease. Some infants with intrauterine CMV infection are severely mentally retarded. Currently there is no method of prevention. CMV infection is frequently unrecognized in the adult.

Because an infected infant sheds the virus, other infants in the nursery should be protected from him and pregnant personnel should not care for him. There is no reason to isolate him from his mother, however. All personnel should be tested for antibody to CMV and care assigned to those who already have CMV antibody (Sever 1978).

Herpes Genitalis

Symptoms of the herpes viruses have been described for nearly 2000 years, but it was not until the 1960s that the two antigenic types, Type 1 and Type 2, were identified. The Type 1 virus causes herpes labialis (cold sores) and a variety of other conditions, including encephalitis, that are usually centered above the waist. Type 2 herpes is associated with herpes genitalis (genital herpes), neonatal herpes, and other herpes infections primarily occurring below the waist. Increasing numbers of Type 1 infections are being found in the genital area, perhaps because orogenital sex play is more frequent. Thus location alone does not always indicate the antigenic type of virus.

As a venereal disease, herpes vaginalis is more prevalent than any condition except gonorrhea. Once a woman is infected with herpes virus, the organism may remain in her system in a latent state, with recurrences over a period of years. There is no known cure, although a variety of palliative measures have been employed. Bahr (1978) reviews the course of the maternal disease.

Unlike the other TORCH diseases, there is no proven relationship between herpes infection and congenital anomalies, although there have been some published studies of malformations due to transplacental infection (South 1969; Florman 1973). Herpes is believed to cause both abortion and premature births.

The most common mode of transmission to the newborn is the direct contact of the infant with herpes lesions during vaginal delivery; under these circumstances as many as 50 per cent of infants may be infected. Infant infection is serious; mortality is as high as 50 per cent. In the disseminated form, which includes involvement of the liver and/or nervous system, mortality is from 60 to 90 per cent. Localized and asymptomatic infections are less serious.

While herpes infections cannot be treated, direct contact between an infected mother and her infant can be prevented. A cesarean delivery is planned for any mother with a current infection or an infection within three weeks prior to delivery. The cesarean should be performed prior to or within four hours following rupture of the membranes. Following delivery, the mother should not care for the baby while she remains actively infected, although she can see the baby and should be encouraged to do so.

Chlamydia Trachomatis

Chlamydia trachomatis is a sexually transmitted organism that can inhabit the vagina and, as in herpes simplex, may infect the infant during vaginal birth. In the infant chlamydia infection may result in an eye infection, inclusion conjunctivitis of the newborn (ICN), which has been recognized for many years, or in pneumonia, which was first recognized as related to *Chlamydia* in 1974. From 40 to 50 per cent of infants exposed to the organism will develop an eye infection; risk figures for pneumonia have not as yet been developed.

It has been tentatively estimated that the incidence of chlamydia infections in infants is 28 per 1000 live births. This rate far exceeds the infection rate of many of the diseases discussed above (e.g., one per 6000 for herpes simplex, one to six per 1000 for toxoplasmosis). Prenatal screening and treatment of infected pregnant women with erythromycin has been suggested (Schachter et al. 1979). These authors believe that such screening could prevent 42,000 instances of inclusion conjunctivitis and 24,000 cases of chlamydial pneumonia each year.

MEDICATIONS, DRUGS, AND HORMONES AS TERATOGENS

In spite of publicity about the harmful effects of some drugs in pregnant women, the use of medications appears widespread during pregnancy. Doering and Stewart (1978) and Brocklebank and colleagues (1978) reviewed the use of medications in over 3000 pregnant women. The number of drugs taken averaged from four to 11 per woman. In the Brocklebank study, 82 per cent of 2,528 women received prescriptions; pregnant women received as many prescriptions for medications as nonpregnant women.

A variety of factors affect the way in which a specific drug will affect a particular mother and her fetus. Drug characteristics that will influence placental transfer include molecular weight, fat solubility, the degree to which ionization occurs, and the degree to which the drug binds to albumin in maternal blood. Compounds with a molecular weight greater than 1000 do not readily pass to the fetus. Increased fat solubility and decreased binding to albumin enhance the likelihood of transplacental passage. Maternal acid-base balance and placental blood flow also influence transfer. Acid-base balance may be particularly important during labor. If the mother hyperventilates and blood pH rises (alkalosis), the fetus becomes acidotic; drugs may cross the placenta and become trapped in the fetus. Certain genetic characteristics of the mother or fetus can also be important; for example, nitrofurantoin (Furadantin) may cause hemolytic anemia in mothers with G-6-PD deficiency.

Specific Drugs that May Cause Problems in the Fetus or Newborn

Thalidomide is probably the best known of the teratogenic drugs and is the one that alerted many individuals to the possibility of teratogenicity.

Propranolol (Inderal), which is considered a safe drug for nonpregnant women with thyrotoxicosis and cardiac arrhythmias, may be associated with intrauterine growth retardation, hypoglycemia, respiratory depression, and bradycardia in the newborn if the drug is present in the infant at the time of birth.

Glucocorticoids (e.g., methylprednisolone, dexamethasone) may inhibit cell growth or cause cell death in a variety of tissues. In a study by Renish and colleagues (1978), women receiving as little as 10 mg of prednisone per day delivered infants weighing 200 to 300 g less than those of control mothers. Further research is necessary to evaluate the mechanism and long-term effects of prednisone and related compounds.

Trimethadione and *paramethadione* have been associated with multiple malformations and mental retardation as well as abortion (Zackai et al. 1975).

Hydantoin anticonvulsants (e.g., phenytoin, Dilantin) appear to produce a constellation of defects in some infants called the "fetal hydantoin syndrome." Signs include craniofacial, digital, and nail anomalies, intrauterine growth retardation, and mental deficiency. It has been suggested that folate deficiency may be related to the use of phenytoin as well as phenobarbital and alcohol, and thus mothers who receive anticonvulsants should begin folic acid supplementation prior to conception so that adequate folic acid will be available during implantation and organogenesis.

Phenobarbital may also cause fetal growth retardation and may, in addition, potentiate the teratogenicity of phenytoin. Until recently, phenobarbital was frequently prescribed as a treatment for preeclampsia.

Metronidazole, a drug used to treat Trichomonas infection, is considered potentially teratogenic in the United States but is used in Great Britain, usually after the sixteenth week of pregnancy.

Oral contraceptives, discontinued in the cycle immediately prior to pregnancy, have been suspected as teratogens (Janerich, Piper, and Glebatis 1974). Ovulation is commonly delayed in the first cycle after oral contraceptives are stopped, and it is suspected that fertilization of an aging ovum leads to malformation. This problem might be avoided if the couple used another form of contraception for one or two cycles after discontinuing oral contraceptives.

Benzodiazepines, of which diazepam (Valium) is the most widely used, have been associated with cleft lip and palate (Safra and Oakley 1975). Diazepam in the third trimester may lead to thrombocytopenia, hypothermia, and hypotonia in the infant. Lithium, also used as a tranquilizer, has been related to irritability and goiter in the newborn.

Thiazide diuretics, given in the third trimester, have been associated with thrombocytopenia and neonatal death. *Indomethacin* (Indocin), an antiinflammatory drug, may also cause thrombocytopenia.

When *magnesium sulfate*, frequently given to mothers with preeclampsia or eclampsia, is used the baby should be observed for hypocalcemia.

Although *immunization vaccines* are not medicines or drugs, they should not be given during pregnancy. Both measles and mumps vaccines may infect the fetus; rubella vaccine can produce congenital rubella syndrome.

Just as the thalidomide experience taught the sad lesson that medication that did not harm the mother could have devastating effects on the fetus, findings associated with *diethylstilbestrol* (DES) show that those effects may appear many years after maternal drug ingestion. Of more than 200 case histories of young women with clear-cell adenocarcinoma of the genital tract, more than 80 per cent were daughters of mothers who had been given DES or a related synthetic hormone to reduce the incidence of spontaneous abortion. Although the number of women in whom adenocarcinoma has been detected and reported is small in relation to the total number of mothers receiving DES or related hormones, the actual incidence may be higher (the discrepancy due to the failure to detect or report the adenocarcinoma or its development later in the daughter's lifetime).

Most women who develop adenocarcinoma of the genital tract have symptoms of abnormal bleeding or discharge; approximately 10 per cent have no symptoms, however. Since a Pap smear may fail to identify the cancer cells, Schiller's test, in which the walls of the vagina are coated with an iodine stain, and colposcopy are essential for women at risk (Stafl et al. 1974).

Other effects include nonneoplastic tissue changes and possible decreased fertility, believed to be a result of disturbed development of the paramesonephric ducts. Changes in the upper genital tract, which may increase the risk of certain pregnancy complications (e.g., spontaneous abortion, prematurity, breech presentation), have been found by Kaufman and colleagues (1977). Women exposed to DES should be closely followed during pregnancy. Genital tract abnormalities have also been detected in 41 of 163 *men* whose mothers received DES during pregnancy, compared with 11 of 168 male controls. Further studies have shown reduced sperm counts, lowered sperm mobility, and abnormal appearance of sperm (Offspring 1977).

DES may also produce the more immediate effect of masculinization of the female fetus, as may synthetic progestins (methyltestosterone), 17-alpha-ethynyl-19-nortestosterone (Norlutin), progesterone, 17-alpha-ethynyl-testosterone (Progestoral), and androgens. Labial fusion and clitoral enlargement are also associated with androgens.

Four antimicrobial drugs may cause problems. *Chloramphenicol* in the third trimester may cause "gray syndrome," an anemia due to bone marrow suppression in the newborn infant. *Tetracycline* inhibits bone growth and stains teeth. Brocklebank found, in his study of drug prescribing during pregnancy, that tetracycline was prescribed to 6.2 per cent of pregnant women. *Streptomycin* may cause damage to the eighth cranial nerve and skeletal anomalies. It has already been noted that in mothers with G-6-PD deficiency, *nitrofurantoin* (Furadantin) may cause a hemolytic anemia in the fetus and the mother. Given at term, *sulfonamides* may decrease bilirubin binding and lead to hyperbilirubinemia in the newborn.

It has been estimated that *acetylsalicylic acid* (aspirin) is taken at some time during pregnancy by approximately 80 per cent of women. The role of aspirin in congenital anomalies in humans has not been proved, although salicylates do cause anomalies in animals. However, salicylates taken within 10 days before delivery can cause platelet dysfunction and thereby interfere with clotting in the newborn. An FDA advisory panel has suggested that no aspirin-containing compound be used during the third trimester of pregnancy.

Sodium warfarin, a coumarin anticoagulant, may cause congenital anomalies if given in the first trimester (Shaul and Hall 1977). "Warfarin embryopathy" includes hypoplastic "saddle" nose, abnormalities of bones and hands, eye problems, and mental retardation. Warfarin adminis-

tered during the third trimester has been associated with increased perinatal mortality.

Narcotics and Illegal Substances

When mothers are addicted to heroin, withdrawal symptoms in the newborn may be severe (Chapter 8). Infants born to mothers receiving methadone are at high risk for sudden infant death syndrome (Chavez, Stryker, and Ostrea 1978; Finnegan and Reeser 1978) and other developmental problems (Kaltenbach, Grazion, and Finnegan 1978).

LSD has been shown to cause chromosomal damage in vitro; there are no good clinical studies showing teratogenicity.

There is conflicting evidence on anomalies related to exposure to amphetamines; certainly pregnant women should not take amphetamines to control diet or alleviate depression.

Epidemiologic studies in both the United States and the United Kingdom have shown an increase in spontaneous abortion and congenital abnormalities not only among women working in operating rooms but among the children of male anesthetists (Table 3–1). Similar findings have been reported when dentists who use anesthetic gases in their practice are compared with those who do not. A 16 per cent rate of spontaneous abortion in 887 pregnancies in wives of exposed dentists compares with a rate of 9 per cent in 1,541 pregnancies in wives of unexposed dentists (Cohen et al. 1975).

Nurses who are exposed to anesthetic gases in their own practice need to consider this information and follow closely the research that is likely to occur in the next decade.

Behavioral Teratogens

Although teratogenesis was originally thought of in terms of major physical malformation, drugs taken by the mother may also affect behavior in the infant or child. Phenytoin (Dilantin), heroin, and

Table 3–1 Adjusted Rates of Miscarriage and Congenital Abnormalities in Anesthetists and Controls in United States and United Kingdom*

	Miscarriages/ Pregnancies (%)	Congenital Abnormalities/ Live-Born Children (%)
Females		
Exposed	16.7 ± 1.0	5.5 ± 0.7
Control	13.3 ± 0.7	4.0 ± 0.4
Significance	p < .001	p = .04
Males		
Exposed	12.6 ± 0.5	5.0 ± 0.3
Control	11.7 ± 0.5	3.7 ± 0.3
Significance	p = .10	p < .001

*From Spence, Cohen, Brown et al.: JAMA 238:955, 1977.

alcohol are the examples discussed in this chapter. Because many behavioral difficulties are not recognized until several years after birth, it is difficult to establish a cause-and-effect relationship. Ongoing research with animal models, however, suggests that certain drugs may produce behavior abnormalities without any physical changes (Vorhees, Brunner, and Butcher 1979). As a general principle this work, along with the findings related to DES, strongly suggests that immediately discernible effects are not the only ones with which responsible professionals must be concerned.

Advising Pregnant Women About Medications

What is our nursing responsibility in relation to medications taken during pregnancy? Assessment at the initial prenatal visit and at subsequent visits of medications a woman may be taking is necessary. Questions must often be specific. What do you do when you have a headache? Do you take medicine when you are nauseated? When you have diarrhea? A general question about drug use is of limited value because the word "drug" has a different meaning for each woman questioned. For example, "drug" may mean only an illegal

drug; a woman would never think of the aspirin and cough syrup in her medicine cabinet as drugs. When asked, "Do you take any medicines?" she may think only of those obtained through prescriptions.

Continuing education is essential not only for prenatal patients but for all individuals about the potential dangers of medications other than those for which there is a specific need. This is particularly important for women during the childbearing years because medications may be taken early in pregnancy before the existence of the embryo is even recognized.

Other Teratogens

LEAD

Around the beginning of the century it was recognized that women employed in the lead trades often produced infants who were small, weak, and neurologically damaged. It was discovered that lead crossed the placental barrier, resulting in retarded intrauterine growth and postnatal failure to thrive. Industrial exposure is now controlled, but lead poisoning can result from other substances such as moonshine liquor, which is still commonly used in the southeastern United States. In a 16-month period at the University of Alabama Medical Center 26 adult women, none of whom happened to be pregnant at the time, were admitted for various forms of lead poisoning related to drinking moonshine. Not all moonshine contains lead — only that produced in stills that use lead pipes or vats — but the buyer has no way of telling how the moonshine was produced.

PICA

Pica, the ingestion of unusual substances such as clay, starch, and flour, is a cultural practice fairly widespread among blacks living in the southeastern United States and those who have migrated from these areas to northern cities. Counseling a mother about the dangers of clay eating is much like counseling about smoking hazards; it may not cause her to stop. In the case of clay eating, her traditions suggest that she is helping her baby. The anemia that is believed to result from clay eating cannot be relieved by oral iron preparations because the clay interferes with the absorption of iron from the gastrointestinal tract. Parenteral iron is essential.

Starch eating is even more common than clay eating because the starch is both inexpensive and easily available at the grocers. The starch comes in small chunks and is eaten as a snack, often with a soft drink, like pretzels or potato chips. Unlike clay, starch does not interfere with iron metabolism, but it does add "empty calories" to the diet and gives a full feeling, which may keep the mother from eating the food she and her baby need (see also Chapter 11).

RADIATION

Radiation was one of the first recognized teratogens. Prior to implantation, the effect is "all or none," i.e., either the dose is lethal or there is no effect at all, because cells are undifferentiated at that stage. Radiation between two and six weeks, the period of organogenesis, is likely to result in neonatal death. Radiation between six and 30 weeks may result in growth and/or mental retardation, with the nervous system being the most radiosensitive.

Stewart and Kneale (1970) suggest that radiation during pregnancy may increase the risk of cancer in children younger than 10. After a statistical analysis of 15,000 children they felt that "among one million children exposed shortly before birth to one rad of ionizing radiations there would be an extra 300 to 800 deaths before the age of 10 due to radiation induced cancer."

The role of radiation in causing spontaneous genetic mutations that would in turn lead to congenital malformation has been postulated but not yet proved.

The Role of the Father in Teratogenicity

Research has focused attention on the effects of the mother's practices on the fetus. In the late 1970s animal studies at the University of Vermont College of Medicine investigated and found some association between drug intakes in male rats and adverse effects on offspring such as low birth weight and increased mortality. Methadone, morphine, caffeine, and propoxyphene (Darvon) have been used in experiments. The process by which drug use in males affects the fetus is unknown; speculated causes include changes in sperm or seminal fluid or alterations in male mating behavior that may affect female hormonal levels (Joffe 1979). Sperm mobility has been found to be lower in men who use heroin and methadone (Cicero et al. 1975).

In humans, the teratogenicity of anesthetic gases when the father alone has been exposed has already been noted. The birth of an infant with fetal alcohol syndrome, with the father rather than the mother as the alcohol consumer, has been reported.

Fetal Alcohol Syndrome

In 1973, Jones and colleagues first reported a "pattern of craniofacial, limb, and cardiovascular defects associated with prenatal onset growth deficiency and developmental delay" that has become known as *fetal alcohol syndrome.* In addition to this specific pattern of defects, maternal alcohol consumption appears to be related to more general conditions such as intrauterine and infant growth retardation and delays in behavior development.

In a study of 305 women in Boston, five of 15 babies born to women who drank heavily had congenital anomalies (Ouellette and Rosett 1977). Forty-four per cent of the surviving children of 23 alcoholic women in a perinatal collaborative project showed mental deficiency (Hanson, Jones, and Smith 1976).

Alcohol compromises maternal nutrition by interfering with the absorption and utilization of a number of nutrients and with the synthesis of proteins. The alcoholic woman is frequently malnourished before she becomes pregnant and may continue to be malnourished during pregnancy. Because thiamine is metabolized at an accelerated rate, the need for that vitamin is increased. Alcoholic women often have iron deficiency or macrocytic anemia. A high protein–high iron diet, appropriate for the woman with iron deficiency anemia, also aids in preventing growth retardation. Folic acid is the therapy for macrocytic anemia. Increased intake of vitamin C enhances therapy in both anemias.

Questions about the type, frequency, and amount of alcohol intake should be part of the initial prenatal assessment for every patient. Not only will these questions help in the early identification of mothers at risk, but they may also alert all mothers to the dangers of alcohol consumption during pregnancy. The presence of alcohol-related diseases, such as hepatitis and cirrhosis, suggests the possibility of alcoholism and the need for further assessment (Luke 1977).

MATERNAL NUTRITION AND THE FETUS

A relationship between nutritional inadequacy and the intrauterine growth of the fetus and long-term growth of the infant has been found in animal studies and suggested by human studies.

In several rat studies, maternal nutritional deficiencies led to fetal growth retardation, increased mortality (Churchill 1977; Dobbing 1968), a decrease in the weights of the placenta and brain, a decrease in the amount of cerebral DNA and protein (Zamenof, van Marthens, and Grauel, 1971), and a deficit in brain cell number at weaning (Winick 1970). Comparable results in humans have been difficult to demonstrate, in part because of the relatively slow growth of the human fetus and also because of the difficulty in

regulating experimental conditions when the subjects are human mothers. Because human malnutrition is often associated with a variety of other factors (poverty, limited education, etc.) it is not easy to identify the effects of nutrition per se. Human studies that do provide evidence of the significance of nutrition are summarized in Table 3–2. Note that in a

Table 3–2 Research on Nutrition in Pregnancy

Study	Findings
Naeye (1969)	Women with low family incomes had increased incidence of stillborn infants and infants who died within 48 hours of birth. Women with low family incomes had infants with lower birth weights.
Winick (1967)	Placental growth was more limited in pregnant women with nutritional deprivation.
Ferguson et al. (1975)	Lymphocyte deficiency in undergrown infants.
Delgado (1977)	High association between maternal nutrition during pregnancy and birth weight. Birth weight associated with performance on three variables in Brazelton assessment and with motor development. Improved maternal nutrition during pregnancy associated with decreased infant mortality. Maternal nutrition (caloric) during pregnancy associated with infant mental development at six months of age.
Moghissi et al. (1975)	Maternal amino acid levels associated with birth weight, length, and cranial volume. Birth weight associated with cranial volume and motor development. Motor development associated with mental development.
Mora et al. (1978)	Supplementation, beginning in the sixth month of pregnancy, decreased perinatal mortality.
Mora et al. (1979)	Supplementation, beginning in the sixth month of pregnancy, increased maternal weight gain and the birth weight of males.
Vuori et al. (1979)	Supplementation, beginning in the sixth month of pregnancy, significantly affected newborn behavior and had a significant effect on visual attention and habituation at 15 days, suggesting increased maturation.
Herrera (1979)	Supplementation, beginning in the sixth month of pregnancy, resulted in infants less apathetic at four and eight months.

number of the studies, not only perinatal factors but later development have been examined and maternal nutrition has been a significant factor.

Animal experimentation has produced a variety of malformations from deficiencies of nutritional elements such as vitamin A, riboflavin, zinc, and manganese. The only proven congenital malformation related to a specific dietary deficiency in humans is cretinism, which is related to a lack of iodine in the diet. Cretinism and the adult form of iodine deficiency are prevalent in several areas of the world where soil and water do not contain sufficient iodine. Recently there have been reports that goiter is increasing in some parts of the United States because of a decrease in the use of iodized salt. Since mountainous and inland areas are most likely to be affected, pregnant women in these areas should use iodized salt.

A general level of malnutrition has been correlated with low birth weight babies who are less likely to thrive after birth and have a considerably higher incidence of infant mortality. There are two general sources of fetal malnutrition. The mother may be adequately nourished but because of an abnormality at the point of placental transfer (due, for example, to faulty implantation), the fetus is not adequately nourished. Or the mother herself may be so inadequately nourished that the fetus is affected. Physiological and cultural factors interact in maternal malnutrition. Changes in maternal metabolism, the expansion of maternal blood volume with the associated reduction in the concentration of hemoglobin and plasma albumin, pulmonary and cardiovascular adjustments — all put increased demands on the mother's nutritional status. On the cultural side, diet patterns, particularly those of teenage and economically poor mothers, and the rather common tendency of medical professionals to limit calories to reduce the possibility of toxemia and produce a smaller infant so that delivery will be easier, have contributed to the incidence of low birth weight babies. The Committee on Maternal Nutrition of the National Research Council in a report,

Maternal Nutrition and the Course of Pregnancy, recommends a weight gain of 24 pounds for the mother. Iron and folate supplementation is also recommended as well as the use of iodized salt in those geographical areas deficient in iodine.

More than a decade of research at the Montréal Diet Dispensary demonstrated that careful assessment of nutritional status coupled with increased protein and calorie intake tailored to the needs of individual mothers resulted in increased birth weight when infants born to mothers with intensive nutritional counseling were compared to siblings born prior to maternal counseling. Perinatal mortality (14.3), prematurity (6.8 per cent), and mean birth weight (3,274 g) were similar to the parameters for private patients and represented a marked improvement over these parameters in other public clinic patients (Higgins 1976).

An underlying principle of the Montreal program is derived from the work of Burke (1948) and Oldham and Sheft (1951), which showed that when caloric intake was low, nitrogen retention and the efficient utilization of protein in the diet were also low. Thus, maternal diets are supplemented with both calories and protein. Criteria for supplementation are summarized in Table 3–3. Basic requirements, to which supplementation is added, are

Table 3–3   Caloric and Protein Supplementation[1]

Criteria	Additional calories/day	Additional protein/day (g)
20 weeks gestation or more	500	25
Protein deficit*	10/g of deficit	equal to deficit
Underweight by 5% or more†	500‡	20
Nutritional stress (per condition)		
Pernicious vomiting	200	20
Less than 1 year between pregnancies	200	20
Poor previous obstetrical history	200	20
Failure to gain 10 lbs by week 20	200	20
Serious emotional problems	200	20

[1]Adapted from Higgins: J Can Diet Assoc *37*:17, 1976.
*Difference between actual dietary intake and requirement.
†Metropolitan Life Insurance weight tables.
‡Permits gain of 1 lb/week; mother is to gain the difference in her weight and the norm for her height.

Table 3–4 Perinatal Outcome in Relation to Maternal Prepregnancy Weight*

	Thin	Normal	Moderately Obese	Obese
Fetal loss (%)	10	5	3	5
Mean placental weight (g)	586	626	679	575
Incidence of preeclampsia (%)	17	9	18	21

[1]Adapted from Higgins: J Can Diet Assoc 37:17, 1976.

based on the Dietary Standard for Canada for mothers 20 years of age or older and Recommended Dietary Allowances (1958) of the Food and Nutrition Board of the National Research Council in the United States for mothers under 20.

Further substantiation of the role of nutrition in perinatal outcome comes from the data of Hollingsworth (1978), who reported that when adolescents were underweight before pregnancy, both fetal loss and the birth of infants with birth weights below 2500 g were increased, even though weight gain during pregnancy was adequate (11.9 to 12.2 kg, 26 lbs). Preeclampsia was as common in thin girls as in the moderately obese. Higgins (1976) also demonstrated a relationship between prepregnancy weight and preeclampsia (Table 3–4).

MATERIAL SMOKING AND THE FETUS

Since Simpson first reported an association in 1957 between birth weight and smoking during pregnancy, a large body of subsequent research has confirmed his findings. Results have been consistent from a wide variety of nations, races, and cultures and in both prospective and retrospective studies. Results are independent of race, parity, maternal size, socioeconomic status, infant sex, and other variables.

Infants born to women who smoke are, on the average, 200 g lighter than infants born to control women who do not smoke. Smokers have twice as many babies weighing less than 2500 g than nonsmokers. Moreover, decreased birth weight is dose-related; the more a mother

smokes, the greater the reduction in fetal size, body length, and head and chest circumference as well as weight. Since gestation is not shortened by smoking, lower birth weights are due to intrauterine growth retardation rather than decreased gestational age.

The mechanism by which smoking inhibits intrauterine growth has not been discovered. Wilson (1972), Wingerd and colleagues (1976), and others have noted a significantly higher ratio between placental weight and infant birth weight and suggested that the increase may be a response by the placenta to chronic hypoxia. Like birth weight, the placental weight was related to the level of maternal smoking. Other research has focused on the effects of smoking on placental metabolism, carbon monoxide, maternal vitamin B_{12} and vitamin C levels, and vascular damage.

The effects of maternal smoking on long-term growth, development, and behavior are less clear. The largest long-term follow-up, of 17,000 births in the British Perinatal Mortality Study, did find differences in physical and mental growth at ages seven and 11 ($p < 0.001$) when social and biological factors were controlled.

Additional studies suggest a relationship between maternal smoking and placenta previa (Underwood et al. 1965), abruptio placentae (Andrews and McGarry 1972; Naeye et al. 1977; Meyer and Tonascia 1977), bleeding during pregnancy (Russell, Taylor, and Maddison 1966), premature rupture of membranes (Underwood et al. 1967), and preeclampsia (Andrews and McGarry, 1972).

In a study of 51,490 births, 701 fetal deaths, and 655 neonatal deaths, perinatal mortality rates per thousand births were

23.5 for nonsmokers, 28.2 for smokers of less than a pack per day (a 20 per cent increase), and 31.8 smokers of more than a pack per day (a 35 per cent increase). Maternal smoking during pregnancy has also been associated with sudden infant death syndrome — SIDS (Steele and Langworth 1966; Bergman and Wiesner 1976; Rhead 1977).

One troublesome question is whether fetal outcome is improved when the mother stops smoking during pregnancy; the answer is unclear at this time. With even a slim possibility that ceasing to smoke would benefit the baby, it seems important to encourage each mother to stop or reduce her smoking. Educating the public so that women who smoke stop prior to pregnancy is even more valuable.

THE MOTHER'S BODY AS FETAL ENVIRONMENT

Most of the environmental teratogens discussed so far enter the mother's body and then the body of the fetus through the placenta. Sometimes conditions exist in the mother's body itself that either alone or in interaction with the fetus become a source of danger to the unborn child.

DIABETES MELLITUS

From 1 to 2 per cent of all pregnant women have diabetes mellitus. Pregnancy places a "diabetogenic stress" on all mothers by altering the response of the mother's pancreas to the stimulus of glucose. In women without sufficient pancreatic reserve, diabetes may become manifest for the first time during pregnancy. Women who are already insulin-dependent diabetics require meticulous care during pregnancy. White's classification is used to describe the extent of diabetes mellitus during pregnancy (Table 3–5).

Perinatal mortality and morbidity have traditionally been from five to 10 times higher in infants of diabetic mothers. With excellent prenatal care, however, that rate can be reduced. Over a four-year period (1971 to 1975), Gabbe (1977) reports a perinatal mortality of 46 per 1000 in 260 women with Classes B to R diabetes mellitus. But, excluding those infant deaths related to congenital malformations, which are two to three times higher in infants of diabetic mothers, the perinatal mortality in the population studied was no greater than that of nondiabetic women in that population.

Other than congenital malformation, the principal causes of mortality in infants of diabetic mothers (IDM) are *intrauterine death*, which is commonly sudden and may occur in 70 per cent of mothers who become acidotic, *prematurity*, which is frequently iatrogenic, and *birth injury* from the vaginal delivery of a macrosomic infant. Careful prenatal care has reduced mortality from each of these causes.

Care begins with the screening of all pregnant women for potential diabetes, since mortality and morbidity are increased in gestational diabetes (abnormal glucose tolerance during pregnancy — Class A) as well as in Classes B to R insulin-dependent diabetes. Screening factors are summarized in Table 3–6.

Table 3–5   White's Classification of Diabetes in Pregnancy*

Group A	Abnormal glucose tolerance test only
Group B	Onset of clinical diabetes after age 20, duration less than 10 years, no demonstrable vascular disease
Group C	Onset between ages 10 and 20, duration 10 to 19 years, no x-ray evidence of vascular disease
Group D	Onset before age 10 or duration over 20 years, x-ray diagnosis of vascular disease in legs, retinal changes
Group E	Same as Group D with addition of calcifications of pelvic arteries by x-ray examination
Group F	Diabetic nephropathy
Group R	Active retinitis proliferans

*Adapted from White: Med Clin North Am 49:1015, 1965.

Table 3–6   Screening Prenatal Women for Diabetes Mellitus

Assessment from health history
  Family history of diabetes
  Previous infant weighing more than 4000 g (9 lbs)
  Repeated preeclampsia in previous pregnancies
  Unexplained stillbirth or neonatal death
  Previous infant with congenital anomalies

Assessment from physical findings
  Polyhydramnios
  Macrosomic infant
  Retinopathy
  Hypertension

Urinalysis for glycosuria at each prenatal visit

Two-hour postprandial blood glucose*

*Not part of routine screening in all clinics

Because the fetus is dependent on the maternal pancreas to regulate fetal glucose supply, careful control of maternal glucose levels is the key to care. Figure 3–1 summarizes the pathway through which major fetal problems arise. Another source of high fetal morbidity and mortality is iatrogenic prematurity, i.e., prematurity because the infant was delivered by cesarean section too early. Tests for assessing fetal maturity, described in Chapter 4, have helped to reduce iatrogenic prematurity.

In addition, the earlier the mother begins prenatal care, the more easily one can correlate gestational age with uterine fundal height.

Contemporary care of diabetic mothers commonly involves a period of hospitalization as soon as pregnancy is confirmed, followed by close out-patient surveillance. Mothers are asked to check double-voided urines for both sugar and acetone daily. Some mothers also use Dextrostix at home to record blood glucose levels. At each clinic visit a fasting blood glucose level is obtained; fasting glucose levels are maintained between 100 and 110 mg per 100 ml and two-hour postprandial glucose levels at 140 to 150 mg per 100 ml. Early detection of urinary tract infections, which can lead to maternal acidosis, and hypertension, which can further compromise the fetus, is particularly important for the mother with diabetes.

During the third trimester fetal growth, well-being, and maturity are carefully assessed. This assessment intensifies from 34 weeks until the time of delivery, utilizing measures described in Chapter 4. Many mothers are hospitalized at 34 weeks whereas others may not enter the

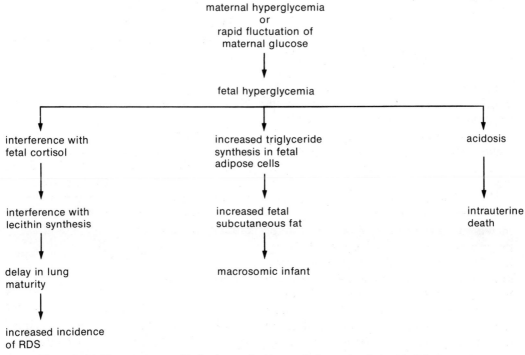

Figure 3–1.   Consequences of lack of control of internal glucose levels in the diabetic mother.

hospital until one to two weeks prior to delivery.

At one time cesarean delivery at 37 weeks was the standard for diabetic mothers, but with close maternal and fetal assessment and care most mothers now deliver at 38 weeks, and many may deliver vaginally if the fetus is not macrosomic.

The special needs of the infant of a mother with diabetes are discussed in Chapter 8.

CHRONIC HYPERTENSION

The infants of mothers with chronic hypertension are at risk of fetal growth retardation. Care for the mother that may enhance fetal development includes bed rest and medication. Hydralazine (Apresoline) is commonly used because it dilates peripheral blood vessels and therefore does not reduce uterine blood flow. Thiazide diuretics, which decrease intravascular volume and possibly compromise placental perfusion, are avoided. As in pregnancy-induced hypertension (described below), fetal and maternal status must be carefully monitored.

RENAL DISEASE

Intrauterine growth retardation has been associated with chronic renal disease, but with close supervision most women with mild to moderate renal disease tolerate pregnancy well. When renal function is decreased by more than 50 per cent (evidenced by a nonpregnant serum creatinine of 3 mg/100 ml), normal pregnancy is rare.

The major renal problem of pregnancy is urinary tract infection. Because of the increased nutrient content of the urine of pregnant women, bacterial growth is enhanced and bacteriuria progresses to pyelonephritis in approximately 40 per cent of women. Diagnosis is important; urine should be collected at midstream after three vulval washings. A bacterial count of greater than 100,000/ml indicates asymptomatic bacteriuria.

Aggressive antibiotic treatment is employed because acute pyelonephritis is associated with intrauterine growth retardation, prematurity, congenital abnormalities, and fetal death. Sulfonamides are not given to mothers near term because of the possibility of hyperbilirubinemia and kernicterus in the newborn.

PULMONARY DISEASE

Mothers with acute or chronic pulmonary disease may have deficits in oxgyen transport that may, in turn, result in fetal hypoxia and growth retardation. Included in this group of conditions are asthma in which symptoms are significant, emphysema, active tuberculosis, inactive tuberculosis with a residual of impaired function, and the presence of a lobectomy or pneumonectomy. Pulmonary function, rather than the presence or absence of disease, is the significant factor.

OTHER HEALTH CONDITIONS THAT MAY AFFECT PREGNANCY

A variety of other health-related conditions may affect mother and fetus. They include lupus erythematosus, multiple sclerosis, thyroid disease, and carcinomas.

Blood Group Incompatibilities

Blood group incompatibilities that may lead to erythroblastosis are another example of fetal/maternal interaction. The two most common types are incompatibility of the Rh$_D$ factors and blood group (ABO) incompatibility. Occasionally, rare blood groups are involved.

RH ISOIMMUNIZATION

When a mother lacks the D factor in her blood, she is said to be Rh negative. If her fetus has D factor and is thus Rh positive, Rh isoimmunization is possible.

In about 10 per cent of all pregnancies, an Rh negative mother is carrying an Rh positive fetus. Theoretically, each Rh positive fetus of an Rh negative mother is a candidate for erythroblastosis fetalis, in which the red blood cells of the fetus and newborn are destroyed. However, only in 5 per cent of pregnancies in which there is a potential problem does the mother develop antibodies to the fetal red blood cells. Erythroblastosis occurs in from four to 10 pregnancies in every 1000. The problem could be eliminated in the vast majority of these babies by application of our current knowledge.

The physiological basis of erythroblastosis is an antigen-antibody reaction. The Rh_D negative mother (genotype dd) has no Rh_D antigen in her body. When her fetus is Rh_D positive, any fetal blood (containing D antigen) that enters her system is treated as a foreign substance, i.e., she develops antibodies to protect her system against the "intruder." Her antibodies attach themselves to the fetal red blood cells and thus mark the cells. The marked cells are then destroyed by phagocytes and other maternal cells.

Since fetal and maternal blood do not mix, fetal red blood cells do not normally enter the maternal system during the prenatal period. Thus the first D positive infant of a D negative mother does not usually have problems unless at some prior time the mother was transfused with D positive blood (rare) or has had a spontaneous or induced abortion of a D positive fetus without the use of passive antibody (Rho-GAM), as described below.

At the time of delivery (or abortion), fetal red blood cells do enter the maternal circulation. The mother's immune system develops anti-Rh_D antibodies. Once the immune response begins, antibody production may continue for many years without additional stimulus.

When the Rh_D negative mother next becomes pregnant with an Rh_D positive fetus, those antibodies cross the placenta, coat the red blood cells of the fetus, and cause their destruction.

In the most severe form, red blood cell destruction in the fetus results in marked anemia and an attempt to raise red cell production and subsequently in heart failure as the heart tries harder and harder to oxygenate the body with a limited number of red blood cells. The fetus develops edema with pleural effusion and ascites. In addition to the anemia, intrauterine hypoxia, hypoproteinemia, and lowered oncotic pressure are probably factors in edema. This condition is known as *hydrops fetalis*. The fetus may die in utero; if born alive, it usually dies in the first days after birth. Once a mother has delivered a stillborn infant because of Rh sensitization, the chances are less than 30 per cent that she will ever be able to deliver a living child.

Fortunately, not every infant of a sensitized mother is so seriously affected. With a more moderate course, the infant may be delivered and may develop *erythroblastosis fetalis* postnatally, with characteristic jaundice and anemia due to the breakdown of red blood cells. The needs and care of the infant with erythroblastosis are discussed in Chapter 8.

Caring for the sensitized mother during the antenatal period   Promethazine (Phenergan), an immunosuppressant, has been given to mothers to decrease maternal antibody production. Phenergan is never given until after 16 weeks gestation because of the possibility of causing a cleft palate. Mothers receiving Phenergan may be drowsy and should be warned to take appropriate safety precautions.

Amniocentesis to determine the level of bilirubin in the amniotic fluid by means of spectrophotometric analysis is the chief method of fetal assessment. The amount of bilirubin in amniotic fluid more accurately reflects fetal involvement than the mother's antibody titer. The optical density (expressed as ΔOD_{450}) of the amniotic fluid indicates the amount of bilirubin and thus the severity of fetal disease. Normally, bilirubin levels in amniotic fluid decrease as the fetal liver matures.

If the ΔOD_{450} is low, the fetus will probably be only mildly affected. If the ΔOD_{450} is moderate at the time of the first amniocentesis, amniotic fluid analysis will be repeated every two to three weeks thereafter. It may subsequently (1) fall to a low zone, with a mildly affected infant delivered at or near term; (2) fall slowly but remain in a middle zone, with a moderately affected infant delivered at approximately 37 weeks; or (3) increase to a high level.

When the ΔOD_{450} is at a level deemed critical on initial or subsequent examination, one of two courses is chosen. If the parameters of gestational age indicate that the baby could survive, he is delivered, with preparations made for a very sick infant. When it is at all possible, the mother should be transferred to a major medical center for delivery. This is safer than attempting to transfer a very sick newborn after delivery.

If the baby is too immature for extrauterine survival, he may receive an intrauterine transfusion. Intrauterine transfusion does not always save the baby's life. If the fetus already has hydrops fetalis, the infused blood is not absorbed. Fetal organs such as the liver or bladder may be perforated. However, since intrauterine transfusion is used only for a fetus already severely sick and in danger of death, any success is welcome.

Radiopaque material is injected into the amniotic fluid approximately five hours prior to the transfusion. Because the fetus is continually swallowing amniotic fluid, the radiopaque material will concentrate sufficiently in the fetal bowel to outline it. A needle is then inserted into the fetal peritoneal cavity, more dye is injected, and the position of the needle is verified by x ray. From 80 to 150 ml of fresh O negative packed red blood cells that have been cross matched with the mother's serum are injected, approximately 15 per cent of the estimated fetal weight.

It is believed that the injected red blood cells enter the fetal circulation by way of the lymphatics below the diaphragm. Fetal hemoglobin rises. The procedure can be repeated every one to two weeks, if necessary, until the fetus has reached a gestational age at which extrauterine existence is possible.

The prevention of sensitization Techniques for treating the affected fetus and newborn of sensitized mothers have certainly improved in the past decade. Far more significant in terms of eliminating the problem is the successful prevention of antibody formation.

Anti-D immunoglobulin (Rho-GAM), already mentioned, is gamma globulin containing anti-D antibody. Remember that when the fetal Rh_D positive cells enter the mother's circulation, she produces antibodies to destroy the positive cells. If she is given antibodies to destroy these cells, her system will not produce antibodies. The antibodies given in this way are not permanent; the positive red blood cells are destroyed and the antibodies, as in all passive immunization, are short-lived. With certain exceptions, sensitization can be prevented and each pregnancy for an Rh_D negative mother can be as safe as a first pregnancy.

Treatment with Rho-GAM is given within 72 hours of delivery. The exact time at which the mother's body begins to produce anti-D antibodies is not known; it is apparently longer than 72 hours. Some researchers believe that if the mother has not been given Rho-GAM in the first days following delivery it may be given up to three to four weeks later. Mothers should be tested for the presence of antibodies four to six months postpartum (or postabortion). Once a mother has been sensitized, Rho-GAM is of no value. Rho-GAM can only prevent sensitization; it cannot eliminate actively acquired anti-D antibodies.

Two types of problems prevent the elimination of Rh sensitization as a cause of infant mortality and morbidity. One is physiological; the second, a problem of the utilization of Rho-GAM.

Physiologic problems About 10 per cent of women given Rho-GAM are sensitized nevertheless. This may be because of bleeding from the mother to the fetus prior to delivery (e.g., in a threatened abortion) or in amniocentesis when the placenta is entered by mistake. A massive hemorrhage at the time of delivery, so large that the amount of Rho-GAM given is inadequate to destroy the large numbers of cells that have entered the circulation, may also result in sensitization.

The Rh_D negative daughter of an Rh_D positive mother may become sensitized at the time of her own birth if some maternal cells enter her bloodstream; there may be no indication that she has been sensitized until Rh titers are performed, perhaps 20 years later when she herself becomes pregnant.

Some women may become sensitized without even knowing they are pregnant. For example, a woman may have a spontaneous abortion during the early weeks of pregnancy and believe she has had a delayed, heavy menstrual period.

Problems in utilization of Rho-GAM It is estimated that 15 to 20 per cent of the women who should receive Rho-GAM each year do not. The rate of utilization is poorer in women postabortion than in women postpartum. Nurses play a vital role in making certain that every woman who should get Rho-GAM is treated.

ABO INCOMPATIBILITY

If the husband is blood type A or B and the wife type O, ABO incompatibility is possible. Severe anemia, hydrops, and stillbirth are rare in ABO incompatibility. This is because the antibody formed in response to the A or B antigen may be either IgM or IgA. If the antibody is IgM, it does not cross the placenta and thus the fetus is unaffected. No specific antenatal care is necessary.

If both Rh_D and ABO incompatibility exist in a mother-infant, the ABO incompatibility may act as a protection for Rh sensitization. This mechanism may destroy the fetal red cells in the mother before they can stimulate Rh antibody formation.

Unlike Rh incompatibility, which becomes progressively more severe at each pregnancy, ABO incompatibility may affect the infant of one pregnancy and not be a problem in a subsequent pregnancy. One reason is that IgA antibody may be involved during one pregnancy and IgM antibody during another.

Age

From a biological perspective, and in many ways from a social and psychological perspective, the ideal age range for reproduction is the twenties to early thirties. Although many women, both younger and older, may successfully bear and care for children, there is evidence that at both ends of the reproductive years both mortality and morbidity are increased. For this reason, the particular needs of adolescents and women over 35 require special attention.

THE ADOLESCENT MOTHER

From a physiologic perspective, adolescents have higher rates of several pregnancy complications. These include preeclampsia and eclampsia, anemia, prolonged labor, preterm delivery, and delivery of a low birth weight infant. The higher incidence of preterm and low birth weight infants, in turn, leads to higher infant mortality and morbidity rates.

One factor that many of these complications appear to have in common is nutrition. The role of nutritional inadequacy in iron deficiency anemia is direct. Although the causes of preeclampsia, eclampsia, and prematurity are not known, the incidence is higher in low-income groups of people who may also eat nutritionally inadequate diets.

When the nutritional demands of pregnancy are imposed upon the nutritional demands of adolescence, it is not surprising that they go unmet unless they are a specific focus of attention in a program designed for adolescent or high-risk mothers.

THE MOTHER OVER 35

Although it is certainly possible for a mother older than 35, and even older than 40, to deliver a healthy infant, the mathematical probability that there may be a problem is increased.

As the hormonal control of the menstrual cycle becomes less regular, the internal environment becomes less optimal for the development of both egg and endometrium. The incidence of multiple pregnancy increases because more than one egg is released. The egg itself may be defective with chromosomal abnormalities.

Down's syndrome, described in Chapter 2, is due to chromosomal abnormality. The risk increases dramatically with maternal age. Because of this, some physicians suggest that all mothers over 35 have an amniocentesis to screen for Down's syndrome (Chapter 4).

MATERNAL OBSTETRICAL CONDITIONS AFFECTING THE FETUS

Placenta Previa

Placenta previa is a condition in which the placenta is attached low in the uterus (Fig. 3–2) in contrast to its normal high position. The mother has painless vaginal bleeding generally beginning after the thirty-second week of gestation because of the physiological changes that begin to occur in the uterus in preparation for labor. As the cervix shortens and dilatation begins there is a partial separation of the placenta from the uterus. The bleeding that occurs is strictly maternal.

Prior to 1945, pregnancy was terminated at the first indication of placenta previa, with a resulting fetal mortality of 50 per cent due chiefly to prematurity. Today, in the absence of continuous or severe hemorrhage the kind of treatment is determined largely by the age of the fetus. Before the thirty-sixth week of gestation the obstetrician will try to minimize the risk of prematurity by allowing the

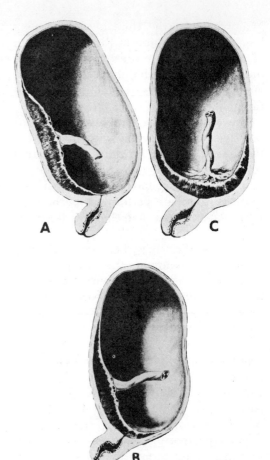

Figure 3–2. Some variations of placenta previa: *A,* low implantation of the placenta; *B,* total placenta previa; *C,* total and central placenta previa. (From Danforth: Textbook of Obstetrics and Gynecology. Hoeber Medical Division, Harper & Row.)

mother to rest and by correcting any deficiency brought about by bleeding. All vaginal examinations are avoided.

After 36 weeks, vaginal examination may be performed in an operating room that is completely prepared for both vaginal delivery and cesarean section. With the exception of multiparas with low-lying partial placenta previa, most deliveries will be abdominal. Perinatal mortality from placenta previa remains near 25 per cent.

Abruptio Placentae

The incidence of abruptio placentae (the premature separation of a normally implanted placenta) remains high. When the separation is sudden and severe, fetal mortality is close to 100 per cent, the fetus dying of intrauterine asphyxia and shock. Reports on the incidence of abruptio vary from one in 85 to one in 200 pregnancies. Reducing the high mortality from abruptio depends on both prevention and prompt diagnosis and treatment.

Total prevention is probably not possible, but since in approximately 40 per cent of the cases abruptio is associated with either toxemia or hypertension, early recognition and treatment of these conditions should reduce the incidence and subsequent perinatal death rate from abruptio.

Prompt treatment, which may save the baby, is dependent on swift diagnosis. Uterine tenderness and pain bring the mother to the hospital. There is uterine bleeding but it may be concealed (Figs. 3–3, 3–4). When the detachment is severe

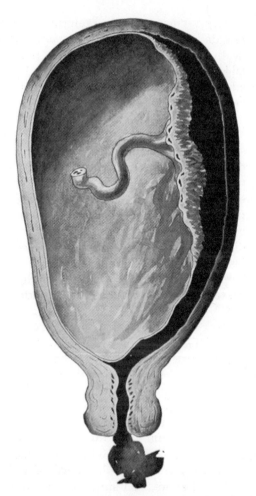

Figure 3–4. Abruptio placentae with external hemorrhage. (From Greenhill and Friedman: Biological Principles and Modern Practice in Obstetrics. 14th Edition. W. B. Saunders, 1974.)

fetal mortality is almost inevitable. Usually a fetal heart beat cannot be detected when the mother reaches the hospital. But in mild to moderate cases immediate delivery, either vaginal or abdominal depending on the condition of the cervix, may save the baby. Unlike placenta previa, in which watchful waiting is often indicated, immediate delivery is essential in abruptio placentae before additional separation further limits the baby's oxygen supply.

Pregnancy-Induced Hypertension (PIH)

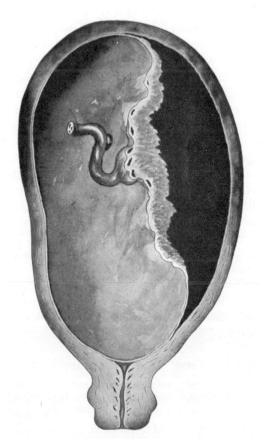

Figure 3–3. Abruptio placentae with internal or concealed hemorrhage. (From Greenhill and Friedman: Biological Principles and Modern Practice of Obstetrics. 14th Edition. W. B. Saunders, 1974.)

Infants of mothers with pregnancy-induced hypertension (preeclampsia,

eclampsia) may suffer intrauterine growth retardation, fetal morbidity, and fetal death. PIH is the leading cause of perinatal loss in the United States, a loss estimated at 25,000 fetal and neonatal deaths per year.

While the etiology of PIH is unclear, we can identify mothers at risk in many instances (Table 3–7). Most risk factors are derived from correlations in the population; just why a specific factor (e.g., poverty) is related to a higher incidence of preeclampsia remains unclear. A common finding in several conditions is an over-distended uterus and/or a large placenta (as in diabetes, multiple gestation), but here again the etiology is unclear. Blood vessel spasm is postulated as the underlying mechanism. When vessels are in spasm, less blood perfuses all body tissues. This problem leads to a number of other physiological changes that account for the classic symptoms of edema, hypertension, and proteinuria.

1. The delivery of oxygen and glucose is decreased in all tissues.

2. Fluid shifts from the vascular compartments (i.e., from within the blood vessels) to the intracellular spaces. Protein and electrolytes also shift into the intracellular space. Particularly significant is the leakage of sodium.

3. Because of this fluid shift, the blood becomes thicker; i.e., there is a tendency for blood to sludge and coagulate. Intravascular coagulation leads to diminished blood flow to all organs including, of course, the uterus, placenta, and fetus. In addition, peripheral resistance is increased when blood is thicker; the heart must work harder and the blood pressure rises. The increased workload of the heart in the presence of a decreased blood supply leads to heart failure.

4. Decreased blood supply to the maternal kidney leads to a loss of integrity in the glomeruli and a consequent spillage of protein in the urine. Acute renal failure is a severe complication.

5. In the brain, loss of fluid from the blood vessels leads to cerebral edema and, if untreated, cerebral hemorrhage.

6. Decreased blood supply to the maternal liver results in abnormal liver enzymes in maternal blood. Hepatic failure and rupture may occur.

7. Decreased blood supply to the uterus is responsible for the fetal distress previously described.

PIH usually occurs after 30 weeks gestation except in the case of trophoblastic disease. Because of the potentially serious effects for both mother and fetus, attention has been directed to screening that may identify women who are at risk for developing PIH. Two screening tools, sensitivity to angiotensin II (preeclamptic women have increased sensitivity beginning at 20 to 22 weeks) and dehydroepiandrosterone (DHEA) clearance, are considered by many to be too cumbersome for widespread screening (for descriptions of these tests, see Gant 1974 and 1976).

Two screening tests, the roll-over test and the evaluation of mean arterial pressure, are noninvasive and simple to perform.

Table 3–7 Risk Factors for Developing Pregnancy-Induced Hypertension

Demographic
  Low income
  Limited education
  Teenage
Nutritional
  Decreased protein intake
Familial
  Daughters of women with preeclampsia
Health-related
  Diabetes mellitus
  Chronic hypertension
  Renal disease
  Trophoblastic disease
Obstetrical
  Primigravida
  Polyhydramnios
  Erythroblastosis
  Multiple gestation
  Preeclampsia in a previous pregnancy
    (25% recurrence)

Roll-over test In a prospective study of 710 women, carried out in several different clinics, the roll-over test was found to be a good predictor of PIH. Of those women who had a positive response, 76 per cent ultimately developed PIH; of those women with a negative response, 91.5 per cent remained normotensive throughout pregnancy (Gant 1978). The roll-over test is performed at 28 to 32 weeks gestation. A gravida first lies in the left lateral position and her blood pressure is measured until it is stable. She then turns to her back and blood pressure is again measured. If there is an increase by 20 to 30 mm Hg in systolic pressure or 15 to 20 mm Hg in diastolic pressure, the test is considered positive and the likelihood of later hypertension is significantly increased.

Mean arterial pressure Mean arterial pressure (MAP) is derived by determining pulse pressure (the difference between systolic and diastolic pressures), dividing pulse pressure by 3, and adding the diastolic pressure:

$$\frac{\text{pulse pressure}}{3} + \text{diastolic} = \text{MAP}$$

At 18 to 26 weeks of pregnancy the normal MAP is 80 to 85. MAP greater than 85 is considered high; levels greater than 90 are unusual. If MAP is greater than 90 on two or more occasions in the second trimester (when there is normally a fall in blood pressure) or greater than 105 on two or more occasions in the third trimester, the mother is considered hypertensive.

When a woman is identified as at risk for hypertension, she should have weekly care from that time on until she gives birth. She is generally advised to take a leave from job or school to remain at home and limit her activity. Bed rest on her side will decrease blood pressure and edema, if it is present, and increase renal and uterine blood flow. She may be given some sedation to encourage rest.

The emotional and social problems that can be associated with weeks of confinement to home are massive. Interference with income, family life, isolation from friends and social life, frequent feelings of inadequacy because of an "abnormal pregnancy" are only a few potential problems. A high level of support and positive reinforcement is needed from all members of the team caring for the mother. Frequently she receives negative rather than positive messages. "If you don't do what we ask, you'll be hospitalized" or "Your baby might die." And then, if she is hospitalized, or in spite of everything her baby does die or requires extensive hospitalization, the health care team has compounded inevitable feelings of guilt.

Preeclampsia

Positive signs of preeclampsia are described in Table 3–8. Once frank preeclampsia develops, hospitalization is considered mandatory. Care of the mother includes bed rest, sedation, and administration of magnesium sulfate. Antihyper-

Table 3–8 Positive Indications of Preeclampsia

	Moderate	Severe
Blood pressure	140/90 Elevation of 30 mm Hg systolic Elevation of 15 mm Hg diastolic Loss of fall in blood pressure at night	Systolic greater than 160 Diastolic greater than 110
Proteinuria	Greater than 0.5 g/24 hours	Greater than 5 g/24 hours 3 to 4 + protein in catheterized specimen
Edema Liver	Hands and face	Pulmonary (with or without cyanosis) Persistent epigastric pain (distended liver) Signs of liver failure Jaundice
Urine volume		Less than 400 to 600 ml/24 hours
Visual symptoms		Blurring, spots before eyes
CNS symptoms		Hyperreflexia Headache Clouding of consciousness

tensive agents (e.g., hydralazine hydro-chloride, Apresoline) are given when diastolic blood pressure is greater than 110 mm Hg, with the goal of maintaining the diastolic pressure near 100 mm Hg. Blood pressure is lowered to protect the mother from a cerebral vascular accident; however, too low a pressure level may decrease uteroplacental perfusion.

Since the only "cure" for PIH is delivery, the fetus is carefully monitored with the nonstress test (NST), the oxytocin challenge test (OCT), fetal movement assessment, and estriol determination (Chapter 4). Lung maturity is assessed (Chapter 4) and the fetus delivered when mature. If fetal or maternal deterioration is evident, delivery may be necessary before the baby's lungs mature.

THE OUTCOME OF INTENSIVE CARE FOR MOTHER AND FETUS

Does the intensive level of care described above result in healthier babies? Are the many hours, the hospitalization, the costs to individual families and society (through tax-supported and other third-party reimbursement) justified? A lot of energy and time from nurses as well as other health professionals are necessary for each mother. One review of 625 multiparous women with PIH found a perinatal mortality of nine per 1000, contrasted with a rate of 129 per 1000 in women in the same unit who left against medical advice prior to delivery. A perinatal mortality rate of nine per 1000 is commendable even in a normal population, so the effort does seem worthwhile.

One way of alleviating costs is hospitalization in a unit at a progressive care level. While mothers with severe preeclampsia require intensive care, mothers with mild preeclampsia have been successfully treated in units that allow bed rest for much of the day and continuing assessment of both fetus and mother, without requiring the intensive care of the severely ill mother. When the cost of maternal care is compared with the cost of neonatal intensive care required by the infants of mothers with PIH who do not receive

specialized care, meticulous maternal care can be shown to be cost effective.

Anemia

When the mother is anemic during pregnancy the hazard to the developing fetus is one of chronic intrauterine asphyxia. One of the real values of early prenatal care is the prompt recognition and subsequent treatment of anemia. Not only is iron deficiency anemia prevalent, particularly in mothers from lower socioeconomic classes and in teenage mothers, but megaloblastic anemia due to folic acid deficiency has been recognized in 10 to 20 per cent of pregnancies. Some researchers feel that there may be a connection between folic acid deficiency and abruptio placentae (Hubbard 1963).

The anemia of pregnancy differs from anemia occurring at other periods of life in that it is due not to a decrease in the number of red blood cells but to an increase in plasma volume, which affects the relative proportion of red blood cells to plasma. For the woman whose iron stores are borderline (because of teenage growth needs, marginal nutrition, or frequent pregnancies), this increase in blood volume lowers hemoglobin levels below acceptable limits. Iron therapy (or folic acid therapy in the instance of megaloblastic anemia) can help increase production of red blood cells. Unfortunately many of those mothers most in danger of marked anemia — the very young and the very poor — are also those least likely to have early prenatal care and long-term supplementation.

It must be added that although all the available knowledge points to the theoretical conclusion that iron supplementation improves the oxygen supply of the fetus, there is no direct clinical evidence that this is so.

MATERNAL STRESS: A TERATOGEN?

Anxiety produces a variety of physiological changes in mammals because of the response of the sympathetic division of the autonomic nervous system: changes in heart rate, the constriction of blood vessels, dilation of coronary vessels, decrease in gastrointestinal motility, and so on. Generally the greater the anxiety, the more severe the response. In addition, anxiety also affects the adrenal cortical hormonal system as indicated in the following flow chart:

STRESS
activates
HYPOTHALAMUS
which stimulates
ANTERIOR LOBE OF PITUITARY
to produce
ACTH
(ADRENOCORTICOTROPIC HORMONE)
which activates
ADRENAL CORTEX
to produce
CORTISONE
which enters
MATERNAL BLOOD STREAM

It has been known for some time that hormones such as cortisone can cross the placental barrier and affect the fetus.

Animal studies indicate that stress-producing situations do tend to affect the fetus. In a study subjecting one group of rat mothers to stress and then observing the behavior of their offspring as compared with the behavior of the offspring of a control group at 30 to 40 days and at 130 to 140 days, a definite behavior difference was noted in the two groups (Thompson 1957).

Similar studies have demonstrated that changes in emotional states as well as in learning activity levels can be produced in rat offspring by exposing mothers to such stimuli as intense sound, x rays, and anxiety-causing conditions during pregnancy. Even when offspring were immediately removed from their anxious mothers after birth to eliminate the possibility that the mothers would transmit anxiety postnatally, the young of stressed mothers responded differently from controls in that they were more timid and "unforthcoming" when placed in strange environments (Dubos 1965).

Still other research has demonstrated that when mice are intensely crowded during pregnancy, behavorial abnormalities are evident in their offspring as compared to the young of uncrowded mothers. Crowding apparently leads to changes in hormonal secretion which are then reflected in behavior.

As was true of drugs and nutritional deficiencies, these studies cannot be considered directly analogous to human pregnancy, but they can suggest possible directions for research. Stott (1957) did find some indication that maternal illness or stress during pregnancy affected young children. Seventy-six per cent of the children of mothers stressed during pregnancy had nonepidemic illness in their first three years compared with 29 per cent of the children of mothers with no trouble in pregnancy. The association was statistically significant at the .001 level; that is, the probability that these findings could have occurred by chance if there was no relationship between the two factors in the population was less than one in 1000. Moreover, when variables such as social class, premature and abnormal births, and possible neglect by mothers in a state of physical or nervous breakdown were controlled, the statistical significance held. An analysis of the types of stress to which the mothers were subjected showed that matrimonial difficulties, illness or death of the husband or another child, difficulties with relatives, eviction, and similar psychological stresses predominated.

Bibliography

Abernathy, J., Greenberg, B., Wells, H. et al.: Smoking as an independent variable in a multiple regression analysis upon birth weight and gestation. Am J Public Health 56:626, 1966.

Andrews, J., McGarry, J.: A community study of smoking in pregnancy. J Obstet Gynaecol Br Commonw 79:1057, 1972.

Bahr, J.: Herpesvirus hominis Type 2 in women and newborns. MCN 3(1):16, 1978.

Bergman, A., Wiesner, L.: Relationship of passive cigarette-smoking to sudden infant death syndrome. Pediatrics 58:665, 1976.

Brocklebank, J., Ray, W., Federspiel, C., Schaffner, W.: Drug prescribing during pregnancy. Am J Obstet Gynecol 132:235, 1978.

Burke, B.: Nutritional needs in pregnancy in relation

to nutritional intakes as shown by dietary histories. Obstet Gynecol Surv 3:716, 1948.

Butler, N., Goldstein, H., Ross, E.: Cigarette smoking in pregnancy: its influence on birth weight and perinatal mortality. Br Med J 2:127, 1972.

Chavez, C., Stryker, J., Ostrea, E.: Sudden infant death syndrome (SIDS) among infants of drug-dependent mothers (IDDM) (abstract). Pediatr Res 12:403, 1978.

Cicero, T., Bell, R., West, W. et al.: Function of the male sex organs in heroin and methadone users. N Engl J Med 292:882, 1975.

Churchill, J.: Factors in intrauterine impoverishment. In Nutritional Impacts on Women, K. Moghissi and T. Evans (eds.). Hagerstown: Harper & Row, 1977.

Cohen, E., Brown, B., Bruce, D. et al.: A survey of anesthetic health hazards among dentists. J Am Dent Assoc 90:1291, 1975.

Davie, R., Butler, N., Goldstein, H.: From Birth to Seven. The second report of the national child development study. London: Longman, 1972.

Davies, D., Gray, O., Ellwood, P. et al.: Cigarette smoking in pregnancy: associations with maternal weight gain and fetal growth. Lancet 1:385, 1976.

Davison, J., Lindheimer, M.: Renal disease in pregnancy. Clin Obstet Gynecol 21:411, 1978.

Delgado, H., Lechtig, A., Yarbrough, C., Martorell, R., Klein, R., Irwin, M.: Maternal nutrition: its effects on infant growth and development and birthspacing. In Nutritional Impacts on Women, K. Moghissi and T. Evans (eds.). Hagerstown: Harper & Row, 1977.

Dobbing, J.: Effects of experimental undernutrition on development of the nervous system. In Malnutrition, Learning and Behavior, N. Scrimshaw and J. Gordon (eds.). Cambridge: MIT Press, 1968.

Doering, P., Stewart, R.: The extent and character of drug consumption during pregnancy. JAMA 239:843, 1978.

Donovan, J.: Effect on child of maternal smoking during pregnancy. Lancet 1:376, 1973.

Dubos, R.: Man Adapting. New Haven: Yale University Press, 1965.

Dunn, H., McBurney, A., Ingram, S., Hunter, C.: Maternal cigartte smoking during pregnancy and the child's subsequent development. Can J Public Health 67:499, 1976.

Edwards, M.: Venereal herpes: a nursing overview. JOGN Nurs 7(5):7, 1978.

Ferguson, A., Lawlor, G., Neuman, C. et al.: Decreased rosette-forming lymphocytes in malnutrition and intrauterine growth retardation. J Pediat 85:717, 1975.

Finnegan, L., Reeser, D.: Incidence of sudden death in infants born to women maintained on methadone (abstract). Pediatr Res 12:405, 1978.

Florman, A.: Intrauterine infection with herpes simplex virus: resultant congenital malformations. JAMA 225:129, 1973.

Gabbe, S.: Congenital malformations in infants of diabetic mothers. Obstet Gynecol Surv 32:125, 1977.

Gant, N., Chand, S., Worley, R. et al.: A clinical test useful for predicting the development of acute hypertension in pregnancy. Am J Obstet Gynecol 120:1, 1974.

Gant, N., Madden, J., Daniels, J. et al.: The metabolic clearance role of dehydroisoandrosterone sulfate. IV. Acute effects of induced hypertension, hypotension, natruresis in normal and hyperten-

sive pregnancies. Am J Obstet Gynecol 124:143, 1976.

Gant, N., Worley, R., Cunningham, F., Whalley, P.: Clinical management of pregnancy-induced hypertension. Clin Obstet Gynecol 21:397, 1978.

Greenberg, G., Inman, W., Weatherall, J., Adelstein, A.: Hormonal pregnancy tests and congenital malformations (letter). Br Med J 2:191, 1975.

Hanson, J., Jones, K., Smith, D.: Fetal alcohol syndrome. JAMA 235:1458, 1976.

Hawkins, D. F.: Teratogens in the human: current problems. J Clin Pathol 29:150, 1976.

Herbst, A., Ulfelder, H., Poskanzer, D.: Adenocarcinoma of the vagina: association of stilbestrol therapy with tumor appearance in young women. N Engl J Med 284:878, 1971.

Herrera, M.: Malnutrition and psychologic development. The section on nutrition and growth of the clinical nutrition and early development branch. In A Report to the National Advisory Child Health and Human Development Council. Washington, D.C., 1979.

Higgins, A.: Nutritional status and the outcome of pregnancy. J Can Diet Assoc 37:17, 1976.

Hollingsworth, D.: Data reported in Ob Gyn News 13(3):43, 1978.

Howard, I., Hill, J.: Drugs in pregnancy. Obstet Gynecol Surv 34:643, 1979.

Hubbard, B. M., Hubbard, E. D.: Aetiological factors in abruption placentae. Br Med J 2:1430, 1963.

Janerich, D.T., Piper, J., Glebatis, D.: Oral contraceptives and congenital limb reduction defects. N Engl J Med 291:697, 1974.

Joffe, J.: Influence of drug exposure of the father on perinatal outcome. Clin Perinatol 6:21, 1979.

Jones, K., Smith, D., Ulleland, C., Streessguth, A.: Pattern of malformations in offspring of chronic alcoholic mothers. Lancet 1:1267, 1973.

Jones, K., Smith, D.: Recognition of the fetal alcohol syndrome in early infancy. Lancet 2:999, 1973.

Kaltenbach, K., Grazioni, L., Finnegan, L.: Development of children born to women who received methadone during pregnancy (abstract). Pediatr Res 12:372, 1978.

Kantor, G.: Addicted mother, addicted baby–a challenge to health care providers. MCN 3(5):281, 1978.

Kaufman, R., Binder, G., Gray, P., Adam, E.: Upper genital tract changes associated with exposure in utero to diethylstilbestrol. Am J Obstet Gynecol 128:51, 1977.

Krugman, S.: Rubella immunization: progress, problems and potential solutions. Am J Public Health 69:217, 1979.

Lewis, B.: The action of drugs on the uteroplacental circulation and the developing fetus. In Obstetric Therapeutics, D. F. Hawkins (ed.). London: Bailliere Tindall, 1974.

Luke, B.: Maternal alcoholism and fetal alcohol syndrome. AGN 77:1924, 1977.

Maternal Nutrition and the Course of Pregnancy. National Research Council, Washington, D.C., National Academy of Sciences, 1970.

McLaughlin, M., Gold, L.: The New York rubella incident: a case for changing hospital policy regarding rubella testing and immunization. Am J Public Health 69:287, 1979.

Meyer, M., Jonas, B., Tonascia, J.: Perinatal events associated with maternal smoking during pregnancy. Am J Epidemiol 103:464, 1976.

Meyer, M., Tonascia, J.: Maternal smoking, pregnancy complications, and perinatal mortality. Am J Obstet Gynecol 128:494, 1977.

Moghissi, K., Churchill, J., Frohman, C.: Relationship of maternal amino acid blood levels to fetal development. In Perinatal Factors Affecting Human Development. Washington: Pan American Health Organization, Scientific Publication No. 185, 1969.

Moghissi, K., Churchill, J., Kurrie, D.: Relationship of maternal amino acids and proteins to fetal growth and mental development. Am J Obstet Gynecol 123:398, 1975.

Mora, J., Clement, J., Christiansen, N., Suescun, J., Wagner, M., Herrera, M.: Nutritional supplementation and the outcome of pregnancy. III. Perinatal and neonatal mortality. Nutritional Reports International 18:167, 1978.

Mora, J., Paredes, B., Wagner, M., Navarro, L., Vuori, L., Suescun, J., Christiansen, N., Herrera, M.: Nutritional supplementation and the outcome of pregnancy. I. Birth weight. Am J Clin Nutr 32:455, 1979.

Naeye, R., Diener, W., Dillinger, W. et al.: Urban poverty: effects on prenatal nutrition. Science 166:1026, 1969.

Naeye, R., Harkness, W., Utts, J.: Abruptio placentae and perinatal death: a prospective study. Am J Obstet Gynecol 128:740, 1977.

Offspring of women given DES remain under study. JAMA 238:932, 1977.

Oldham, H., Sheft, B.: Effect of caloric intake on nitrogen utilization during pregnancy. J Am Diet Assoc 27:847, 1951.

Ouellette, E., Rosett, H.: The effect of maternal alcohol ingestion during pregnancy on offspring. In Nutritional Impacts on Women, K. Moghissi and T. Evans (eds.). Hagerstown: Harper & Row, 1977.

Povar, G., Maloney, M., Watson, W., McBean, A., Giguere, G.: Rubella screening and follow-up immunization in Vermont. Am J Public Health 69:285, 1979.

Pregnancy: In The Health Consequences of Smoking. Washington, D.C.: U. S. Department of Health, Education and Welfare, 1973.

Pregnancy and Infant Health. A reprint of Chapter 8 In Smoking and Health: A Report of the Surgeon General. Rockville, Md.: U. S. Department of Health, Education and Welfare; Office on Smoking and Health, 1979.

Redmond, G.: Effect of drugs on intrauterine growth. Clin Perinatol 6:5, 1979.

Reinisch, J., Simon, N., Karow, W. et al.: Prenatal exposure to prednisone in humans and animals retards intrauterine growth. Science 202:436, 1978.

Rhead, W.: Smoking and SIDS. Pediatrics 59:791, 1977.

Rubella vaccine. Recommendation of the U.S. Public Health Service Advisory Committee on Immunization Practices. MMWR 27:451, (Nov. 17) 1978.

Russell, C.S., Taylor, R., Maddison, R.: Some effects of smoking in pregnancy. J Obstet Gynecol Br Commonw 73:742, 1966.

Sadovsky, E., Yaffe, H.: Daily fetal movement recording and fetal prognosis. Obstet Gynecol 41:845, 1973.

Safra, M., Oakley, G.: Association between cleft lip with or without cleft palate and prenatal exposure to diazepam. Lancet 1:478, 1975.

Schachter, J., Grossman, M., Holt, B. et al.: Prospective study of chlamydial infection in neonates. Lancet 2:377, 1979.

Sever, J.: Viral infections in pregnancy. Clin Obstet Gynecol 21(2):477, 1978.

Shaul, W., Hall, J.: Multiple congenital anomalies associated with oral anticoagulants. Am J Obstet Gynecol 127:191, 1977.

Simpson, W.: A preliminary report on cigarette smoking and the incidence of prematurity. Am J Obstet Gynecol 73:808, 1957.

South, M.: Congenital malformations of the central nervous system associated with genital type (type 2) herpes virus. J Pediatr 75:13, 1969.

Spence, A., Cohen, E., Brown, B. et al.: Occupational hazards for operating room-based physicians. JAMA 238:955, 1977.

Stafl, D., Dattingly, R. et al.: Clinical diagnosis of vaginal adenosis. Obstet Gynecol 43:118, 1974.

Steele, R., Langworth, J.: The relationship of antenatal and postnatal factors to sudden unexpected death in infancy. Can Med Assoc J 94:1165, 1966.

Stewart, A., Kneale, G.: Radiation dose effects in relation to obstetric x-rays and childhood cancers. Lancet 1:1185, 1970.

Stott, D.: Physical and mental handicaps following a disturbed pregnancy. Lancet 272:1006, 1957.

Thompson, W.: Influence of prenatal maternal anxiety on emotionality in young rats. Science 125:698, 1957.

Underwood, P., Hester, L., Laffitte, T., Gregg, K.: The relationship of smoking to the outcome of pregnancy. Am J Obstet Gynecol 91:270, 1965.

Underwood, P., Kesler, K., O'Lane, J., Callagan, D.: Parental smoking empirically related to pregnancy outcome. Obstet Gynecol 29:1, 1967.

Vorhees, C., Brunner, R., Butcher, R.: Psychotropic drugs as behavioral teratogens. Science 205:1220, 1979.

Vuori, L., Mora, J., Christiansen, N., Clement, J., Herrera, M.: Nutritional supplementation and the outcome of pregnancy. II. Visual habituation at 15 days. Am J Clin Nutr 32:463, 1979.

Whitelaw, A.: Subcutaneous fat in newborn infants of diabetic mothers: an indication of quality of diabetic control. Lancet 1:15, 1977.

Wilson, E.: The effect of smoking in pregnancy on the placental coefficient. NZ Med J 74:384, 1972.

Wingerd, J., Christianson, R., Lovett, W., Schoen, E.: Placental ratio in white and black women: relation to smoking and anemia. Am J Obstet Gynecol 124:671, 1976.

Winick, M.: Cellular growth of the human placenta. III. Intrauterine growth failure. J Pediatr 71:390, 1967.

Winick, M.: Cellular growth in intrauterine malnutrition. Pediatr Clin North Am 17:333, 1970.

Zackai, E., Millman, M., Neiderer, B. et al.: The fetal trimethadione syndrome. J Pediatr 87:280, 1975.

Zamenhof, S., Marthens, E. van, Grauel, L.: DNA (cell number) in neonatal brain: Second generation alteration by maternal dietary protein restriction. Science 172:850, 1971.

MATERNAL/FETAL ASSESSMENT

4

Assessment of the Fetus In Utero

As the chapters on embryology and genetics have indicated, it is possible today to gather data about the fetus many weeks before birth. Fetal assessment will be considered in two general categories: prior to the twentieth week of pregnancy, and during the third trimester.

Prior to the twentieth week of pregnancy, assessment is principally for the purpose of detecting abnormalities in the fetus with the thought that the parents may choose to terminate the pregnancy if a fetal defect is discovered. Methods of assessment are amniocentesis, maternal blood sampling, fetoscopy, and ultrasonography.

After 20 weeks the purposes of fetal assessment are to determine fetal well-being and assess fetal maturity.

Although many of the techniques used in assessment are performed by physicians (e.g., amniocentesis, fetoscopy), parents frequently seek the counsel of nurses as they consider decisions they must make. The ability to describe the tests as well as their purposes and possible benefits and risks is important in obstetrical nursing.

ASSESSMENT PRIOR TO 20 WEEKS

Amniocentesis

Amniocentesis involves the withdrawal of amniotic fluid from the intrauterine sac that surrounds the baby. Before the procedure is carried out, the placenta is located, by means of ultrasonography in most instances, so that it can be avoided when the needle is inserted. In addition, ultrasonography aids in the identification of any uterine abnormality such as a bicornuate uterus, that might complicate the amniocentesis. It also provides oher kinds of information.

After the site is chosen, the abdominal skin is prepared and a local anesthetic is injected into the skin surrounding the site. Approximately 15 to 30 ml of amniotic fluid is withdrawn through a spinal needle. This volume of fluid is replaced within three to four hours following the amniocentesis.

RISKS

The potential risks of amniocentesis include miscarriage, fetal injury, infection,

64

subsequent leakage of amniotic fluid, and Rh sensitization. In a prospective study evaluated by the National Institute of Child Health and Human Development, no difference was found in the rate of fetal loss between 1,040 women who had amniocentesis and 922 matched controls who did not. There were no cases of fetal injury. The probability of risk is considered to be less than 1 per cent.

Although amniocentesis is not advocated for mass screening, when family history or maternal age suggests there may be a potential problem it is considered a safe procedure.

When amniocentesis is performed on a mother who is Rh_D negative, the administration of anti-D immunoglobulin (RhoGAM) following the procedure is currently recommended to prevent sensitization.

DETECTION OF GENETIC DEFECTS

Amniocentesis is performed at 16 to 18 weeks gestation (menstrual age) to detect genetic defects. It is possible to detect all the fetal chromosomal anomalies, approximately 75 serious inborn errors of metabolism (e.g., galactosemia), levels of alpha-fetoprotein (see below), and fetal sex (useful when there is an increased risk of an X-linked disease in the male child such as Duchenne muscular dystrophy or X-linked mental retardation). Accuracy in detecting chromosomal problems and inborn errors of metabolism exceeds 99 per cent. In approximately 95 per cent of amniocenteses, the fetus does not have the condition for which the test is performed. The fetus may, however, have another genetic problem, just as any fetus may, which will not be detected, because testing is specific for each defect.

Alpha-fetoprotein In 1972 Brock and Sutcliffe first recognized that the level of alpha-fetoprotein (AFP), a protein produced by the yolk sac and the fetal liver, is as much as eight times higher when the fetus has an *open* neural tube defect (NTD) — most commonly spina bifida or anencephaly — as when there is a closed NTD. The AFP moves from the fetal serum to the fetal cerebrospinal fluid and then through the open lesion into the amniotic fluid. When there is a closed defect of the neural tube, such as hydrocephalus, the AFP cannot get into the amniotic fluid. Therefore, the level of AFP is higher with an open NTD than with a closed NTD. The level of AFP in amniotic fluid increases until 15 weeks gestation and then decreases until term; hence, studies are done at 14 to 16 weeks gestation.

Screening for neural tube defects by amniocentesis is a highly reliable procedure. Milunsky (1979) reports experience with more than 14,000 pregnancies in which 110 NTDs were detected and none were missed. The false-positive rate (i.e., diagnosing a NTD when none is present) was below 0.1 per cent.

Amniocentesis for the detection of NTD is reserved for women who have previously delivered an infant with this anomaly. Because the probability of risk of amniocentesis, even though less than 1 to 2 per cent, is greater than the risk of having a child with a NTD (approximately 0.2 per cent for women in general), the procedure is inappropriate for mass screening. The development of a method for determining maternal serum levels of AFP makes mass screening likely. In normal adults, serum AFP levels are very low; AFP from fetal sources, however, can be detected in maternal blood after the tenth week of pregnancy, with maximum levels between 16 and 18 weeks. Maternal blood is drawn for AFP testing at this peak time.

In a large collaborative study in the United Kingdom (1977), serum studies were 79 per cent accurate in predicting myelomeningocele and 88 per cent accurate in predicting anencephaly. Screening for AFP is not widespread at this time in the United States; many still consider the procedure experimental. Large studies are currently in progress.

Elevated AFP levels may be related to factors other than open NTD. Abortion, intrauterine fetal demise, and multiple gestation are recognized causes. False-positive results are relatively common. When serum AFP is elevated further evaluation is indicated before an open NTD is confirmed; included are a repeat of the serum AFP analysis, ultrasound evaluation, and amniocentesis.

PREGNANCY TERMINATION

It has been the practice of many centers to offer amniocentesis only if the parents agree that if the fetus is abnormal, the pregnancy will be terminated. Those who believe that amniocentesis should be offered even if the parents do not feel they would terminate the pregnancy suggest that (1) finding evidence of normality in the fetus can be reassuring to the parents, and (2) if there is evidence of abnormality, parents who choose not to terminate the pregnancy can begin to plan for their infant's special needs.

In regard to the first reason, consider mothers over 40 who are screened for Down's syndrome. Even with the high probability (one in 40) of having an infant with Down's syndrome, 39 mothers out of 40 will *not* be carrying a fetus with Down's syndrome. Knowing this at 20 weeks gestation can relieve a great deal of anxiety. However, *parents must understand that amniocentesis is specific for the condition under consideration and is not a general test of fetal normality.*

Fetoscopy

Fetoscopy is an experimental procedure by which a fetoscope is introduced into the amniotic cavity through the abdominal wall. Depending on the preference of the examiner, ultrasound examination to locate the fetus and placenta is done before and/or during the procedure. Three uses of fetoscopy at present are fetal blood sampling, fetal skin sampling, and direct visualization of the fetus.

The seventeenth week of pregnancy is the preferred time for fetoscopy. The pro-cedure is difficult to perform before this time. The seventeenth week allows three weeks for cell growth, examination and therapeutic abortion, if indicated, by the twentieth week.

Prior to fetoscopy, the mother may be given Demerol, which will cross the placenta and quiet the fetus, because excessive fetal activity makes the procedure more difficult.

Through fetal blood sampling, sickle cell anemia, β thalassemia (a type of hemolytic anemia), and hemophilia may be diagnosed in the fetus, as well as certain immunologic disorders including Rh incompatibility. Fetal skin biopsies may indicate the presence of certain primary skin disorders such as ichthyosis, a condition in which the skin is harsh and dry with adherent scales. Through direct visualization, the diagnosis of certain severe malformations or the confirmation of others, such as neural tube defects, is possible.

Fetoscopy is available almost exclusively in large medical centers. It is a technically difficult procedure and is not without risk. As in amniocentesis, spontaneous abortion is possible following the procedure; less common is the occurrence of a stillborn infant. Amnionitis has also occurred; prophylactic antibiotics may be prescribed for 10 days following examination.

Ultrasound

Ultrasound is based on the piezoelectric effect; sound too high to be heard causes the movement of crystals, which generates electrical impulses. These impulses are directed toward the surface tissue and reflect back onto a screen, where a photograph of the tissue (a visualization of the reflection of the ultrasonic impulses) may be taken (Fig. 4–1).

Two types of ultrasound are used in fetal assessment, real time and gray scale — B-scan (Tables 4–1, 4–2). Real time is used most frequently; it is rapid, portable, and inexpensive in both initial cost and maintenance and therefore less expensive to the patient. It is possible to

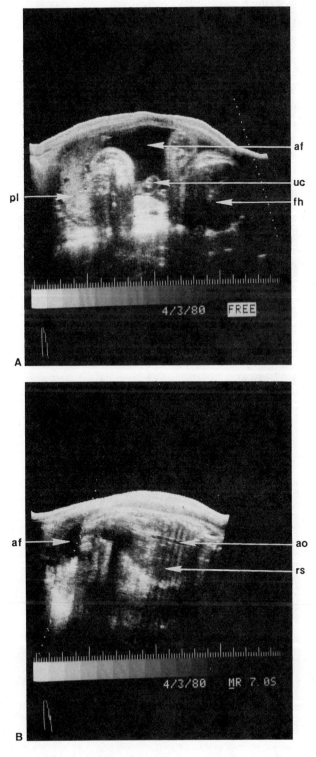

Figure 4–1. Varying views of the same fetus as seen on ultrasound at 32 weeks. Ultrasound and photography by Dr. Lewis Nelson. (pl = placenta, af = amniotic fluid, uc = umbilical cord, fh = fetal head, ao = aorta, rs = rib shadows, ab = arm bone, f = fist, k = kidney, sc = spinal cord, sp = spine).

Illustration continued on following page

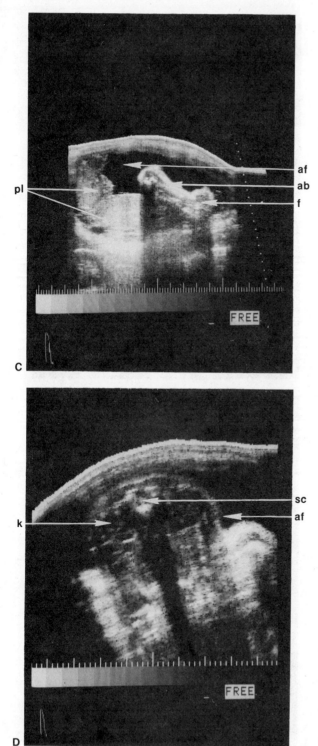

Figure 4–1. Continued.

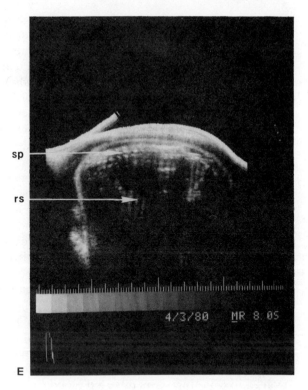

Figure 4–1. Continued. E

Table 4–1 Uses of Real Time Ultrasound

Biparietal diameter
Crown-rump length
Placental localization
Fetal presentation
General screening for congenital anomalies
Prior to amniocentesis
Multiple gestation
Early signs of fetal life (after nine weeks)
Early absence of fetal life
Bleeding (e.g., possible placenta previa)
Pelvic masses

observe movement during the later stages of pregnancy, including cardiac and respiratory movements, with real time scanning. The chief disadvantage of real time sonography is that distinctions between adjacent areas are more difficult to make.

Many mothers say that seeing their baby move on the screen, perhaps sucking a thumb, makes the baby seem very real to them. Mothers are frequently given pictures of their fetuses after ultrasound.

A number of fetal anomalies have been diagnosed by ultrasound in the second or early third trimester including anencephaly, meningomyelocele, hydrocephaly, renal agenesis and dysplasia, diaphragmatic hernia, gastroschisis, and omphalocele (Hobbins et al. 1979). Current research projects are investigating diagnosis prior to 20 weeks for a variety of conditions including cardiac defects and kidney abnormalities.

RISKS

Any procedure must be evaluated in relation to potential fetal risks. The vast majority of experiments on animals and

Table 4–2 Uses of Gray Scale (B-Scan) Ultrasound

Genetic screening
Some instances of placenta previa
Posterior placenta
When real time ultrasound is not available
Observation of gestational sac by six weeks
Early localization of the placenta (nine weeks)

human observations do not indicate any harmful or permanent effects using ultrasound at diagnostic levels. In one study (the outcome of 1,952 pregnancies, 303 that included exposure to ultrasound), no physical or developmental differences were found in exposed and control groups of infants at one year of age. It is always possible, of course, that differences might appear at some future time (Scheidt and Lundin 1977). No research has reported any harm from diagnostic ultrasound.

Antepartum Fetal Heart Rate Monitoring

The development of antepartum fetal heart rate (FHR) monitoring arose from the observation that the heart rate dropped in the fetus of some women after they had climbed one or more flights of stairs. Observers wondered if the stress involved in climbing stairs diverted blood from the placenta. In Europe, antepartum monitoring focused on spontaneous FHR utilizing the nonstress test (NST); in the United States the contraction stress test (CST) was initially employed. The CST is frequently called an oxytocin challenge test (OCT), but this is not quite correct; although oxytocin is usually given to the mother to stimulate uterine contractions, it does not challenge either mother or fetus. NSTs are widely used in the United States as well as in Europe at present.

NONSTRESS TESTING (NST)

The NST evaluates a complex response of the fetal central nervous system. Babies born within seven days of fetal heart rate acceleration in response to either fetal movement or uterine contractions are almost invariably in good health.

An NST is classified as either *reactive* or *nonreactive* (Table 4–3). Originally, an NST was considered reactive if, five times within a 20-minute period, the fetal heart rate increased 15 beats per minute or more and the accelerations lasted for 15 seconds or longer. Now two accelerations of 15 beats for 15 seconds within any 10-minute period constitute a reactive test. Failure to meet any of these criteria constitutes a nonreactive test. If no reactive pattern is recorded within 40 minutes, the test is also considered nonreactive. A 40-minute period is used because this is the duration of the sleep/wake cycle of the fetus, although the cycle varies considerably. When the fetus appears to be sleeping, stimulation by glucose or sound may induce activity. The result in about two-thirds of NSTs is reactive, which is interpreted as indicating fetal well-being (Paul and Miller 1978). A false-normal test occurs 1 per cent of the time, so that the test is considered highly reliable when it is reactive. However, a nonreactive test does not necessarily indicate that the fetus is in jeopardy. When the NST is nonreactive, it is usually followed by a contraction stress test (CST). In one study of 2,422 patients, 91 per cent of those fetuses with a nonreactive NST also had a negative CST, indicating fetal well-being (Martin and Schifrin 1977).

Directions for Nonstress Test (NST)
1. The purpose of this test and the procedure are explained to the mother.
2. The mother signs a consent form.
3. The mother lies in semi-Fowler's position or in lateral tilt with her right hip elevated 3 to 4 inches to avoid supine

Table 4–3 Nonstress Testing (NST) Results

	Pattern	
	Reactive	*Nonreactive*
Accelerations		
Number in 10 minutes	≥ 2	< 2
Duration in seconds	≥ 15	< 15
Beats per minute	≥ 15	< 15

Table 4–4   Contraction Stress Testing (CST) Results

Pattern	Criteria	Frequency of Occurrence (%)
Negative	Absence of late decelerations in three contractions within 10 minutes	85 to 90
Positive	Repetitive late decelerations	3 to 10
Equivocal	Occasional but not repetitive late decelerations; absence of a positive or negative "window"	5 to 10
Unsatisfactory	Inability to provoke sufficient uterine contractions; lack of adequate FHR data	5 to 10

hypotensive syndrome (decreased maternal blood pressure from pressure on the inferior vena cava).

4. The monitor is applied.

5. Maternal blood pressure is checked initially and at frequent intervals throughout the procedure.

6. The mother is observed for 20 minutes or until two to five fetal movements are present.

7. If no fetal movements are observed in 20 minutes, the mother is observed for a second 20-minute period. Fetal movements may be induced by giving the mother a snack with readily available glucose if they do not occur spontaneously. Glucose in the maternal blood stream crosses the placenta and the fetus becomes active in response.

CONTRACTION STRESS TESTING (CST)

In the contraction stress test uterine contractions are stimulated, usually by the intravenous administration of oxytocin, and the reaction of the fetus to the contractions is assessed by external fetal monitoring. Results are categorized as negative, positive, equivocal, or unsatisfactory (Table 4–4). If fetal oxygen reserve and placental function are satisfactory, there should be no late decelerations in the fetal heart rate and the test result is *negative* (late decelerations are described in relation to intrapartum fetal monitoring in Chapter 5). In a *positive* CST, repetitive late decelerations occur. If there are occasional but not repetitive late decelera-

tions, the test is considered *equivocal* and is repeated, usually 24 hours later.

Recently, the concept of a "10-minute window," i.e., a period of 10 minutes that satisfies the criteria of either a positive or a negative test, has reduced the incidence of equivocal tests. If an occasional deceleration is followed by 10 minutes in which there are no decelerations during three contractions, this is a "negative window" and the test is considered negative. Conversely, a "positive window" is one in which there is a 10-minute period that satisfies the criteria of a positive test. Failure to stimulate sufficient uterine contractions or to collect adequate FHR data results in an unsatisfactory test.

As with a reactive NST, a negative CST is reassuring. The chances of the infant dying in utero are considered to be less than 1 per cent. Although antepartum deaths from 5 of 1000 to 10 of 1000 have been reported, analysis shows that these deaths are usually the result of factors that could not have been predicted, such as abruptio placenta.

A positive CST, while identifying a group of mothers and fetuses who are at risk, is of less value. Evaluation and care of each mother and fetus is individual, combining the results of various fetal assessments.

Directions for Contraction Stress Test (CST)

1. The purpose of this test and the procedure are explained to the mother.

2. The mother signs a consent form.

3. The mother lies in semi-Fowler's position or in lateral tilt with her right hip elevated 3 to 4 inches to avoid supine hypotensive syndrome (decreased maternal blood pressure from pressure on the inferior vena cava).

4. The monitor is applied.

5. Maternal blood pressure is checked initially and at frequent intervals throughout the procedure.

6. Intravenous infusion is started; low-dose oxytocin by infusion pump is "piggy-backed" into IV. The initial rate is 0.5 to 1.0 milliunit per minute.

7. Oxytocin dose is increased, usually every 10 minutes, until there are three 40-second contractions in a 10-minute period.

8. Oxytocin is discontinued if the contractions last longer than 90 seconds.

9. Oxytocin is discontinued; the mother is observed until contractions are at least 10 minutes apart.

ADVANTAGES AND DISADVANTAGES OF NST AND CST AND THEIR USE IN THE CARE OF A MOTHER AND FETUS

The NST offers obvious advantages for initial screening. It is easily administered in any setting where a fetal monitor is available, which can usually be an outpatient clinic or office. This fact alone makes it less expensive than the CST. The time involved may be as little as 10 to 15 minutes and, following protocol, no longer than 40 minutes. If the test is reactive, a CST is unnecessary.

The CST requires at least 90 to 100 minutes and is commonly performed in a hospital setting because of the need to administer intravenous oxytocin. This increase in expense as well as time suggests that the CST is not as valuable in screening but is useful for the approximately 10 per cent of women who have a nonreactive NST. The use of the combination of NST and CST (Fig. 4–2) has been shown to aid in reducing perinatal mortality (Gordon and Schifrin 1979).

Assessment of Daily Fetal Movement: The Count-To-10 Chart

Daily fetal movement begins at approximately the eighteenth week of pregnancy, reaches a peak between 29 and 38 weeks, and then decreases slightly until term. When there is marked placental insufficiency, there is a significant decrease in fetal movement that precedes intrauterine fetal death. However, there is a period of time during which fetal movement is decreased but fetal heart rate remains normal. These observations form the basis of the "count-to-10" chart.

The "count-to-10" chart gives the mother an opportunity to help assess the well-being of her fetus. Beginning at 30 to 32 weeks gestation she is asked to count the number of fetal movements beginning at 9:00 AM. When she has counted 10 discrete instances of fetal movement, she

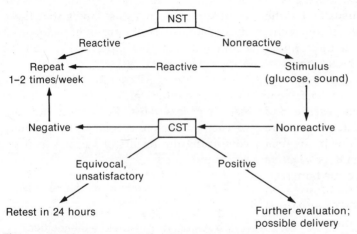

Figure 4–2. Nonstress test and contraction stress test.

marks the time on her chart. If she has not felt 10 fetal movements by 9:00 PM, she records the number of movements actually felt. If, for two days in a row, less than 10 movements are felt for each day, she is to notify her health care provider, thus assessing her fetal well-being at no expense to either family or health care system.

Biochemical Analysis

At present, the focus of biochemical testing is estriol analysis. Because the mother, the fetus, and the placenta contribute to the production of estriol, the concentration of estriol in maternal blood and urine reflects the function of the maternal fetoplacental unit. The fetal hypothalamus and pituitary stimulate the fetal adrenal gland to synthesize dehydroepiandrosterone sulfate (DHEA), which is hydroxylated in the fetal liver to 16α-hydroxydehydroepiandroster-

one sulfate. This compound then moves from fetus to placenta where further biochemical processes result in the production of estriol. Estriol enters the maternal circulation and is conjugated in the maternal liver. Half or more of the conjugated estriol enters the enterohepatic circulation, is hydrolyzed by bacteria in the gut, and is then reabsorbed (Fig. 4–3). Understanding this pathway is important in the interpretation of serum and urinary estriol levels because many factors can influence them (Table 4–5).

Since estriol is present in maternal blood and excreted in maternal urine, both substances are utilized in assessment. When a 24-hour urine specimen is being collected, *all* the urine excreted in 24 hours must be included or the reported estriol level will be inaccurate. The difficulty in accurately collecting urine for 24 hours and the delay in obtaining information when there is reason to suspect that

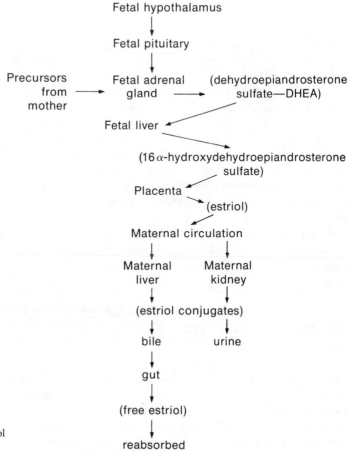

Figure 4–3. The pathway of estriol synthesis.

Table 4-5   Factors that may Influence Estriol Levels in
Maternal Serum and Urine

Condition	Result	Estriol Level
Anencephaly	Stimulatory portions of the brain absent	↓
Maternal corticosteroid therapy Hypoplasia or aplasia of fetal adrenal gland	Fetal adrenal gland suppressed	↓
Reduced function of placenta (e.g., infarction, growth retardation)	Limitation of conversion ability	↓
Maternal hepatic disease	Impaired estriol conjugation in liver	↓
Ampicillin administration	Decreased gut flora Decreased hydrolyzation and limited reabsorption	↓
Maternal obstructive gallbladder disease	Disturbed enterohepatic circulation; estriol lost in feces	↓
Impaired maternal renal function	Decreased excretion of estriol and decreased estriol levels in urine	↓
Increased fetoplacental size	Large baby	↑

the fetus is in jeopardy have led to increasing use of serum estriols.

A single estriol determination is of no value in assessing fetal status; it is the pattern of serial determinations that is helpful. Abnormal patterns include both a progressive downward trend and a rapid fall in values. "Normal" values, which vary from one laboratory to another, are reassuring in that perinatal mortality is rare when these values are found. However, abnormal values do not necessarily indicate fetal distress in a mother. Estriol values are always considered in conjunction with other assessments of fetal well-being.

ASSESSMENT DURING THE THIRD TRIMESTER

During the third trimester, assessment of fetal maturation becomes important if there is reason to interrupt the course of pregnancy. Pregnancy may need to be interrupted because of factors that may put the mother at risk if the pregnancy continues (e.g., severe preeclampsia) or because of indications that the fetus may be in jeopardy. When a cesarean section is to be performed because of a previous cesarean delivery, assessing fetal maturity is important; choosing the date on the basis of maternal history or fundal height may potentially lead to the delivery of a preterm infant.

Amniotic Fluid in the Assessment of Fetal Maturity

Measurement of phospholipids in amniotic fluid through L:S ratio or "shake" tests and the measurement of creatinine are the tests most commonly utilized in the assessment of fetal maturity.

PHOSPHOLIPIDS IN THE ASSESSMENT OF LUNG MATURITY

Assessment of lung maturity is particularly important because a major problem of preterm infants is respiratory distress. A surface active material, surfactant, lowers surface tension in the alveoli. If there is insufficient surfactant, alveoli collapse during exhalation, resulting in atelectasis and respiratory distress syndrome (Chapter 8).

Surfactant is synthesized by Type II cells lining each alveolus beginning at 24 to 26 weeks gestation. Phospholipids are the active components of surfactant; the most abundant of the phospholipid compounds is *lecithin*. After 32 weeks, concentrations of lecithin begin to rise rapidly. The concentration of a second phospholipid, *sphingomyelin*, changes very little. The ratio between the concentrations of lecithin and sphingomyelin in amniotic fluid, the *L:S ratio*, has become a standard measurement of fetal lung maturity.

When the L:S ratio is greater than 2, the chances of respiratory distress syndrome (RDS) are very slight (less than 1 per cent). When the L:S ratio is less than 1.5, the likelihood of RDS is high (78.9 per cent in a 1974 report by Whitfield and Sproule). It is more difficult to predict outcome when the L:S is between 1.5 and 2.0.

These ratio limits do not apply to the mother with diabetes. Lung maturity is frequently delayed in the infant of a diabetic mother, making estimation of maturity even more significant. Yet L:S ratios are less accurate in predicting RDS in infants of diabetic mothers. In some hospitals a higher L:S ratio (> 2.5) is used as the standard of maturity for the infant of a diabetic mother.

A more sensitive indicator of lung maturity, phosphotidyl glycerol (pg), is a phospholipid that appears at 36 weeks and increases until term. If pg is present in amniotic fluid, RDS did not occur (Kulovich, Hollman, and Gluck 1979).

The shake test is also an assessment of surfactant in amniotic fluid, the results of which have been correlated with the L:S ratio and the incidence of RDS. It requires no expensive laboratory equipment, and the results are available in less than 30 minutes. Although the technique is simple, errors can be easily made if care is not taken.

The shake test is based on the principle that the presence of surface active materials (e.g., surfactant) prolongs the stability of an emulsion. When amniotic fluid is diluted with saline and alcohol is added to nullify the action of other surface active materials, the persistence of fine bubbles indicates the presence of surfactant. A positive test result, in which fine bubbles (foam) are present at dilutions greater than 1:2 (amniotic fluid:saline), indicates pulmonary maturity; the accuracy is considered high. If there is no foam in undiluted amniotic fluid, the risk for RDS is high and the test is judged negative. Results between 0 and 1:2 are considered intermediate and a determination of the L:S ratio is indicated to more accurately predict the possibility of RDS.

SOME LEGAL AND MORAL ASPECTS OF FETAL MEDICINE

Technological advances can at times raise moral and legal questions; recent developments in fetal medicine are no exception. The desirability of abortion based on knowledge of a defective fetus and the right of a fetus to prenatal treatment are two current controversial issues.

The concept of therapeutic abortion when there is strong evidence that the fetus is defective, either because of known exposure to a teratogen such as rubella or because of abnormal chromosome findings in the amniotic fluid, is intertwined with religious and philosophical beliefs as well as medical and cultural values. The current trend in the United States undoubtedly points toward acceptance of abortion under these circumstances even by individuals who would not accept legalized therapeutic abortion for other reasons.

The legal rights of the unborn infant were considered at a conference held at the National Institute of Child Health and Human Development in 1969. Legal consensus seems to support the idea that life, and therefore the right of the fetus to protection, begins at five to six months after conception, based on the assumption that at this age the fetus could conceivably exist on its own outside the uterus. Many court decisions have rejected the concept that a fetus is living before this time.

The question of legal rights becomes more direct when intrauterine transfusion is considered in the face of parental objection, such as may arise with members of a religious sect such as Jehovah's Witnesses who believe that no foreign blood should enter the body. In such instances the physician or hospital administrator may go to court to have the guardianship of the unborn child temporarily removed from the parent and assigned to himself. After the transfusion takes place the child is then returned to the legal guardianship of the parents. One consequential problem in this sort of procedure, as pointed out by Professor Sanford Katz of the Boston College Law School, is the future attitude of parents toward a child "hexed" by foreign blood. Would he really be welcomed into the family?

The long-range implications of these procedures are likely to pose many questions for which we have no answers as yet. And as our technological ability to care for the fetus increases, these problems will surely multiply as well.

Bibliography

Antenatal diagnosis: Report of a consensus development conference. Bethesda, National Institute of Health, 1979.

Boehm, F., Somkeart, S., Ishii, T.: Lecithin-sphingomyeline ratio and a rapid test for surfactant in amniotic fluid: a comparison. Obstet Gynecol 41:829, 1973.

Brock, D., Sutcliffe, R.: Alpha-fetoprotein in the antenatal diagnosis of anencephaly and spina bifida. Lancet 2:197, 1972.

Galloway, K.: Placental Evaluation Studies: the procedures, their purposes and the nursing care involved. MCN 1(5):300, 1976.

Gordon, E., Schifrin, B.: Antepartum heart rate monitoring. In New Techniques and Concepts in Maternal and Fetal Medicine, H. Kaminetzky and L. Iffy (eds.). New York: Van Nostrand Reinhold, 1979.

Gortmaker, S.: Effects of prenatal care on the health of the newborn. Am J Public Health 69:653–660, 1979.

Hobbins, J., Grannum, P., Berkowitz, R. et al.: Ultrasound in the diagnosis of congenital anomalies. Am J Obstet Gynecol 134:331, 1979.

Kulovich, M., Hollman, M., Gluck, L.: The lung profile: I. Normal pregnancy. Am J Obstet Gynecol 135:57, 1979.

Martin, C., Schifrin, B.: Prenatal fetal monitoring. In Perinatal Intensive Care, S. Aladjem and A. Brown (eds.). St. Louis: C. V. Mosby, 1977.

Maternal serum-alpha-fetoprotein measurement in antenatal screening for anencephaly and spina bifida. Report of U.K. collaborative study on alpha-fetoprotein in relation to neural-tube defects. Lancet 2:1323, 1977.

Milunsky, A.: Alpha-fetoprotein and the prenatal tube defects. Am J Public Health 69:552–553, 1979.

National Institute of Child Health and Human Development: Amniocentesis Registry Symposium. JAMA 236:171, 1976.

Paul, R., Miller, F.: Antepartum fetal heart rate monitoring. Clin Obstet Gynecol 21(2):375, 1978.

Sadovsky, E., Yaffe, H.: Daily fetal movement recording and fetal prognosis. Obstet Gynecol 41:485, 1973.

Scheidt, P., Lundin, F.: Investigations for effects of intrauterine ultrasound in humans. In Symposium on biological effects and characteristics of ultrasound sources, D. Hazzard and M. Litz (eds.). Washington: DHEW Publication No. (FDA) 78-8048.

Whitfield, C., Sproule, W.: Fetal lung maturation. Br J Hosp Med 12:678, 1974.

5 TRANSITION: THE NEWBORN DURING LABOR AND DELIVERY

Although the precise mechanism that initiates labor is not completely understood, endocrine changes in the fetus, placenta, and mother and the increased size of the uterus appear to be important factors (Table 5–1).

As changes occur in the mother — contractions, effacement, dilatation of the cervix — the baby begins to descend through the vaginal canal. Figure 5–1 illustrates the changes in position that the baby normally undergoes in the process of birth. The nurse in the labor room, while caring for the mother, is also caring for the baby by monitoring and evaluating his condition throughout labor. Everything he or she is able to do for the mother, e.g., relieving the mother's anxiety so that only a minimum amount of analgesia and anesthesia will be needed, is also a boon to the baby.

MONITORING THE FETUS

There are several ways in which the fetus can be monitored during labor:

1. Observation of fetal heart rate (FHR) by auscultation or external fetal heart rate monitoring.

2. Fetal electrocardiogram, particularly

Table 5–1 Factors Believed to Influence Onset of Labor

Factor	Effect
Increased secretion in the fetal pituitary	
ACTH	Stimulates fetal adrenal gland to produce increasing amounts of cortisol
	Mediates initiation of labor
	Stimulates fetal lung maturity
Prolactin	Possibly stimulates cortisol production
	Role in stimulation of milk production
Oxytocin	Crosses placenta; acts in combination with maternal oxytocin
Decrease in maternal progesterone production by placenta	Allows increased excitability of uterine muscles
	Maternal prolactin no longer inhibited
Increase in maternal estrogen production by placenta	Enhances responsiveness of uterine muscles to oxytocin
	Enhances secretion of prolactin
Increase of prostaglandins in amniotic fluid	Stimulates uterine contractions
Increase in contractility and excitability of myometrium as uterine volume increases	Uterus more sensitive to oxytocin

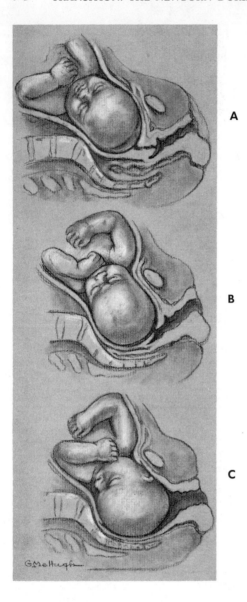

Figure 5–1. The baby undergoes a number of changes in position in the process of birth: *A,* engagement; *B,* descent; *C,* flexion.

in connection with amniotic fluid pressure.

3. The presence of meconium.

4. Fetal movement.

5. Analysis of fetal capillary blood for pH or oxygen concentration.

Physiologic Basis of Fetal Heart Rate Monitoring

The fetus derives oxygen from blood in the intervillous space of the placenta. Normally, the Po_2 of intervillous blood is 30 to 40 mm Hg with a 65 to 75 per cent oxygen saturation, similar to that of capillary blood in adults. Note in Table 5–2 that the blood supply to the fetal brain is lower than the blood supply to the placenta. The fetus is able to tolerate this relatively low Po_2 because of several compensatory mechanisms:

1. A high fetal cardiac output in relation to body weight (three times greater than that of an adult at rest).

2. Fetal hemoglobin (hemoglobin F), which combines with more oxygen at a lower pressure.

3. An increased hematocrit, which increases the oxygen-carrying capacity of fetal blood.

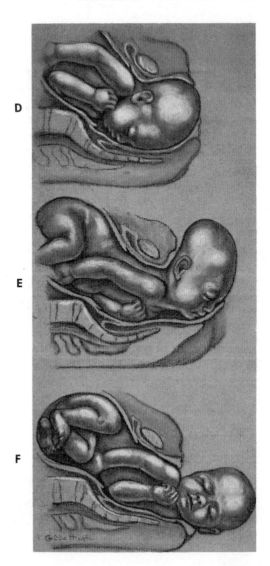

Figure 5–1 *Continued.* *D,* completion of internal anterior rotation; *E,* extension; *F,* external rotation. (From Davis and Rubin: DeLee's Obstetrics for Nurses. 18th Edition. W. B. Saunders, 1966.)

4. Preferential circulation of oxygen-rich blood to the fetal brain.

Several conditions must be met for the fetus to continually receive adequate oxygen: (1) the mother must continuously supply blood to the placenta, (2) oxygen levels must be maintained within the intervillous space of the placenta, (3) the umbilical cord vessels must be patent, and (4) the fetal heart must be able to circulate blood through the placenta.

During labor, uterine contractions in-

Table 5–2 Po_2 and O_2 Saturations in Mother, Placenta, Umbilical Vein, and Fetal Brain*

	Mother (lungs)	Placenta (intervillous space)	Umbilical Vein	Fetal Brain
Po_2 (mm Hg)	100	30 to 40	20 to 30	20 to 30
O_2 (%)	100	65 to 75	60	60

*Adapted from Hochberg *In* Kaminetzky and Iffy: Progress in Perinatology. George F. Stickley Co., 1977.

terfere with the flow of blood in the inter-villous space. At the peak of a contraction, blood flow from uterine artery branches may be interrupted for 10 to 15 seconds as intrauterine pressure temporarily exceeds the pressure within the branches. During this period in which the uterine artery flow is interrupted, the fetus must rely on reserve blood in the intervillous space as a source of oxygen. If this supply is com-promised and fetal oxygenation becomes inadequate, fetal hypoxia occurs. Marked hypoxia in turn results in deceleration of the fetal heart rate. Fetal heart rate (FHR) is also slowed as a reflex response to compression on the baby's head. The rela-tionship between deceleration of FHR and uterine contractions, visible on the fetal monitoring strip, provides information about fetal condition.

The goal of fetal monitoring is to recog-nize situations in which the fetal brain is not receiving adequate oxygen and there-by to prevent fetal brain damage or death.

Terms Describing Fetal Heart Rate and Uterine Contractions

A number of terms are used to describe FHR and uterine contractions. *Baseline fetal heart rate* is the heart rate between contractions or between transient changes unrelated to contractions. *Baseline fetal heart rate variability* refers to fluctuations in the baseline fetal heart rate. Short-term variability occurs between successive pairs of heart beats. Long-term variability is related to fetal activity and averages five to 15 beats per minute when the fetus is active but may be suppressed when the fetus is asleep. The absence of short-term, beat-to-beat variability indicates a need for immediate further evaluation of the fetus. The absence may be related to drugs taken by the mother (narcotics, barbitu-rates, tranquilizers, anesthetics, atropine, scopolamine), or it may be due to fetal hypoxia and acidosis. A smooth baseline may precede the late decelerations that indicate fetal hypoxia. In small premature

infants, absence of baseline variability re-flects immaturity of the cardiac control mechanisms.

Fetal tachycardia is a FHR of more than 160 beats per minute. Rates higher than 180 bpm are classified as *marked tachycar-dia*. Prematurity, maternal fever, mild or chronic hypoxia, intrauterine fetal infec-tion, maternal anxiety, fetal activity, and drugs such as atropine, scopolamine, isoxsuprine hydrochloride (Vasodilan), and ritodrine are potential causes of fetal tachycardia (Table 5–3). When tachycardia is associated with late or variable de-celerations, fetal stress is indicated.

Fetal bradycardia is a FHR of less than 120 beats per minute (Fig. 5–2). Rates be-low 99 bpm are classified as *marked brady-cardia*. Hypoxia, maternal hypothermia, arrhythmias of the fetal heart, and drugs, including agents used for local anesthesia, are potential causes of fetal bradycardia. A transient bradycardia may be seen after vaginal examination, probably owing to pressure on the fetal head. Fetal bradycar-dia does not always indicate severe fetal distress, but it should always be inves-tigated (see Table 5–3).

Deceleration patterns, seen on the fetal monitoring strip, indicate the way in which the fetal heart rate slows in re-sponse to certain stimuli. The timing and configuration of the deceleration in rela-tion to the uterine contractions indicates certain facts about the fetus.

Acceleration patterns involve FHR accel-erations above the baseline.

Table 5–3   Factors Affecting Baseline Fetal Heart Rate*

Causes of Fetal Tachycardia (rate > 160)	Causes of Fetal Bradycardia (rate < 120)
Maternal hyperthermia	Fetal hypoxia (late sign)
Fetal hypoxia (early sign)	Response to vagal stimulus
Fetal sepsis	Maternal hypothermia
Maternal anxiety	Certain drugs (see text)
Fetal arrhythmia	Congenital heart block
Certain drugs (see text)	Idiopathic
Reaction to stimulus (transient)	
Idiopathic	

*From Moore: Realities in Childbearing. W. B. Saunders Co., 1978.

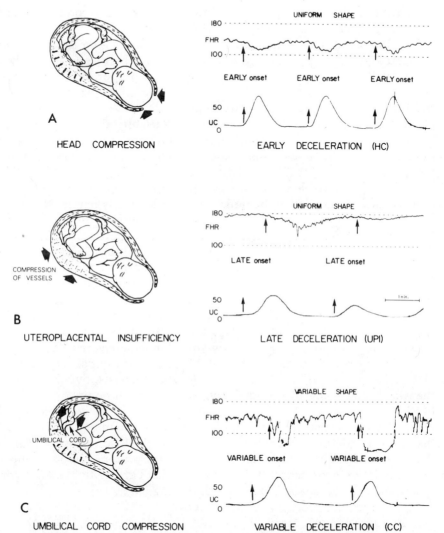

Figure 5–2. Patterns of fetal bradycardia. *A,* early deceleration due to head compression (HC). UC is the tracing of uterine contraction. This is also known as a Type I dip. *B,* late deceleration due to uteroplacental insufficiency (UPI). This is also known as a Type II dip. *C,* variable deceleration due to cord compression (CC). (From Hon: An Atlas of Fetal Heart Rate Patterns. Harty Press, 1968.)

PATTERNS OF FETAL HEART RATE DECELERATION

Deceleration patterns may be early, late, or variable. Some major characteristics of each type are summarized in Table 5–4.

Early decelerations Compression of the descending fetal head during a uterine contraction elevates fetal intracranial pressure and thereby reduces the flow of blood to the fetal brain. Chemoreceptors in the brain are stimulated, and the fetal heart rate is slowed by reflex action. This is the physiological basis of early deceleration.

Although this sequence might appear threatening to the fetus, this transient hypoxia is apparently well tolerated by the fetus. Thus, early decelerations are, in our present state of knowledge, benign.

Late decelerations As described previously, the fetus must rely on blood already in the intervillous space for oxygen during the peak of a contraction. Once that oxygen supply has been depleted by the fetus, if it is not soon replaced and fetal oxygen falls below 18 mm Hg, the direct effect of hypoxia on the fetal myocardium causes FHR to slow. This fall in FHR comes at least 20 to 30 seconds after the contraction when intervillous oxygen has become depleted. The return to normal occurs approximately 30 seconds after the end of a contraction because it takes that long for fresh maternal arterial blood to fill the intervillous space. If the oxygen in the intervillous space is reduced and the fetus does not receive adequate oxygen, late decelerations occur.

Late decelerations with the absence of beat-to-beat variability usually occur when the fetus is *chronically* asphyxiated and acidotic because of a chronic pathological condition involving the placenta or maternal/fetal exchange. For example, one might expect such a pattern in some mothers with hypertensive disease. The depressed FHR is due to the effect of hypoxia on the fetal myocardium.

Late decelerations with normal beat-to-beat variability and a normal baseline fetal heart rate usually indicate *acute* compro-

mise of maternal/fetal exchange. The heart rate slows because of a reflex that is triggered by stimulation of the chemoreceptors within the brain, as in early deceleration. Because the stimulus is acute, intervention (e.g., administering oxygen, turning the mother to her side) may often relieve this second cause of late deceleration.

Hypoxia is the direct cause of late decelerations. The magnitude of the decelerations is in proportion to the degree of oxygen impairment experienced by the fetus.

Variable decelerations Variable decelerations are variable both in timing in relation to uterine contraction and in shape. They are principally reflex in origin. Umbilical cord compression causes a lack of oxygen in the fetal blood from compression of the umbilical vein and fetal hypertension from compression of the umbilical arteries. Baroreceptors are activated by the former and chemoreceptors by the latter; as a result, the vagus nerve is stimulated and fetal heart rate slows.

If the source of cord compression is immediately relieved, FHR promptly returns to the baseline rate. If the obstruction persists, hypoxia with prolonged deceleration occurs.

Occasional variable decelerations are not uncommon; approximately 25 per cent of all fetuses have a *nuchal cord* (umbilical cord wrapped around the neck), which may become tightened at some point during labor.

PATTERNS OF FETAL HEART RATE ACCELERATION

Acceleration in fetal heart rate above the baseline level between contractions usually indicates fetal well-being. Tactile stimulation, such as given during an examination, may cause fetal heart rate acceleration as may the touch of the uterine lining during a contraction. Fetal activity and FHR acceleration are the basis of the nonstress test (Chapter 4).

Acceleration may be a danger sign

Table 5-4   Relation of Deceleration of Fetal Heart Rate to Uterine Contractions*

Deceleration Pattern	Configuration	Onset	Low Point	Return to Baseline	Comments	Mechanism
Early	U-shaped	Early in contraction cycle	Corresponds to peak of contraction	By end of contraction	The stronger the contraction, the greater the fetal heart rate; slowing rarely below 110 to 120 beats/min Occurs in vertex presentation only Appears after 6 to 7 cm cervical dilatation	Compression of fetal head (see text)
Late	U-shaped	20 to 30 seconds or more after onset of contraction	After peak of contraction	After end of contraction	Degree of fetal heart rate deceleration reflects intensity of contraction	Fetal hypoxia (see text)
Variable	Irregular	Variable relation of fetal heart rate to uterine contraction	Variable relation of fetal heart rate to uterine contraction	Variable relation of fetal heart rate to uterine contraction	Variable in every aspect including magnitude and occurrence with successive contractions	Umbilical cord compression
Prolonged	Wide U-shaped	Variable relation of fetal heart rate to uterine contraction			Cannot predict when or whether deceleration will end	Maternal hypotension Uterine hyperactivity Paracervical block Umbilical cord compression

*From Moore: Realities in Childbearing. W. B. Saunders Co., 1978.

when it occurs late in the contraction cycle and when beat-to-beat variability has been lost. This acceleration pattern may precede a late deceleration pattern. Partial obstruction of the umbilical cord may lead to acceleration before a variable deceleration.

Methods of Fetal Heart Rate Monitoring

Four methods of continuous fetal heart rate monitoring are by phonocardiography, abdominal electrocardiography, Doppler ultrasonography, and use of scalp electrodes. The first three methods are indirect, i.e., the fetus is monitored through the abdominal wall. In the fourth method an electrode is attached directly to the fetus's scalp; this is possible only after the membranes have ruptured.

PHONOCARDIOGRAPHY

A *phonocardiogram* is a graphic recording of fetal heart sounds. However, it also picks up other sounds including any sound the mother makes when she moves. The high noise level makes this monitoring method impractical for labor. Phonocardiography is valuable, however, in evaluating the fetus prior to labor.

If the FHR is very slow, the phonocardiographic reading may be doubled; if the FHR is very fast, the reading may be halved. No fetal monitor currently available can count rates slower than 30 to 60 beats per minute or faster than 240 to 250 beats per minute.

ABDOMINAL WALL ELECTROCARDIOGRAPHY

An *abdominal wall electrocardiogram* uses electrodes placed on the mother's abdomen. Maternal QRS complex and P waves and fetal QRS complex are recorded. Usually the maternal QRS complex is larger and can be identified. Each brand of

abdominal electrocardiograph monitor offers its own method for separating maternal and fetal patterns; more methods will undoubtedly become available in the future because at present no totally satisfactory method has been found.

DOPPLER ULTRASONOGRAPHY

The principle of ultrasound has been described in Chapter 4. When used to monitor the fetal heart, ultrasound waves are "bounced off" the walls of the moving heart or heart valves. Because two sets of heart valves are moving at different times (the bicuspid and tricuspid valves), the system is designed so that once the movement of one valve is detected, the system will not respond for a specific period of time. Understanding this is important because (1) if the FHR is very rapid, every beat may not be detected, and (2) if the FHR is very slow, the movement of both valves may be indicated on the monitor, thus doubling the rate.

Because monitors vary in range of response, one must know the specifics of the particular instrument used in the practice setting.

DIRECT MONITORING WITH FETAL SCALP ELECTRODES

The most reliable technique for measuring fetal heart rate is a stainless steel spiral electrode inserted into the fetal scalp after the membranes are ruptured (either spontaneously or artificially). The electrical signal detected is the QRS complex, which denotes the passage of an electrical impulse through the heart. The machine computes the fetal heart rate on the basis of the time interval between each QRS complex.

Monitoring Uterine Contractions

Uterine contractions may be monitored externally or internally.

EXTERNAL TOCOGRAPHY

The external *tocograph* converts the force of each uterine contraction into an electrical signal which is then displayed on a strip of paper. External monitoring is useful only in indicating the timing of contractions not their intensity. To function properly, the external tocograph must be moved during labor. External monitoring is less comfortable for the patient than internal monitoring.

INTERNAL MEASUREMENT OF INTRAUTERINE PRESSURE

Changes in intrauterine pressure can be measured by inserting a small, open-ended plastic catheter filled with fluid through the cervix into the uterus. The catheter is attached to a strain gauge that sends out an electrical signal reflecting the pressure placed against it (Fig. 5–3). Through this internal system one can monitor not only rate but baseline tone and intensity of contractions. This capability is particularly important if oxytocin is used to stimulate contractions.

In internal monitoring, it is important to remember that (1) any break in the system, such as an air bubble, a leak, or a meconium plug will impair accuracy, and (2) the height of the strain gauge must match the height of the catheter tip.

Fetal Scalp Blood Sampling

When the fetus becomes hypoxic, fetal acidosis occurs; the duration of the fetal hypoxia is reflected in the degree of acidosis. The level of acidosis at birth correlates with the condition of the newborn and with the Apgar scores. These observations have led to the use of fetal scalp sampling as a method of fetal assessment when there is reason to suspect hypoxia (e.g., late decelerations). A series of studies suggests that a fetal scalp pH of 7.20 to 7.24 or lower represents a state of preacidosis and is generally considered to indicate a need for intervention. That intervention might include the cessation of oxytocin administration, administration of oxygen, change in maternal position, or immediate delivery. As with other methods of assessment, the results of fetal scalp sampling are evaluated in conjunction with other parameters in deciding the appropriate care for mother and baby.

The technique for obtaining scalp blood is as follows: the fetal scalp is exposed with a sterile speculum, vaginal retractors, or a conical amnioscope, and a small incision is made (Fig. 5–4). Blood is collected in microtubes that are immediately clamped at both ends to keep it anaerobic. The blood is placed on ice and analysis is done immediately.

Following scalp sampling the incised area is observed for bleeding during at

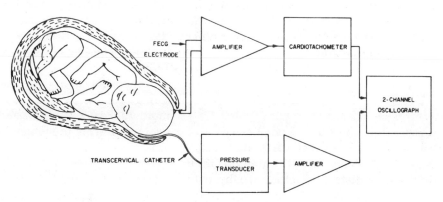

Figure 5–3. The placement of an electrode on the fetal scalp and a transcervical catheter to measure amniotic fluid pressure. (From Willis: Canad Nurse Dec. 1970, p. 28.)

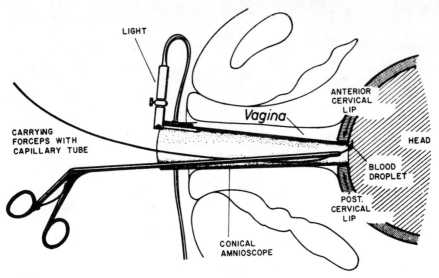

Figure 5-4. Diagram showing method of obtaining a fetal blood sample. (From Willis: Canad Nurse Dec. 1970, p. 28.)

least one contraction. Usually the site bleeds very little after initial blood collection.

Fetal Movement

A fetus deprived of oxygen is likely to be initially hyperactive and may have fetal tachycardia. Mothers who have a severe abruptio placentae, for example, may report that for a period of time following the initial pain (when the placenta became detached) the baby was unusually active before becoming unusually quiet. Unusual activity of this type during labor or the mother's report of strenuous activity should be noted, and the mother should be even more carefully observed for other signs of fetal distress.

Meconium in the Amniotic Fluid

Even before the time of our Civil War, a German physician, Schwartz, had recognized that meconium in the amniotic fluid indicated a distressed fetus. A baby with both bradycardia and meconium in the amniotic fluid requires rapid assessment followed by appropriate intervention.

The Fetal Monitoring Debate

The issue of intrapartum fetal monitoring has been widely debated by the public and in the lay press. In preparing parents for childbirth, the nurse will find it of concern to many, although not all, parents.

Intrapartum fetal monitoring was initially reserved for women considered at high risk for fetal distress during labor. However, it has been estimated that from 60 to 70 per cent of all labors are monitored (Dilts 1976). A major impetus for the increased use of monitoring has been a strong desire to decrease perinatal mortality and morbidity coupled with the recognition that some women who are at low risk during the prenatal period develop high risk conditions during labor (Aubrey 1978).

Controversy about the use of fetal monitoring centers on its use in low risk mothers. Few argue the need and value of fetal monitoring in women known to be at risk.

The discussion in this chapter will focus on the need for fetal monitoring in women who do not appear to be at risk for perinatal complications. The basic question is, Should 1000 women who are apparently normal and healthy be monitored to find a few infants who are at risk? Do the risks of monitoring these women outweigh the benefits?

AREAS OF CONTROVERSY

A basic argument against monitoring is the idea that childbirth is a normal experience for the vast majority of women; fetal monitoring is viewed as one of several examples of interference with the natural birth process. For example, monitoring confines the mother to a bed. Since vertical positions (standing, walking, or sitting) have been shown to facilitate labor by increasing contractions and the rate of cervical dilatation and have been associated with less pain (Caldeyro-Barcia 1979), confining a mother to bed with a monitor may indeed affect the course of her labor, although that effect may not be evident in perinatal morbidity and mortality statistics.

The two belts required by the external monitor can interfere with the coping techniques couples have learned, specifically effleurage (light stroking of the abdomen) and back rubs. The very presence of the belts, which must fit snugly if monitoring is to be effective, is irritating to some women.

Several objections relate to internal (direct) fetal monitoring with scalp electrodes rather than monitoring per se.

Technically, direct monitoring is generally considered more reliable. However, direct monitoring with scalp electrodes requires rupture of the amniotic sac. Caldeyro-Barcia (1975) has suggested that intact membranes allow the pressure of the uterine contraction to be evenly distributed to all parts of the fetus. He believes that early rupture may be a factor in traumatic brain damage.

Fetal scalp abscess is an occasional complication at the site of fetal monitor attachment, but several studies, including a prospective study by Okada and colleagues (1977), have found that the abscesses are usually small, the infection is generally mild, requiring only topical treatment, and hospitalization is only very rarely prolonged. Nevertheless, for the occasional baby more seriously affected, it is important to ask if the risk is worth the benefit.

Because the rate of *cesarean births* has more than doubled in the United States between 1968 and 1976 (the same period in which fetal monitoring has become increasingly widespread), the question quite naturally arises, Has fetal monitoring been the cause of the rise in cesarean births? A number of studies have attempted to answer that question. In Table 5–5, comparison is made between cesarean delivery rates in women who were not monitored and women who were. In Table 5–6, comparison is made between the rates of cesarean delivery before and after the in-

Table 5–5 Cesarean Delivery Rates in Patients With and Without Electronic Fetal Monitoring (EFM)

Study	Patients Without EFM (N)	CDR Without EFM (%)	Patients With EFM (N)	CDR With EFM (%)
Haverkamp et al. 1976	241 (HR)	6.6	242 (HR)	16.5
Haverkamp 1979	232 (HR)	5.6	233 (HR) 230 (HR)*	17.6 11.0
Renou et al. 1976	175 (HR)	14.0	169 (HR)	20.0
Kilso et al. 1978	253 (LR)	4.4	251 (LR)	9.5

CDR = cesarean delivery rate
HR = high risk patients
LR = low risk patients
*with fetal scalp sampling

Table 5–6   Cesarean Delivery Rates Before and After the Introduction of
Electronic Fetal Monitoring (EFM)

Study	Before EFM (%)	Year	After EFM (%)	Year
Koh et al. 1975	6.4	1971	12.5	1973
Lee and Baggish 1976	7.3	1969 to 1971	10.4	1972 to 1974
Gabert and Stenchever 1977	3.2	1970	10.5*	1975
Hughey et al. 1977	2.6	1968, 1969	6.9*	1974 to 1975

*primary cesarean delivery

troduction of electronic fetal monitoring. Questions that must be asked include the following: (1) Are the groups being compared comparable? (2) Is the increase in the cesarean rate related to a higher rate of births involving fetal distress? (The incidence of breech presentations and midforceps deliveries that were subsequently delivered by cesarean section increased between 1968 and 1976. This increase cannot be attributed to fetal monitoring.)

In Kilso's research (1978), no increase in cesarean deliveries due to fetal distress was shown, but in two studies by Haverkamp (1976, 1979) there was a difference. Multivariate analysis, in which many variables are controlled simultaneously, suggests that the difference in rates for monitored and unmonitored groups is primarily due to differences in the characteristics of women in the groups. When these differences are controlled, the association between monitoring and cesarean birth is negligible in the populations studied (Antenatal diagnosis 1979).

Two studies report a decrease in cesarean delivery because some potentially high risk mothers who at one time would have routinely delivered by cesarean section (e.g., the diabetic mother) may now be monitored and may deliver vaginally (Kelly and Kulkarni 1973; Beard, Edinger, and Sabanda 1977).

The cost of electronic fetal monitoring has been compared with the possible benefits in a low risk population. The estimated cost of electronic fetal monitoring per delivery was $30 to $60 in 1978. For those who argue an increase cesarean birth rate,

additional costs accrue. The prevention of cerebral palsy or mental retardation in a *single* person has been estimated to save over $170,000, the lifetime cost of maintaining and rehabilitating a severely handicapped person (Conley 1973). One might also consider the cost of a lifetime of lost income and the family grief that cannot be measured in dollars. It is not known at this time what the impact of fetal monitoring on mental retardation might be, but more questions must be raised and data gathered.

SPECIAL HAZARDS OF LABOR AND DELIVERY

Obstetrical Analgesia and Anesthesia and the Newborn

Because analgesia or anesthesia is used in the majority of deliveries in the United States (more so than in many other nations), it is important to understand how each type of drug affects the fetus. *All drugs* used during labor and delivery for the relief of apprehension and pain can pass through the placenta and affect the infant. Moreover, animal studies suggest that the fetus is far more sensitive to depressant drugs than an adult would be.

Barbiturates   Barbiturates, once widely used to relieve apprehension during early labor, tend to depress the newborn, particularly in the following circumstances:

1. If the drug was used in large doses in a mistaken attempt to relieve pain (barbiturates will only relieve pain in overdosage).

2. If the drug was used in combination with a general anesthetic.

3. If the baby was unusually asphyxiated for some other reason.

The better the mother's preparation for delivery during the prenatal period and the better her care in the labor room the less apprehensive she will be, thereby eliminating the need for barbiturates. Since there is no reliable barbiturate antidote, the baby depressed from these drugs will have to be resuscitated (page 102).

Tranquilizers Tranquilizers, such as diazepam (Valium), are also used to alleviate apprehension and, like barbiturates, tend to depress the baby, particularly if they are combined with narcotics or sedatives. Diazepam is not given in premature labor because buffers in the solution may increase the susceptibility of the baby to hyperbilirubinemia and kernicterus.

Morphine and meperidine Morphine and meperidine hydrochloride (Demerol) are the two narcotics most often used to relieve pain during labor. Again the possibility of respiratory depression exists. Giving larger than usual doses (generally 50 mg) or giving the drug intravenously or in combination with a barbiturate increases the chance that the newborn will be depressed.

Unlike depression caused by barbiturates, much of the depression caused by morphine and Demerol can be overcome through the use of the narcotic antagonist naloxone hydrochloride (Narcan) in a dose of .01 mg/kg of the baby's weight. Given intramuscularly, naloxone begins to take effect in two to three minutes, acting by competing with the narcotic and binding sites. When naloxone is given, nurses who care for the baby following delivery must be informed; as the drug is metabolized, the baby may again become depressed.

The narcotic antagonists formerly used, nalorphine (Nalline) and levallorphan tartrate (Lorfan), reversed narcotic-induced respiratory depression in many instances but contributed to respiratory depression from other causes.

Regional anesthesia With regional anesthesia the chief hazard to the infant is the possibility of hypotension that will, in turn, interfere with uterine blood flow and hence with fetal oxygenation. Prevention of hypotension includes the rapid infusion of intravenous fluids at the time the anesthesia is being given and positioning the mother on her side for five minutes or more after the drug has been injected to take the pressure of the heavy uterus off the inferior vena cava, which in itself would cause hypotension. Frequent checks of maternal blood pressure should detect hypotension promptly.

One additional danger in the use of caudal anesthesia is the accidental penetration of the fetal scalp, which introduces the anesthetic directly into the fetus with resultant severe bradycardia and generalized convulsions. The treatment in this case is gastric lavage combined with prompt exchange transfusion.

General anesthesia General anesthesia is infrequently used for vaginal delivery today. General anesthesia for the mother in labor involves several problems that reflect the anatomical and physiological changes that differentiate her from the nonpregnant woman. Her residual lung volume is decreased because of her enlarged uterus, which means that she will quickly build up higher alveolar concentrations of anesthetic (there is less air to dilute it). Because of a tendency toward hyperventilation in labor she will become anesthetized more quickly — in three minutes as compared to 10 to 12 minutes for nonpregnant women. The emptying time of the stomach is delayed during labor; once labor has begun, no solid foods can pass through the stomach. Moreover, pressure on the fundus can cause the mother to aspirate stomach contents even if she has eaten nothing for many hours. Thus, if the mother has eaten within six hours of the onset of labor, general anesthesia will be avoided if at all possible.

All of these factors can affect the baby. "The depression produced in the baby is directly related to the depth and the duration of the mother's anesthesia" (Abramson 1966). It takes only about two minutes for gases to reach the baby. Since the mother will be anesthetized very quickly, so will the infant. The shorter and lighter the anesthesia, the better. There should always be at least 25 per cent oxygen in any gaseous mixture given for delivery.

Aspiration of stomach contents is the chief hazard to the mother when general anesthesia is used for delivery, and obviously any such serious problem in the mother is a potential danger to the baby as well.

LONG-RANGE EFFECTS OF ANESTHESIA AND ANALGESIA

Most early research that evaluated the depressant effect of drugs on infants used Apgar scores at one minute and five minutes but rarely followed the infant beyond this period. Several later studies involved observation of the baby during the first four days of life.

In a test of visual attentiveness of 20 term infants between the second and fourth days of life there was a significant relationship indicating that "the more drugs administered closer to delivery, the less attentive is the infant likely to be" (Stechler 1964).

Behavioral impairment, defined as failure to have sustained movement after stimulation, and EEG changes, were found at 36 hours more frequently in a group of babies whose mothers received medication during labor than in a control group whose mothers were not medicated (Borgstedt and Rosen 1968).

Infants born to mothers who were sedated during labor consistently demonstrated depressed sucking activity during the first four days of life (Kron et al. 1966).

Standley and colleagues (1974) evaluated 60 first-born, healthy infants (48 to 72 hours old) born to white, middle-class mothers with medically uneventful pregnancies and deliveries. The mothers received commonly used analgesics (chiefly Demerol with Phenergan or Vistaril) and anesthetic agents such as lidocaine, tetracaine, and mepivacaine via saddle block (42 of the 52 women receiving anesthesia), pudendal block, paracervical block, etc. Babies of the mothers receiving anesthesia demonstrated decreased motor maturity and greater irritability when tested.

Scanlan and colleagues (1974) tested 41 infants during the first eight hours of life. The 28 infants whose mothers had received continuous lumbar epidural blocks showed significantly lower scores on tests of muscle strength and tone and demonstrated less vigorous rooting behavior (but no differences in sucking behavior).

Because the baby's early behavior is felt to be a significant factor in the early relationship between parents and infant, these differences may prove to be important. It is also necessary to discover if there are differences at later periods — one week or one month, for example. Techniques for behavioral assessment (Chapter 6) have increased our ability to evaluate the effect of anesthesia on the newborn.

Abnormal Position of the Fetus in Utero

BREECH POSITION

In about 2 or 3 per cent of all deliveries the baby is in a breech position (Fig. 5–5), either complete or frank (incomplete) breech (Fig. 5–6). Although there is no clear reason why the baby assumes or maintains this position at birth, several theories exist. At 30 weeks gestation about one fetus in four will be in a breech position; thus the incidence of breech delivery is considerably higher in premature than in term deliveries. At approximately 34 weeks most infants will shift position and will present head first at delivery. But if the fetus's legs are extended and for some reason cannot be flexed, the fetus will be unable to turn.

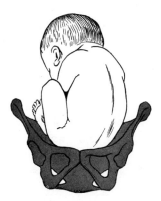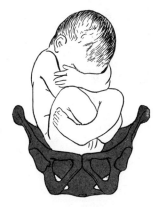

Figure 5-5. Complete breech presentations. (From Davis and Rubin: DeLee's Obstetrics for Nurses. 18th Edition. W. B. Saunders, 1966.)

At delivery the baby's body will emerge first, and difficulties may arise if the head is delivered either too quickly or too slowly. In the first instance, intracranial hemorrhage may result from a tear in the tentorium cerebelli and lead to the infant's death. Considering how many hours it takes the head to pass through the pelvis in a normal vertex delivery and how quickly it must pass through the pelvis in a breech delivery (usually 10 minutes or less), it is not difficult to see why this problem can develop. The pressure on the head tends to pull the cranium away from the base of the skull, thus pulling the falx cerebri away from the tentorium cerebelli with resultant tear and hemorrhage.

If delivery is too slow the danger is one of asphyxia rather than hemorrhage. Once the head enters the pelvis, the cord is squeezed between the unborn head and the bony pelvis and cervix. Until the nose and mouth are delivered the baby has no means of oxygenation. However, this is much less commonly a cause of death than hemorrhage.

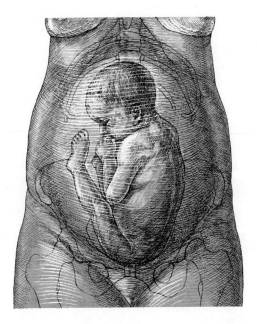

Figure 5-6. One type of incomplete breech presentation. The legs are extended. (From Davis and Rubin: DeLee's Obstetrics for Nurses. 18th Edition. W. B. Saunders, 1966.)

Babies presenting in a breech position are also more likely to have fractures of clavicle or long bones and injuries to the brachial plexus or the sternocleidomastoid muscle. Injuries to the spinal cord may result from forceful traction on the feet during extraction. For all of these reasons, many infants today with a breech presentation are delivered by cesarean section.

TRANSVERSE POSITION

In one delivery out of 200 the baby lies in a transverse position in the uterus (Fig. 5–7). If vaginal delivery is attempted in this situation perinatal mortality is approximately 30 per cent. Early diagnosis and abdominal delivery reduce the rate of mortality.

FACE AND BROW PRESENTATION

There is usually no difficulty when there is an anterior face and brow presentation; babies with a posterior face and brow presentation are generally delivered by cesarean section.

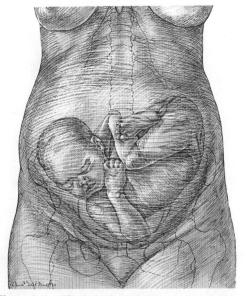

Figure 5–7. The baby lies in a transverse position in approximately one delivery out of 200. (From Davis and Rubin: DeLee's Obstetrics for Nurses. 18th Edition. W. B. Saunders, 1966.)

Multiple Gestation

Perinatal mortality in multiple gestation is double that of single births for the following reasons:

1. The increased frequency of toxemia.

2. The increased frequency of prematurity (80 per cent of all twin deliveries are premature).

3. Hazards to the second twin during delivery. Perinatal loss of the second twin is 100 per cent greater than that of the first twin; both breech delivery and version of the fetus in breech position carry a high rate of loss.

Delivery Following Rapid Labor

When labor lasts less than three hours the chief hazard to the infant is subdural hematoma from a tear in the tentorium cerebelli which is turn ruptures veins in the tentorium. The tear is due to the rapid descent of the head through the birth canal, which leaves no time for the gradual molding that normally takes place during delivery. Less frequently there is cranial bleeding because the sudden compression of the skull causes one cranial bone to override the other, catching veins as if they were between the blades of scissors.

Delivery Using Forceps

Occasionally the baby is found to have a cephalohematoma (Chapter 6) or a linear skull fracture following a low forceps delivery. Neither condition is serious nor requires treatment.

However, a mid- or high forceps delivery is associated with an increased incidence of both perinatal mortality and neonatal morbidity. This is due in part to the conditions that require a mid- or high forceps delivery, such as prolonged labor or uterine inertia. Among the hazards of forceps delivery are depressed skull fracture, intracranial hemorrhage, and brachial plexus injuries.

CARE IMMEDIATELY FOLLOWING DELIVERY

Clearing the Respiratory Tract

Following delivery, the baby's head is placed in a dependent position in relation to the rest of his body to facilitate the drainage of mucus from his mouth and to prevent mucus, and in some instances blood and meconium, from entering the respiratory tract. Suctioning, if it is necessary, must be gentle and brief; prolonged and deep suction may cause reflex bradycardia.

Although infants are commonly placed in a warm bed in the head-down position during this initial phase, placing the baby on the mother's uncovered abdomen is effective in keeping the baby warm (below) and, if the baby is in a prone position, allows drainage of mucus (Kliot 1980). This practice has the important advantage of allowing immediate contact between mother and infant and is worth consideration when the infant does not appear to be in danger.

Spontaneous respirations should begin within a few seconds to a minute after birth. If they do not, the delivery-room staff must take immediate steps to initiate respirations (below); there is no time to hope that the baby will eventually begin to breathe on his own.

The Leboyer Approach

With the publication in 1975 of *Birth Without Violence,* the ideas of the French physician Frederick Leboyer about a gentle birth process became a topic of discussion for consumers as well as providers of care. His specific recommendations include a delivery room that is warm, quiet, and dark, placing the infant on the mother's abdomen immediately following delivery, delay in cutting the cord for approximately five minutes, and the use of a warm bath in which the baby is placed after the cord is severed. Many parents who have chosen to incorporate Leboyer's principles into their own birth

experiences report great feelings of satisfaction from participation in such a birth.

It was suggested by Leboyer that this approach to delivery could have significant long-term developmental effects on the infant. Rappoport (1976) reported that children delivered by the Leboyer method had less colic, marked ambidexterity, and higher than average IQs and walked at an earlier age, among other differences. However, no control group was used, so it is not really possible to attribute these differences to the Leboyer method per se. Nelson and colleagues (1980) found no differences among 56 births randomly assigned to Leboyer and more conventional delivery methods in newborn deaths and infant behavior in the first hour, between 24 and 72 hours, and at eight months. In the conventional deliveries, however, the newborns were treated gently and were encouraged to interact with their parents. One might also assume that attention was paid to thermoregulation. Thus, there were not the sharp contrasts in the manner of delivery that probably existed at the time Leboyer first proposed his idea of gentle birth. Leboyer's concepts of a gentle, controlled delivery with support for the baby's head, neck, and sacrum, the avoidance of cold, and the avoidance of painful stimuli are essentials. Moreover, if there are no differences in infant behavior or condition, there seems no valid reason to deny the experience to parents who desire this approach when the infant is healthy.

Leboyer reminds us that the infant is human and worthy of gentle handling. This principle deserves incorporation into our concept of neonatal care.

Immediate Evaluation of the Infant

In evaluating the newborn it is advisable to note and record the time at which the baby first gasped and cried and then was able to sustain respiration. A system for recording this kind of information was devised by Dr. Virginia Apgar and is now widely used in the evaluation of the new-

Table 5–7   The Apgar Scoring Method*

Sign	0	1	2
Heart rate	Absent	Below 100	Over 100
Respiratory effort	Absent	Minimal; weak cry	Good; strong cry
Muscle tone	Limp	Some flexion of extremities	Active motion; extremities well flexed
Reflex irritability (response to stimulation on sole of foot)	No response	Grimace	Cry
Color	Blue or pale	Body pink; extremities blue	Pink

*From Apgar: Anes Analg 32:260, 1953. Apgar et al.: JAMA 168:1985, 1958.

born (Table 5–7). The first recording is made at one minute after delivery, this time having been chosen because in a large series of observations it was found to be the point at which the lowest score was likely to be obtained. A second Apgar evaluation is then made at five minutes after delivery.

Although each item scored — heart rate, respiratory effort, muscle tone, reflex irritability, and color — is numerically equivalent, some signs are actually more significant than others. For example, and Apgar 9 newborn who is scored 2 in every area except color is in less distress than an Apgar 9 infant who is scored 2 in every area except heart rate or respiratory effort. However, it is likely that an infant with cardiac or respiratory distress would also have a low score on other items. Only about 15 per cent of infants will score 2 in color at one minute after delivery.

Statistically significant correlations have been found between mortality and low Apgar scores at one minute, and even more significant correlations have been found at five minutes. The incidence of neurological defects is also high in infants with low five-minute Apgar scores.

Providing Warmth for the Newborn

A most crucial need for the infant during the first minutes and hours after birth is warmth. Chilling increases the baby's need for oxygen and aggravates the metabolic acidosis that is present to some extent in all infants during the first hour of life. In addition, recent evidence indicates that hypothermia may increase the possibility of hyperbilirubinemia in newborns.

In the average delivery room there is a 15-degree difference between room temperature and the temperature of the intrauterine environment from which the baby has been delivered. A wet, small newborn loses up to 200 calories per kilogram per minute in the delivery room through evaporation, convection, and radiation. Realizing that an adult generates only about 90 calories per kilogram per minute at full compensation makes it easier to appreciate the severity of this heat loss.

The conservation of heat is directly related to the several processes of heat loss. Loss by evaporation occurs because the baby is wet; the single act of drying him immediately cuts heat loss in half. Convective heat loss, caused by air blowing across the baby, causes a transfer of heat from baby to environment. We deliberately use cool air to cool ourselves on a hot day or to reduce temperature in a febrile patient. But no newborn should be accidentally cooled by a current of air blowing across his body.

A third mechanism of heat loss is radiation. The baby will radiate heat to the nearest object. It he is swaddled in a blanket, he will radiate to the blanket and his environment will be warm. If he is left uncovered and unclothed he will radiate heat in an attempt to raise the temperature of the entire delivery room — rather like trying to raise the temperature of an entire house by means of a single fireplace.

To counterbalance heat loss, the newborn has mechanisms through which he strives to retain heat (vasoconstriction and insulation) and produce heat.

Vasoconstriction is the most important of the mechanisms of heat retention. However, if the mother has been treated with magnesium sulfate for toxemia, the baby's vasoconstrictive mechanisms may not function at peak capacity. Insulation is a second way in which the body conserves heat. But even the term infant in this regard is at a relative disadvatage in comparison with older children and adults because of his limited amount of fat. The baby weighing less than 2500 g has almost no subcutaneous fat and will thus have difficulty conserving heat. The third way in which the baby conserves heat is by assuming a position similar to his position in utero.

Besides conserving heat, the baby will also produce heat. Although older individuals do this predominantly by shivering, newborns rely primarily on nonshivering thermogenesis; they raise their temperature by an increase in their rate of metabolism. This increases oxygen consumption, but if for some reason the baby has difficulty delivering oxygen to his cells, he will be unable to increase his metabolic rate and nonshivering thermogenesis will be compromised.

Research indicates that term infants held by their mothers in the delivery room (Phillips 1974) or placed on the mother's undraped abdomen (Kliot 1980) are able to maintain body heat well within an acceptable range. Phillips demonstrated that infant temperature dropped further when delivery room temperature was 72°F (22.0°C) than when environmental temperature was 75°F (24°C), suggesting the importance of further research into temperature regulation. Delivery rooms with more comfortable environmental temperatures would seem to offer a decided advantage in this respect.

If all the preceding principles are implemented in the nursing care of the baby it will not be too difficult to keep the full-term, apparently healthy newborn warm. The problem arises when a baby having difficulties needs resuscitation or other medical attention that requires exposure. This baby, who may be of low birth weight and who is probably not oxygenating adequately, is even more in need of warmth than the healthy newborn. The best available solution to this dilemma at present is an overhead warmer that utilizes radiant heat to keep the baby warm yet allows free access for resuscitation. If possible, the baby's extremities can be covered to further minimize heat loss.

Several points need to be kept in mind in relation to these warmers:

1. Hyperthermia, as well as hypothermia, is a stress, leading to increased oxygen consumption. When the baby is under a warmer for more than a few minutes, his temperature should be monitored. The temperature on most warmers can be easily adjusted.

2. Burns are a possibility though they are infrequent.

3. The warmer should be turned on before the baby is delivered; in this way the blankets will be warm and the baby will not have to be placed on a cold surface on which he will immediately lose heat.

Identifying the Infant

The identification of the infant should be carried out in the delivery room before the baby is taken to the nursery. Occasionally, because of severe illness, a baby may not be footprinted in the delivery suite. The nurse in the nursery must always be aware of this so that he or she can complete these tasks as soon as possible. Identification is carefully checked before transferring the infant to a regional center.

Identification bands for mother and child, with matching numbers as well as names and the sex of the baby, are one way in which mother and baby can be identified. These bands should be checked each time the baby is removed from his crib or taken to this mother as well as at the time of discharge.

Footprinting, another widely used means of identification, has been subject to much criticism. In a study by the Chicago Board of Health, policemen who were accustomed to interpreting finger prints found that 98 per cent of footprints submitted by most of the Chicago hospitals were valueless and could not serve as a means of identification. However, two minutes of instruction to the hospital personnel responsible for taking footprints produced prints from which positive identification could be made in 99 per cent of the cases (Gleason 1969).

To produce reliable and meaningful prints, Gleason suggests the following procedure for footprinting:

1. Proper equipment should be used, preferably a disposable footprinter ink plate and a smooth, high-gloss type of paper.

2. Immediately after the baby is received from the physician and wrapped in a warm blanket his foot should be wiped so that the vernix will not dry on it. This will make it easier to clean the foot when the actual footprinting is done.

3. At footprinting time (immediately before the baby is to be taken from the delivery room) the following technique is used:

   a. The foot is cleaned thoroughly but gently. Scrubbing it too hard will make the baby's skin peel.

   b. The foot is dried thoroughly.

   c. The baby's knee is flexed so that his legs are close to his body; his ankle is grasped between the thumb and middle finger; the nurse's index finger is pressed on the upper surface of the foot just behind the baby's toes to prevent his toes from curling.

   d. The footprinter is pushed gently to the baby's foot.

   e. The baby's foot is gently touched to the footprint chart; the chart should be attached to a hard surface such as a clipboard.

   f. The heel is placed on the chart first; then the baby's foot is walked gently onto the chart with a heel-to-toe motion. The foot should not be rolled back and forth on either the inking pad or the footprint chart.

The footprint should be checked to see if the ridges are discernible. Any excess ink can then be wiped from the baby's foot. Usually the mother's fingerprints are placed on the same sheet as the baby's footprint.

Prophylactic Eye Care

Prior to the use of silver nitrate prophylaxis, 25 per cent of the children in schools for the blind in the United States were blind because of *ophthalmia neonatorum*, a gonococcal infection of the eye contracted during labor and delivery by direct contact with *gonococcus* in the cervix or, occasionally, during the first days of life, possibly through contamination from the mother's fingers.

The occurrence of ophthalmia neonatorum dropped dramatically both in the United States and in Europe as Credé's prophylaxis with silver nitrate and, later, antibiotic prophylaxis (used less commonly), became legally mandatory in many areas. In the United States, silver nitrate must be used in 15 states; silver nitrate or an "other equally effective agent" is specified in the laws or regulations of 33 other states and the District of Columbia.* However, as the worldwide incidence of gonorrhea has increased to epidemic levels, so too has the incidence of ophthalmia neonatorum.

Careful instillation of prophylactic silver nitrate in the eyes of each infant within the first hour following birth is therefore extremely important. Because silver nitrate is irritating and causes the baby to shut his eyes, it is preferable to delay instillation until after the initial meeting of parents and baby. The packaging of silver nitrate in wax ampules, which prevent both evaporation and overconcentration, has virtually eliminated serious chemical eye injury. Chemical irritation, however, does occur; a mild chemical conjunctivitis *should* result if prophylaxis is properly performed. This is a

---

*A summary of the laws and regulations requiring use of a prophylactic for the prevention of ophthalmia neonatorum in effect as of August 1968 is available from the National Society for the Prevention of Blindness, Inc., 79 Madison Avenue, New York, New York, 10016.

transient condition with no permanent sequelae.

An antibiotic ointment has been used as an alternative to silver nitrate in those states where the law permits, largely because of the chemical irritation caused by the silver nitrate. However, it is currently believed that (1) antibiotic preparations offer no better prevention, (2) penicillin may lead to sensitivity or untoward reaction, (3) there is an increase in the number of gonococci resistant to penicillin, and (4) antibiotics could encourage the colonization of antibiotic-resistant organisms in babies in the nursery.

These measures do not always prevent gonococcal infections. There are a number of possible reasons why, several of which are directly related to nursing care. The medication may inadvertently be overlooked or improperly administered. One drop should be placed in each conjunctival sac. The lids must be separated so that the medication touches the cornea. If it touches only the lids and lid margins, instillation should be repeated. After the first drop is administered, there may be severe blepharospasm, which makes it difficult to place the drop in the second eye. Wait to be sure that both drops are effectively instilled. The Committee on Ophthalmia Neonatorum of the National Society for the Prevention of Blindness *does not recommend irrigating the eye* following silver nitrate administration.

In addition to those factors related to the procedure itself, prophylaxis may fail because the disease has become established before birth because of premature rupture of the maternal membranes or because the disease was acquired by the baby subsequent to prophylaxis by contamination from the hands of the mother or hospital personnel. Silver nitrate will not prevent newborn conjunctivitis caused by other infectious agents.

THE TIMING OF EYE INFECTION
PROPHYLAXIS

If silver nitrate is instilled immediately following birth, the usual quiet alert state of the baby, in which he gazes at his mother and father, is disrupted. Since this period appears to be important in the attachment process, prophylaxis is frequently delayed until late in the first hour of life, after parents and baby have had an opportunity to become acquainted.

Assessment of Gestational Age

The gestational age of a baby is the number of weeks since the first day of his mother's last normal menstrual period. Accurate estimation of gestational age is important in planning care that best meets the needs of each newborn. Until recently, maternal history, obstetrical evaluation, and the size of the baby had been the principal criteria in estimating gestational age. But many mothers are unsure of menstrual dates or have irregular periods. Some have first trimester bleeding that may be mistaken for a period. The obstetrical evaluation of the height of the fundus is only a rough estimate of gestational age because it assumes normal fetal growth. When mothers receive no prenatal care, parameters such as the height of the fundus and fetal heart tones are obviously not available. The baby's weight can be misleading, as some babies weigh less than might be expected for their age and others are large in size yet are delivered before term.

A *term* infant has a gestational age of from 38 weeks to 41 weeks, 6 days. An infant born prior to 38 weeks is called *preterm*; an infant of 42 or more weeks gestation is called *postterm*. When estimated gestational age is compared with birth weight, preterm, term, and postterm babies are classified as small for gestational age (SGA), appropriate for gestational age (AGA), or large for gestational age (LGA), respectively. SGA infants may be intrauterine growth retarded (IUGR). These concepts are discussed more fully later in this chapter.

Because babies in every combination of age and weight have particular characteristics and needs within the first 24 hours as well as later, an immediate assessment of age is very important.

The accurate assessment of gestational

age is based on the fact that a number of physical characteristics and neurological signs vary with the gestational age of the baby. However, it has been recognized that estimating age on the basis of one or two characteristics (e.g., ear cartilage and breast tissue) is not sufficiently accurate because of individual variations. But when a number of criteria are scored, the total score is a reasonably reliable index of the infant's gestational age. The criteria for scoring physical characteristics and neuromuscular assessment and their use in determining gestational age are shown in Figure 5–8.

Scoring should be done as soon as possible after birth. Skin criteria are not accurate after 24 hours; if assessment is delayed beyond that time a more accurate estimate is obtained by eliminating the external criteria and doubling the neurological score. Scoring can usually be done regardless of the baby's state, i.e., awake or asleep, hungry or recently fed, etc.

EXTERNAL PHYSICAL CHARACTERISTICS

The lower the gestational age, the thinner the infant's *skin* will be. Because of the thinness of the skin, blood vessels are closer to the surface in the preterm infant. Veins and venules are distinctly seen, particularly on the abdomen, and the skin

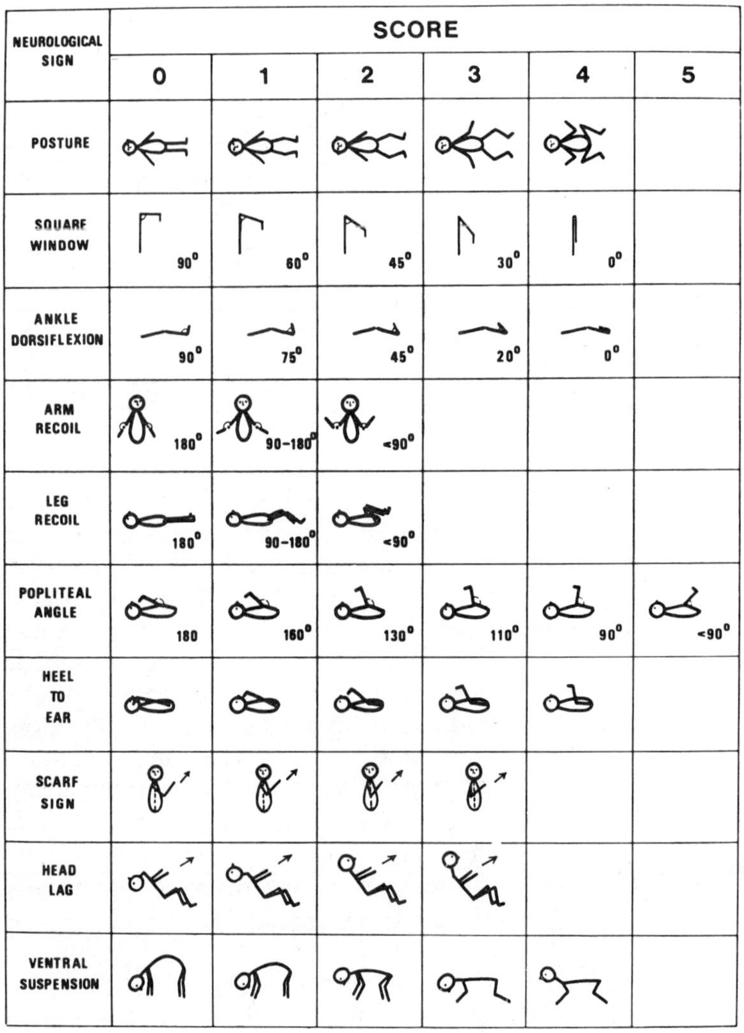

A

Figure 5–8A. Scoring system for neuromuscular criteria. Add scores for all signs and apply score to Figure 5–8B. (From Dubowitz, Dubowitz, and Goldberg: J Pediatr 77:1, 1970.)

Score   **Units**

	0	1	2	3	4	5	6	7	8	9
0						26.0	26.0	26.5	26.5	27.0
10	27.0	27.5	27.5	28.0	28.0	28.5	29.0	29.0	29.5	29.5
20	30.0	30.0	30.5	30.5	31.0	31.0	31.5	31.5	32.0	32.0
30	32.5	33.0	33.0	33.5	33.5	34.0	34.0	34.5	34.5	35.0
40	35.0	35.5	35.5	36.0	36.0	36.5	36.5	37.0	37.5	37.5
50	38.0	38.0	38.5	38.5	39.0	39.0	39.5	39.5	40.0	40.0
60	40.5	40.5	41.0	41.0	41.5	42.0	42.0	42.5	42.5	43.0
70	43.0									

B

Figure 5–8B. To determine gestational age in weeks, take score from examination, find on chart, and read off value in weeks. For example, for a score of 44, find 40 in the far left column. Then read across to the column headed by 4. The gestational age is 36.0 weeks. (From Dubowitz, Dubowitz, and Goldberg: J Pediatr 77:1, 1970.)

is much redder than in the term baby. With each successive week the skin become thicker and paler and abdominal veins less clearly visible.

Prior to 28 weeks *lanugo*, a fine downy hair, covers the entire body. In each subsequent week until term some of the lanugo disappears, first from the face and later from other areas of the body. At term it is slight, if present at all.

Transverse creases on the sole of the infant's foot are absent prior to 32 weeks. From approximately 32 to 36 weeks the creases are found only on the anterior third of the foot; two-thirds of the foot are covered at 38 weeks. By 40 weeks the entire sole is a series of complex crisscrosses (Fig. 5–9).

There is usually no *breast nodule* before 33 weeks. Until 36 weeks the nodule will usually be no larger than 3 mm; at term the nodule is from 4 to 10 mm surrounded by a full areolar area.

Because ear cartilage is not developed before 36 weeks, the pinna of the ear is flat and stays folded. Term babies have a firm ear that recoils when folded.

In both males and females the genitals continue to develop during the last weeks of gestation. Prior to 28 weeks the testes are undescended and no rugae are present on the scrotum. From 28 to 36 weeks the testes are normally descending and are

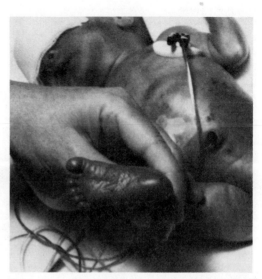

Figure 5–9. Creases on the anterior two thirds of this baby's foot suggest a gestational age of more than 38 weeks. Score 3 for plantar creases. Photography by Bill Moore.

first found high in the inguinal canal and subsequently lower in the canal. Rugae also develop during these weeks. The testes are in the scrotum by approximately 36 weeks, which by that time has well-developed rugae. Testes remain undescended in approximately 3 per cent of term infants, illustrating why no one criterion is adequate in determining gestational age.

In female infants the relative size of the labia majora and labia minora change as the fetus becomes more mature. Before 28 weeks the clitoris and labia minora are prominent. In the weeks that follow the labia majora grow, covering the labia minora by 36 to 38 weeks.

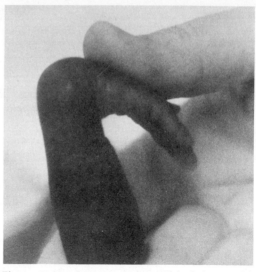

Figure 5–11. Square window. This baby would receive a score of 2 for a 45° angle. The examiner's fingers were placed in a slightly different position to facilitate photography. Photography by Bill Moore.

SIGNS OF NEUROMUSCULAR MATURITY

Muscle tone is flaccid at 28 weeks, accounting for many of the criteria associated with neuromuscular maturity. *Posture* should be observed with the baby lying quietly on his back. Flexor muscle tone increases as the baby approaches term and is strong in an infant of 40 weeks gestation (Fig. 5–10).

The *square window* refers to the 90-degree angle at the wrist when the infant's hand is flexed (Fig. 5–11). The examiner's thumb is placed on the dorsal aspect of the baby's hand with the index and third fingers on the dorsal aspect of the baby's forearm. As the baby increases in gestational age, the angle at the wrist decreases to 0.

Just as the square window evaluates the

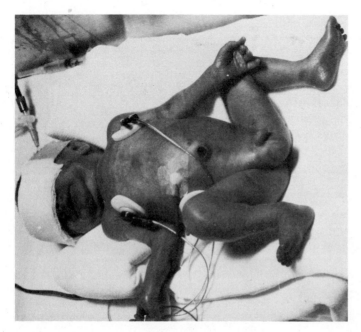

Figure 5–10. Posture. Both legs and one arm are flexed. The baby would receive a score of 4 for posture. Photography by Bill Moore.

flexibility of the wrist joint, *ankle dorsiflexion* (Fig. 5–12) evaluates the flexibility of the ankle joint. Early in gestation the joints are relatively stiff; they become more relaxed closer to term, an accommodation that allows the larger infant to mold himself to the small space available within the uterus.

Arm recoil is measured with the baby supine. The arms are extended by pulling on the hands. The angle of the elbow is measured after the release of the hands. *Leg recoil* is also measured with the baby supine. The hips and knees are fully flexed for five seconds then extended by traction on the feet and released.

The *popliteal angle* (Fig. 5–13) is also measured with the infant supine and the pelvis flat on the examining table. The baby's thigh is held in the knee-chest position by the examiner's left index finger and thumb. The leg is then extended by gentle pressure behind the ankle from the examiner's right index finger and the popliteal angle measured.

Assessment of the *scarf sign* is based on the position of the elbow when the baby's hand is drawn across his body to the other shoulder as far as it will go without resistance.

In the *heel-to-ear maneuver* the baby's foot is drawn toward his head, and the distance from his foot to his ear is assessed. The knee is left free; it will fall alongside the abdomen.

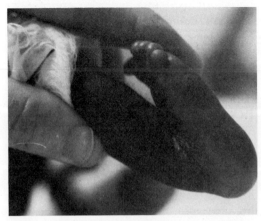

Figure 5–12. Ankle dorsiflexion. The angle between the dorsal aspect of the foot and the tibia approximates 20°, rating a score of 3. Photography by Bill Moore.

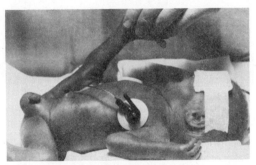

Figure 5–13. The popliteal angle is 180°, rating a score of 0. Photography by Bill Moore.

Head lag is measured with the infant supine. The forearms are grasped just above the wrist, and the baby is gently pulled to a sitting position. To what extent he supports his head is a measure of active muscle tone that increases with gestational age. The position of the infant when he is held in *ventral suspension* is another measure of active tone. The baby is held with his chest in the palm of the examiner's hand, and the increasing muscle tone is observed.

COMPARING GESTATIONAL AGE AND BODY MEASUREMENTS

Either before or after gestational age is ascertained the baby is weighed and length and head circumference are measured. The baby's measurements can then be compared with the norms of the Colorado Growth Charts (Fig. 5–14). (Although the Denver norms may not be totally accurate for all parts of the country — babies born at sea level are somewhat larger — they are considered the best standard of reference currently available.)

If length, weight, and head circumference are all below the tenth percentile* on the Colorado Chart, the baby is considered both small for gestational age and intrauterine growth retarded. The insult to this baby probably occurred early in pregnancy, perhaps an early viral illness. The long-term prognosis for normal development in these babies is usually poor.

*If the baby's measurements are in the tenth percentile, this means that 90 per cent of the babies of that gestational age are larger.

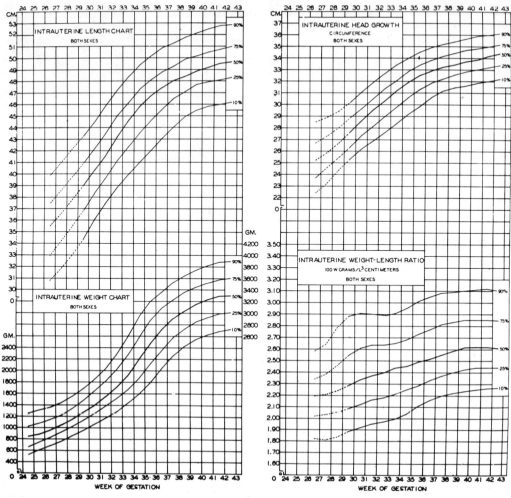

Figure 5–14. Colorado Growth Charts. (From Lubchenco, Hansman, and Boyd: Pediatrics 37:403, 1966. Copyright American Academy of Pediatrics, 1966.)

When length and weight fall below the tenth percentile for the baby's gestational age but head size is normal (approximately the fiftieth percentile), the baby's growth was probably affected in the third trimester. Common causes are toxemia, hypertension, long-term malnutrition, and vascular disease in the mother. Babies below the tenth percentile are small for gestational age and more at risk than babies appropriate for gestational age, but they usually have brighter futures than those infants with intrauterine growth retardation.

Babies whose weight, length, and head circumference fall between the tenth and ninetieth percentiles are appropriate for gestational age. At every age these infants have a better chance for survival than babies of the same age who are SGA or LGA infants. A baby with measurements above the ninetieth percentile is large for gestational age.

CARING FOR THE BABY WHO DOES NOT BREATHE SPONTANEOUSLY

The delivery room nurse plays a central role in preventing death or permanent brain damage in the baby who does not breathe spontaneously and immediately after birth. Even if he or she does not actively participate in resuscitation, it is the nurse who makes sure that both personnel and equipment are ready for emergency use at every delivery.

The following equipment should be available for every delivery:

1. A bulb syringe for suctioning.
2. Suction equipment and suction catheters; suction should be checked prior to each delivery to be sure it is in working order.
3. Oxygen.
4. Mask and bag.
5. Pharyngeal suction catheter.
6. Laryngoscope.
7. Small endotracheal tubes.
8. Drugs and syringes.
9. Umbilical artery catheter.

The Need for Resuscitation

Any infant may require resuscitation because of conditions that cannot be anticipated. Certain risk factors have been identified (Table 5–8) which, if present, require that adequate personnel be available in the delivery room to assure care for both infant and mother. (Although some hospitals still feel uncomfortable about the presence of the father or another support person in the delivery room during a high risk delivery, this is a time when the mother needs even more support than when all is well. Obviously, there are individual circumstances when the mother's support person contributes in a negative rather than a positive way to a difficult situation, but judgments should be made on an individual rather than a general basis.)

Apgar scoring, described previously, is a rough but rapid guide to the need for active resuscitation. Infants with Apgar scores of 7 or above require no extraordinary measures. Infants with Apgar scores from 3 to 6 have mild to moderate asphyxia and require attention and some efforts at resuscitation. An Apgar score of 0 to 2 indicates severe asphyxia.

The causes of failure to breathe spontaneously (in order of frequency of occurrence) are medications given to the mother, intrauterine hypoxia, trauma, sepsis, and congenital anomalies.

MEDICATIONS GIVEN TO THE MOTHER

The infant may be easily depressed by medications given to the mother because

Table 5–8 Prenatal and Intrapartal Factors that Increase the Risk of a Need for Resuscitation*

Maternal Factors	Placental Factors	Fetal Factors
Preeclampsia or eclampsia	Placenta previa	Abnormal presentation
Polyhydramnios or oligohydramnios	Abruptio placentae	Multiple pregnancy
Amnionitis	Gestation longer than	Persistent FHR less than 160 bpm
Rupture of the uterus	42 weeks	Persistent fetal tachycardia
Premature rupture of membranes		Loss of beat-to-beat variability of
(more than 12 hours before birth)		FHR on monitor
Vaginal bleeding other than "show"		Persistent abnormal FHR pattern
Fever		on monitor
Diabetes mellitus		Fetal acidosis (fetal scalp sample)
Cesarean birth		Prolapsed cord
Prolonged labor and/or prolonged		Estimated fetal weight less than
second stage (longer than 2½ hours)		2500 g (preterm or intra-
Precipitous labor (less than 3 hours)		uterine growth retardation)
		Erythroblastosis
		Meconium staining (particularly
		dark staining with vertex
		presentation)
		Abnormal NST, CST, and/or
		estriol
		Immature L:S ratio
		General anesthesia

*Adapted from Hobel et al.: Am J Obstet Gynecol *117*:1, 1973; and Fisher and Patton *In* Klaus and Fanaroff: Care of the High Risk Neonate. W. B. Saunders Co., 1979.

all infants are normally somewhat hypoxic and acidotic and because the blood brain "barrier" in the fetus/newborn is less effective than that in adults, allowing greater central nervous system depression. Table 5–9 summarizes the effects of drugs given to the mother of the fetus/newborn. The prevention of drug-related depression through the careful administration of medication to the mother is far better than correcting that depression.

In drug-related depression, the baby will commonly respond rapidly to resuscitation efforts but become depressed again when active resuscitation ceases. Naloxone (Narcan) is the narcotic antagonist currently used to reverse the effects of narcotic drugs. Naloxone in the dose used in the United States (.01 mg/kg of infant weight) is frequently metabolized more rapidly than the narcotics; thus there may be a recurrence of respiratory distress in the nursery. It is essential that the nursery nurses know that the baby has been given naloxone so the baby can be closely observed for further respiratory distress and given an additional dose of naloxone if necessary.

INTRAUTERINE HYPOXIA

Hypoxia is related to a decrease in placental blood flow; it may be chronic, as in the mother with severe preeclampsia, or acute, as from compression of the umbilical cord or placental accident. Maternal hypotension, which may occur from compression of the vena cava when the mother lies flat on her back (supine hypotension syndrome), can produce fetal asphyxia. A mother in the third trimester or labor should never lie supine; she should lie on her side or tilted to one side. This is especially important when the mother is being prepared for cesarean delivery; in the business of preparation maternal hypotension could be overlooked.

Fetal heart rate and pH changes (described above) and meconium in amniotic fluid are the principal signs of anoxia.

Changing maternal position and administering oxygen are emergency measures used until delivery can be accomplished.

A Basic Approach to Resuscitation

Resuscitation should be approached in a systematic fashion. The sequence is summarized as follows: Airway, Breathing, Circulation, Drugs, Environmental temperature.

AIRWAY

Prior to birth the fetal lungs are filled with lung fluid, which differs from amniotic fluid. The amount is approximately 30 ml of lung fluid per kilogram of the baby's weight. During vaginal delivery, much of that fluid is "squeezed" from the lungs as the baby passes through the birth canal.

At birth, fluid in the mouth and nose must be cleared with a bulb syringe. In a vertex presentation, suction begins when the head is delivered. Drainage of fluid is further facilitated by placing the baby on his side with his head slightly dependent. When the baby is delivered by cesarean section, the vaginal squeeze does not occur, and some fluid remains in the lungs for several days. Such a baby commonly has some degree of respiratory distress during the first day or two of life, which diminishes as the baby's circulatory system "picks up" the excess fluid. (Infants of cesarean birth may have respiratory distress for additional reasons related to the cause of the abdominal delivery.)

Deep oropharyngeal suction with a catheter should be avoided because the larynx may be "tickled," leading to laryngospasm and failure to breathe.

When the baby is delivered through thick, "pea soup" meconium, *meconium aspiration syndrome,* i.e., the aspiration of meconium into the lungs, may occur. This baby requires insertion of an endotracheal tube and suction before his first breath forces the meconium further into the respiratory tree. Today, many physicians

Table 5–9   Some Commonly Used Medications

Route	Drug	Effect on Mother	Effect on Newborn
Systemic	Barbiturates Pentobarbital (Nembutal) Secobarbital (Seconal) 100 mg IM 100 to 200 mg PO	Central nervous system depression Dulls participation in labor process Do not relieve pain; sedative only Maximum effect: 30 min IM, 60 min PO May impair uterine activity and prolong labor in large doses	Delayed interest in breast-feeding Depressed response to auditory and visual stimuli Metabolized slowly; effects may last 24 to 48 hours Delay in parent-infant interaction
	Diazepam (Valium)	Does not relieve pain; sedative only Relief of anxiety Potentiates barbiturates and analgesics; reduces dosage of these drugs	May cause depression, particularly when combined with narcotics or sedatives
IV titration preferred	Meperidine hydrochloride (Demerol) 10 mg IV	Hypotension	Meperidine converted to by-products capable of depressing neonatal respiratory center
	Alphaprodine (Nisentil) 25 mg IV	Analgesia	May affect infant behavior for several days postdelivery and thus affect parent-infant interaction
Regional analgesia	2-Chloroprocaine hydrochloride (Nesacaine)	Short duration of action; does not accumulate in maternal blood; often used initially for rapid onset	Should not be given in premature labor
	Bupivacaine (Marcain)	Longer duration action; does not accumulate in maternal blood	Decreases newborn muscle tone
	Mepivacaine Lidocaine	Long duration; tends to accumulate in maternal blood; less frequently used today	Decreases newborn muscle tone

feel that the baby with thin watery meconium in the amniotic fluid does not require endotracheal intubation and suction.

BREATHING

When the airway is clear but the baby does not breathe, assisted ventilation may be necessary.

Prior to the first breath the wet internal surfaces of the lungs adhere to one another in much the same manner as wet glass slides adhere to each other in the laboratory. Therefore, the first breath requires more pressure than subsequent breaths, from 40 to 100 cm water pressure. The initial puff of air, when it hits the larynx, often stimulates the baby to breathe and will be all that is necessary. If further ventilation is required, the pressure should be from 25 to 45 cm water pressure and the rate from 12 to 20 breaths per minute. This rate is slower than the rate at which a newborn breaths spontaneously (about 30 to 50 bpm) because positive pressure ventilation impedes the return of venous blood to the heart and cardiac refill. Ventilation without circulation is of little value. Ventilation, however, may in itself improve circulation (Fig. 5–15).

CIRCULATION

The clearing of the airway and the initiation of breathing should take less than one minute. If the infant is still cyanotic 60 to 90 seconds following birth, the cause may be low cardiac output, a cyanotic congenital heart disease, or lung abnormality. Polycythemia is an uncommon but possible cause; in polycythemia there is an excess of red blood cells and the baby is unable to oxygenate all of them.

If the heart rate remains less than 50 bpm after 30 seconds of ventilation, cardiac massage is indicated. The thumbs should be on the middle third of the baby's sternum; pressing on the lower third may cause laceration of the liver. The rate of cardiac massage is approximately 80 to 100 chest compressions per minute, slower than a baby's normal rate of 130 to 150 beats per minute to allow the heart to refill so that the cardiac output will be adequate. If cardiac massage is at a rate of 100 and ventilation at a rate of 20, the ratio will be 5:1.

DRUGS

If the baby does not respond satisfactorily to ventilation and cardiac massage, the use of drugs may be necessary. The narcotic antagonist naloxone has already been discussed in the section on drugs as a cause of depression.

Emergency medications are used less frequently than previously because of the recognition that the drugs themselves may be dangerous for the infant. However, used properly in appropriate dosage, they can also be lifesaving. Table 5–10 de-

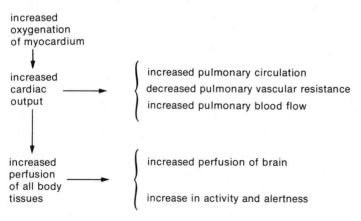

Figure 5–15. Ventilation.

Table 5–10 Drugs and Blood Products for Neonatal Resuscitation Emergencies

Drugs	Dosage and Rate	Reason for Administration	Comments
Sodium bicarbonate (NaHCO$_3$) (1 mEq = 1 ml) Diluted 1:1 (Sterile H$_2$O)	2 to 3 mEq/kg IV; over 1 to 2 min	Metabolic acidosis	Baby must be ventilated during administration
Epinephrine (1:1000) Dilute 1:10,000 (NaCl)	0.1 to 0.5 ml/kg IV	Heart rate falling or below 50 bpm in spite of resuscitation	May be given in cardiac muscle
Calcium gluconate Dilute 1:1 (after every third dose NaHCO$_3$)	100 mg/kg slow IV	Replace calcium depleted during asphyxia	Calcium and bicarbonate cannot be mixed in infusion solutions; causes bradycardia if injected too rapidly; cardiac massage should accompany epinephrine
Atropine sulfate	0.01 mg/kg IV	Severe bradycardia	
Naloxone (Narcan)	0.01 mg/kg IV/IM	Reverse narcotic depression	Observe for later distress
Albumin (may mix 1:1 with NaCl or NaHCO$_3$)	1.0 g/kg IV	Circulatory support	O negative blood is used in emergencies
Fresh frozen plasma	10 to 20 ml/kg IV		
Packed RBC	10 to 20 ml/kg IV		
Whole blood	10 to 20 ml/kg IV		
Glucose (10%)	2 ml/kg for first 5 minutes	Necessary for metabolism	During the first day, continue glucose at 80 mg/kg/day; follow with blood glucose determinations

scribes the most frequently used emergency drugs.

Sodium bicarbonate ($NaHCO_3$) is given so frequently that nurses need to be thoroughly familiar with its use. Several principles are important. One of the chief breakdown products of $NaHCO_3$ is carbon dioxide (CO_2). Retention of CO_2 leads to respiratory acidosis. Therefore (1) when acidosis is purely respiratory, $NaHCO_3$ has no value, and (2) when $NaHCO_3$ is given, *the baby must be continuously ventilated* by either bag and mask or bag and endotracheal tube so that CO_2 does not accumulate.

In relation to the first point, respiratory acidosis, unless corrected by ventilation, leads rapidly to metabolic acidosis (in the absence of oxygen, anaerobic metabolism results in the production of lactic acid). The initial dose of $NaHCO_3$ is 2 to 3 mEq/kg IV. As soon as blood gas values are available, dosage can be calculated as follows:

mEq = wt of the baby in kg $\times$ 0.3 $\times$ base deficit (desired bicarbonate level − actual bicarbonate level)

For example:
   weight of baby = 2000 g
   bicarbonate level (blood gas) = 17
   desired level (blood gas) = 21
   base deficit = 4

$$2000 \times 0.3 \times 4 = 2.4 \text{ mEq}$$

The prepared dose is diluted 1:1 with sterile water and given slowly through an umbilical vein catheter (no faster than 1 mEq/kg/minute).

The possible role of sodium bacarbonate in intracranial hemorrhage in premature infants makes it imperative that the drug be used only in severe life-threatening metabolic acidosis and then in appropriate doses.

ENVIRONMENTAL TEMPERATURE

The critical need for warmth has already been noted. It is crucial that the baby's need for warmth be met during resuscitation or other efforts may be compromised. The environment should allow the baby to maintain an axillary temperature of 97.6° F (36.5° C). This is the thermoneutral temperature, i.e., the temperature at which the least amount of oxygen is required by the baby.

The environmental temperature required to keep the baby's temperature at this level will vary with the size of the baby. Failure to maintain a thermoneutral environment increases the baby's need for oxygen, leading to anaerobic metabolism. Lactic acid, a by-product of anaerobic metabolism, is an important factor in metabolic acidosis.

THE TRANSITION TO EXTRAUTERINE LIFE

From the moment of birth through the first hours of life the newborn adapts to a new way of life. Under normal circumstances both his internal changes and his behavior are characteristic.

The transition from intrauterine to extrauterine life includes an initial period of reactivity, an interval during which the baby is relatively unresponsive and inactive, and then a second, more active period of reactivity. The transition is usually complete in the healthy term newborn by about six hours of age.

The initial period of reactivity lasts for approximately 15 to 30 minutes after birth and is characterized by activity in many body systems. The heart beats rapidly, muscle tone is increased, and the baby is alert and exploring. He may have tremors of the extremities or chin and sudden outcries that stop as suddenly as they begin. He sucks, swallows, grimaces, and moves his head from side to side.

If the mother has not been anesthetized, the baby is generally alert during this period and will look at his mother and father. This period seems designed by nature for the attachment of parents and baby. Then, for approximately an hour and a half, he becomes much more quiet and relatively unresponsive. His color improves as his muscle tone returns to normal. Heart and respiratory rates decline.

Both external and internal stimuli bring little response.

A second period of reactivity completes the transition. By comparing healthy infants with these norms, nurses can recognize more readily what is usual and what is unusual during this significant time.

Physiological Changes at Birth

The physiological functioning of the infant differs from that of the fetus in several important respects. In the moments following birth, the transition to newborn functioning begins but is not completed.

RESPIRATORY CHANGES

Throughout fetal life the lungs are filled with fluid that keeps them partially expanded. What happens to this fluid? In a vertex delivery the pressure of the birth canal on the fetal thorax literally "squeezes" part of the fluid from the lung and out through the baby's nose and mouth. The remaining fluid is picked up by the blood vessels and lymphatics surrounding the lung, a process greatly facilitated by the changes in pulmonary vasculature described below (circulatory changes).

When the baby is delivered in a presentation other than vertex (e.g., by caesarean section or breech presentation), this fluid is not as easily expelled from the lungs. The lungs are stiff and the baby may breathe rapidly for several days, a condition termed *transient tachypnea* of the newborn.

Within 10 minutes after birth the volume of air remaining in the lungs at end expiration is the same as it is at five days of age. Vital capacity reaches values proportional to those of an adult within eight to 12 hours after birth.

CIRCULATORY CHANGES

Fetal circulation is depicted in Figure 5–16. The establishment and maintenance of good respiration influences the changes that occur in the cardiovascular system at the time of birth (Fig. 5–17). Within moments following delivery:

1. Oxygen enters the lungs and pulmonary alveoli expand.

2. The oxygen lowers resistance in the pulmonary vessels, allowing blood to flow more freely to and from the lungs (in the fetus no more than 10 per cent of the total circulating blood flowed through the lungs).

3. Pressure in the right atrium decreases because of the increased flow of blood to the lungs.

4. Pressure in the left atrium increases because of the increased flow of blood from the lungs.

5. The ductus arteriosus begins to constrict with oxygenation, becoming functionally closed during the first 24 hours. (If the PaO_2 is low or becomes low during the first days of life, the ductus arteriosus has the capacity to remain open or to reopen.)

6. The umbilical vessels, already clamped in the delivery process, contract.

7. As pressure in the left side of the heart begins to exceed that in the right side (owing to the activation of pulmonary circulation described above) the valve of the foramen ovale becomes "plastered" against the septum secundum, thus functionally closing the foramen ovale.

Although functional changes in circulation take place very shortly after birth, structural changes occur over a period of many months (Table 5–11).

CHANGES IN KIDNEY FUNCTION

Prior to birth the kidney is apparently not essential to life, although it produces urine, which becomes part of the amniotic fluid from about the twelfth gestational week. Even a fetus with total renal agenesis may exist intact because the placenta carries on the necessary regulatory functions. At birth, however, the kidney must immediately begin to function; the infant totally lacking kidneys cannot survive.

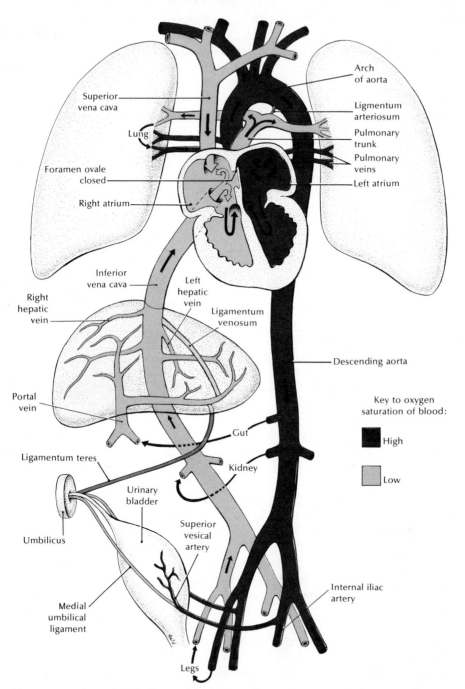

Figure 5–16.   A simplified scheme of the fetal circulation. The arrows show the course of the fetal circulation. The organs are not drawn to scale. (From Moore: The Developing Human. 2nd Edition. W. B. Saunders, 1977.)

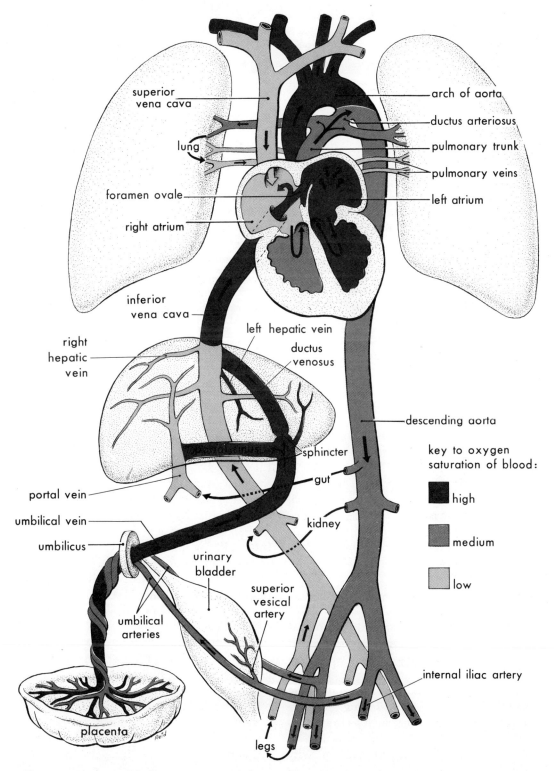

Figure 5-17. A simplified representation of the circulation after birth. The adult derivatives of the fetal vessels and structures that become nonfunctional at birth are also shown. The arrows indicate the course of the neonatal circulation. The organs are not drawn to scale. (From Moore: The Developing Human. 2nd Edition. W. B. Saunders, 1977.)

Table 5–11   Structural Changes in Circulation after Birth

Structures in Fetal Circulation	Approx. Time of Anatomical Obliteration	Resulting Structures
Foramen ovale	1 year	Fossa ovalis
Ductus arteriosus	1 month	Ligamentum arteriosum
Ductus venosus	2 months	Ligamentum venosum of the liver
Umbilical arteries	2 to 3 months	Distal portion: lateral umbilical ligaments
		Proximal portion: internal iliac arteries, which function throughout life
Umbilical vein	2 to 3 months	Ligamentum teres of the liver

Just as pulmonary vascular resistance decreases, allowing more blood to flow to and from the lungs, so also does the vascular resistance of the renal vessels decreases, allowing increased blood flow to the kidneys with a marked improvement in kidney function within a few days.

Kidney function, however, remains immature for many months. The glomerular filtration rate is low, a factor particularly significant in the sick baby because the excretion of drugs by the kidney is limited. Acid-base balance is labile because the bicarbonate threshold is lower. (In adults no bicarbonate is spilled into the urine until serum levels reach 24 to 26 mEq/liter, term newborns lose bicarbonate at levels of 21 to 22 mEq/liter and preterm babies at a level of 19 to 20 mEq/liter.) Newborns also retain hydrogen ion, an additional factor in acid-base metabolism. Because Henle's loop is short, newborns have a limited ability to concentrate urine.

CHANGES IN LIVER FUNCTION

The liver is the chief organ of blood formation in the fetus from the third to the sixth months and continues to produce some cells into the first postnatal week.

Some functions that were handled by the placenta during fetal life must now be undertaken by the liver, such as the excretion of bilirubin. Placental excretion of bilirubin would seem to explain why there is usually a minimal rise of serum bilirubin levels in cord blood in newborns with erythroblastosis fetalis at birth but a rapid increase within a few hours after birth.

Glucuronyl transferase, the enzyme necessary for the conversion of indirect bilirubin to water soluble direct bilirubin, which can then be excreted by the kidneys, is less active in the first days of life; thus even the small degree of hemolysis that normally occurs in the newborn can cause a pronounced degree of hyperbilirubinemia and subsequent jaundice.

Prothrombin and blood clotting Factors VII (proconvertin), IX (plasma thromboplastin component), and X (Stuart-Prower) are synthesized in the liver. Prothrombin is low in cord blood. Prothrombin time, which measures the activity of Factors VII and X,* may be within a normal range or may be low at birth but will become most prolonged at three to four days of life and continue at abnormal levels for two to three additional days. About 75 per cent of term infants and an even larger percentage of preterm infants show this drop in clotting factors. These changes are related to the inability of the baby to synthesize and utilize vitamin K. The drop in clotting factors means that the infant has a greater risk of hemorrhage than those infants who have no drop in clotting factors.

In most nurseries 1.0 mg of vitamin K is given to every newborn shortly after birth. This practice has virtually eliminated hemorrhagic disease of the newborn. Larger amounts of vitamin K do not enhance its therapeutic value; moreover, larger doses predispose the baby to hyperbilirubinemia and kernicterus. Giving vi-

---

*Factor V (proaccelerin) is also measured in prothrombin times but is of normal levels in the newborn.

tamin K to the mother during labor, rather than to the baby, has been found to be less dependable. Natural vitamin K preparations (e.g., AquaMephyton, Konakion) act more rapidly than synthetic preparations (e.g., Hykinone) and are considered a better choice for that reason.

Infants of low gestational age have an even more limited ability to synthesize clotting factors, even in the presence of large amounts of vitamin K.

CHANGES IN THE BLOOD

By the sixth month of fetal life the bone marrow has become the chief site of blood formation. At the time of birth it is highly active, with most of the marrow space involved in red cell production. This means that there is little marrow reserve to increase red cell production if any excess hemolysis occurs. As mentioned above, the liver may continue to produce red blood cells in the first week of life because of this lack of marrow reserve; the spleen is an additional site of extramedullary hematopoiesis.

Hemoconcentration appears to be a major characteristic of the first hours of life. Hemoglobin concentration rises by as much as 17 to 20 per cent in the first two hours, then drops slightly but remains elevated until some time between the first and third weeks. Hemoglobin levels range from 17 to 22 g/100 ml in the term newborn and from 15 to 17 g/100 ml in the preterm baby. Decreasing hemoglobin levels during the first week indicated red cell destruction or blood loss. Hematocrit also rises sharply during the first hours of life and then declines slowly; values at one week of age are close to values in cord blood (57 to 58 for term newborns; 45 to 55 for preterm infants).

Red cells increase in the first hours to a level of more than 500,000/cu mm higher than cord blood. The red blood cells of the newborn infant are usually larger than those of an older infant; by the end of the second month cells are close to adult size in term infants. Most studies seem to indicate that the life span of red blood

cells of term infants is the same or only slightly shorter than that of a normal adult, whereas the life span of red blood cells of preterm infants is definitely shorter. There is not universal agreement on this, however.

A small increase in white blood cell (WBC) count occurs at birth, possibly also owing to hemoconcentration. Following this initial peak, WBC count drops and leukocytes become markedly less efficient at phagocytosis after the first 24 hours and throughout the first month. One study reports the mean number of leukocytes as 18,000 at birth, 12,200 at seven days, and 11,400 at 14 days. This decrease in number and activity of leukocytes is one factor in the newborn's lowered resistance to infection. White cell counts vary widely from infant to infant and even within the same infant from day to day with no apparent reason. Thus, a single elevated WBC count is of little value; two or more tests are needed when sepsis is suspected.

In comparing blood values in the first hours and days of life, it is important to remember that capillary samples, usually obtained from the heel or toe, have higher concentrations of white blood cells than venous samples. This is believed to be caused by the relatively sluggish circulation in the peripheral blood vessels, which in turn leads to transudation of the plasma. Warming the area by wrapping it with a warm towel for a few minutes before the sample is obtained and discarding the first few drops of the sample minimize these differences. Even then capillary samples should not be compared with venous samples.

ACID-BASE BALANCE

All newborn infants are acidotic to some degree at birth. With normal lungs and ventilation, the acidosis corrects itself within the first hour (Table 5–12). Infants who have had a period of apnea or a delay in the onset of respirations will be more acidotic, with pH levels falling below 7.0.

Values will vary with the site from

Table 5–12   Neonatal Acid-Base Balance

	pH	PaO$_2$	PaCO$_2$	HCO$_3$ (Bicarbonate)
Cord blood	7.2	16 to 32*	60 to 70	23
Arterial blood at one hour	7.32	90 to 100	35 to 40	20

*Values vary considerably, even in vigorous newborns.

which the sample is obtained. There is considerably less oxygen and slightly more CO$_2$ in venous blood. If the sample is obtained from a heel stick and the heel is not warmed adequately, the blood obtained may be venous blood. The pH and Pco$_2$ values will vary slightly, but the Po$_2$ of venous blood is normally 40 while the PaO$_2$ of arterial blood is normally 90 to 100. Thus, in high risk babies who need close monitoring, an umbilical artery catheter is usually inserted shortly after delivery (Chapter 8).

METABOLIC CHANGES

Because plasma glucose and calcium are regulated by the placenta during fetal life, even a healthy newborn shows immaturity in glucose and calcium metabolism during his first days. It is one to two weeks before homeostasis is reached. Preterm babies who develop postnatal illness or infants of diabetic mothers or mothers with hyperparathyroidism may have increased difficulty in achieving homeostasis.

Bibliography

Abramson, H. (ed.): Resuscitation of the Newborn Infant. 2nd Edition. St. Louis: C. V. Mosby, 1966.

Antenatal diagnosis: Report of a consensus development conference. Bethesda: National Institute of Health, 1979.

Apgar, V.: Proposal for a new method of evaluation of the newborn infant. Anes Analg 32:260, 1953.

Apgar, V., Holaday, D., James, L. et al.: Evaluation of the newborn infant: second report. JAMA 168:1985, 1958.

Aubrey, R.: Identification of the high-risk perinatal patient. In Perinatal Intensive Care, S. Aladjem and A. Brown (eds.). St. Louis. C. V. Mosby, 1978.

Beard, R., Edinger, P., Sabanda, J.: Effects of routine intrapartum monitoring on clinical practice. Contrib Gynecol Obstet 3:14, 1977.

Borgstadt, A., Rosen, M.: Medication during labor correlated with behavior and EEG of the newborn. Am J Dis Child 115:21, 1968.

Caldeyro-Barcia, R.: The influence of maternal position on time of spontaneous rupture of the membranes, progress of labor, and fetal head compression. Birth Family J 6(1):7, 1979.

Caldeyro-Barcia, R.: Some consequences of obstetrical interference. Birth Family 2(2):34, 1975.

Chaucer-Hatton, M.: Consumer satisfaction with labor and delivery in a birth room. Master's thesis. Yale School of Nursing, 1978.

Conley, R.: The Economics of Mental Retardation. Baltimore; Johns Hopkins University Press, 1973.

Dilts, P.: Current practices in antepartum and intrapartum fetal monitoring. Am J Obstet Gynecol 126:491, 1976.

Dubowitz, L., Dubowitz, V., Goldberg, C.: Clinical assessment of gestational age in the newborn infant. J Pediatr 77:1, 1970.

Duff, R.: Care in childbirth and beyond. N Eng J Med 302:685, 1980.

Fisher, D., Paton, J.: Resuscitation of the newborn infant. In Care of the High Risk Neonate, M. Klaus and A. Fanaroff (eds.). Philadelphia: W. B. Saunders, 1979.

Gabert, H., Stenchever, M.: The results of a five-year study of continuous fetal monitoring on an obstetric service. Obstet Gynecol 50:275, 1977.

Gleason, D.: Footprinting for identification of infants. Pediatrics 44:302, 1969.

Haverkamp, A., Orleans, M., Langendoerfer, S. et al: A controlled trial of the differential effects of intrapartum fetal monitoring. Am J Obstet Gynecol 134:399, 1979.

Haverkamp, A., Thompson, H., McFee, J., Cetrulo, C.: The evaluation of continuous fetal heart rate monitoring in high-risk pregnancy. Am J Obstet Gynecol 125:310, 1976.

Hobel, C., Hyvarinen, M., Okada, D., Oh, W.: Prenatal and intrapartum high-risk screening. Am J Obstet Gynecol 117:1, 1973.

Hochberg, H.: The physiological basis of fetal heart rate monitoring. In Progress in Perinatology, H. Kaminetzky and L. Iffy (eds.). Philadelphia: George F. Stickley Co., 1977.

Hughey, M., La Pata, R., McElin, T., Lussky, R.: The effect of fetal monitoring on the incidence of cesarean section. Obstet Gynecol 49:513, 1977.

Kelly, V., Kulkarni, D.: Experiences with fetal monitoring in a community hospital. Obstet Gynecol 41:818, 1973.

Kilso, I., Parsons, R., Lawrence, G. et al.: An assessment of continuous fetal heart rate monitoring in labor: a randomized trial. Am J Obstet Gynecol *131*:520, 1978.

Kliot, D.: Gentle birth. Presentation at a conference, Childbirth: A Family Experience. Charlotte ASPO, Charlotte, North Carolina, February 22, 1980.

Koh, K., Greves, D., Yung, S., Peddle, L.: Experience with fetal monitoring in a university teaching hospital. Can Med Assoc J *112*:455, 1975.

Kron, R., Stein, M., Goddard, K.: Newborn sucking behavior affected by obstetric sedation. Pediatrics *37*:1012, 1966.

Leboyer, F.: Birth Without Violence. New York: Knopf, 1975.

Lee, W., Baggish, M.: The effect of unselected intrapartum fetal monitoring. Obstet Gynecol 1976, *47*:516, 1976.

Moore, M. L.: Realities in Childbearing. Philadelphia: W. B. Saunders, 1978.

Nelson, N., Enkin, M., Saigal et al.: A randomized clinical trial of the Leboyer approach to childbirth. N Eng J Med *302*:655, 1980.

Okada, D., Chow, A., Bruce, U.: Neonatal scalp abscess and fetal monitoring: factors associated with infections. Am J Obstet Gynecol *129*:185, 1977.

Phillips, C. R.: Neonatal heat loss in heated cribs vs. mothers' arms. JOGN Nurs *3*(6):11, 1974.

Rappoport, D.: Pour une naissance sans violence resultats d'une première enquête. Bull Psychol *29*:552, 1976.

Renou, P., Chang, A., Anderson, I., Wood, C.: Controlled trial of fetal intensive care. Am J Obstet Gynecol *126*:470, 1976.

Scanlan, J., Brown, W., Weiss, J. et al.: Neurobehavioral responses of newborn infants after maternal epidural anesthesia. Anesthesiology *40*:121, 1974.

Shields, D.: Maternal reactions to fetal monitoring. Nurs '78 2110.

Standley, K., Soule, A., Copano, S. et al.: Local-regional anesthesia during childbirth: effect on newborn behavior. Science *186*:634, 1974.

Stechler, G.: Newborn attention as affected by medication during labor Science *144*:315, 1964.

Taft, J.: Consumer birth preferences. Master's thesis, Yale School of Nursing, 1978.

Tatano, C.: Patient's cognitive and emotional responses to fetal monitoring. Master's thesis, Yale School of Nursing, 1972.

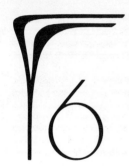

THE UNIQUE CHARACTERISTICS OF THE NEWBORN

The nursing assessment of the newborn and his family has various dimensions. Three modes of assessment (the Apgar score, the assessment of gestational age, and the correlation of gestational age with body weight) have been described in Chapter 5. In this chapter the assessment and significance of infant states and the physical assessment of the infant are described. The assessment of parent-infant interaction will be discussed in Chapter 10.

STATE

State is a concept that describes a way of being. Characteristics that commonly occur together, including activity, breathing patterns, eye movements, and response to stimuli, differentiate one state from another. As adults, we recognize that not only does our sleep state vary from our waking state but we may even be in a variety of states when awake. At one time we may be very alert, our attention intently focused on a specific matter. At other times our minds wander. Some adults train themselves or are trained to achieve certain states (e.g., a state of conscious relaxation).

Weiss, in a paper published in 1934, was the first to recognize that infants are also able to manifest a variety of states.

Prechtl further advanced the concept of state in papers published in the 1950s through the 1970s in both the German and American literature.

In the United States Wolff's 1959 paper is generally considered to be the first to systematically observe states. It stimulated a vast amount of subsequent research involving newborns and infants. Although Wolff (1966) described seven states and Prechtl (1974) described five, the six states described by Brazelton (1973) are most widely utilized in nursing practice today. These include two sleep states — deep sleep and light or rapid eye movement (REM) sleep — and four awake states: drowsy, quiet alert, active alert, and crying (Table 6–1). States are sometimes referred to by number, with the number 1 assigned to deep sleep and the number 6 assigned to crying.

During *deep sleep* the infant scarcely moves except for occasional startles. Breathing is smooth and regular. The infant in deep sleep is difficult to arouse;

Table 6–1   Infant States

Sleep States	Awake States
Deep sleep (1) Light (REM) sleep (2)	Drowsy (3) Quiet alert (4) Active alert (5) Crying (6)

thus it is hard to feed him or elicit other behaviors.

In contrast, the infant may move, smile, and make "fussy" sounds during *light sleep*. Rapid eye movements (REM) may be observed beneath closed eyelids. Infants in light sleep, the predominant sleep pattern of newborns, may respond to either external or internal stimuli by a state change (to deep sleep or drowsiness), or they may remain in light sleep.

In the *drowsy* state infants raise their eyelids at intervals, but the eyes appear dull and glazed. Activity is variable; facial movement may or may not be present. Breathing is commonly irregular during both light sleep and drowsy states. If one desires to further waken a drowsy infant, visual stimuli, such as a face, and/or auditory stimuli such as a voice, may rouse the infant to the quiet alert state.

When in the *quiet alert* state, infants show little general activity but are highly attentive to many types of stimuli. In the first hour after birth the infant is commonly in a prolonged quiet alert state if not affected by medications given to the mother. The quiet alert infant who gazes at his parents with a bright-eyed look has a marked effect on them. Parents make statements such as "He's really looking at me" and "She looks as though she knows us." Nurses who have been caring for mothers and infants for many years find this in sharp contrast to the comments of mothers of previous decades, when mothers were asleep during delivery and infants were drowsy from maternal medication; infrequent opportunities for interaction during hospitalization meant that a baby might be several days old before his mother saw him with his eyes open. Dad rarely saw more than a sleeping baby through the nursery window until discharge.

Active alert infants move both body and face actively. Breathing is irregular. "Fussy" describes this state well; stimuli such as hunger, noise, and too much handling disturb the baby easily. Some infants are able to console themselves quite readily and return to a lower state; others require more frequent intervention from caregivers (see below).

Crying is the last state. The eyes may be open or closed, breathing is irregular, and the baby is very active, with changes in skin color. As in the active alert state, some infants can console themselves or are easily consoled by others, whereas other infants are far more difficult to console.

State-Related Behaviors

An understanding of the concept of state requires a knowledge not only of the states themselves but also of other behaviors characteristic of newborns. These behaviors are called "state-related" because they are not present at all times but are more common during specific states. During infant assessment these behaviors should be noted; they are part of the baby's uniqueness that the parents must recognize to care for him. Although there are wide variations within the range of normal, some behaviors indicate a need for more detailed assessment.

CUDDLINESS

Cuddliness describes the way in which a baby molds himself to the body of the person holding him. Most newborns will "nestle" when they are held, fitting their body into the body of the holder. If held to the shoulder, they may nestle into the holder's neck. All babies are not cuddlers. Some resist being held by becoming active and squirming. Other babies are very passive, neither resisting nor making an attempt to cuddle.

A cuddly baby gives a great deal of positive reinforcement to the parents. They feel rewarded for their efforts. But what happens when a baby is not cuddly? Parents may feel that a baby who resists cuddling does not love them, and their attachment to that baby may be impaired. Similarly, a baby who lies passively in his parents' arms may fail to elicit caregiving or stimulating behavior from the parents.

Nurses can help parents in two ways. First, they can emphasize the uniqueness of each baby's personality. Some babies are active and resist cuddling; this is a part of their personality, not a reflection on the parents' competence. Parents of very passive babies also need reassurance that their baby is not rejecting them. Brazelton's *Infants and Mothers* is a helpful resource for parents in this regard; Brazelton traces the development of an average baby, a quiet baby, and an active baby through the first year.

Nurses can also help parents by encouraging them to experiment with positions their baby finds comforting. While these positions may not represent "cuddling" in the traditional sense, they can be mutually satisfying.

IRRITABILITY

An irritable infant responds to both internal and external stimuli with frequent fussing and crying. Although extreme irritability may be a sign of central nervous system disorder (just as extremes in lack of affect may be), there is a wide range of normality in healthy infants. Irritable infants will need increased consoling (see later in this chapter); they frequently need a somewhat more subdued environment and slower, more careful handling to prevent sudden changes. For example, a baby who is irritable may respond more comfortably to being unwrapped and undressed slowly rather than rapidly.

HABITUATION

Habituation is the ability to shut down one's response to repeated stimuli. For example, if you walk into a quiet room in which a clock is ticking loudly, you may be aware of the clock's ticking. But usually within a few minutes you will no longer hear the ticking; the clock has not stopped but you have shut down your response to that auditory stimulus. Like adults, new-

borns shut down responses to stimuli after initially attending to them. Without habituation, the world would be a constant source of buzzing confusion. By demonstrating examples of habituation to parents the nurse can help them appreciate this ability in their baby. For example, if someone shines a light in the baby's eyes or rings a bell near his ears, he will respond at first, but he will respond less at each successive trial until there is a minimal response or no response at all. Similarly, attempts to elicit the Moro reflex result in a decreasing response on successive trials (see later in this chapter).

An understanding of habituation is of value to the parents because it suggests that their baby is able to cope with his environment and thus does not need to be isolated from the normal noises in his home. As noted above, some highly irritable babies may have a need for a reduced level of stimulation.

CONSOLABILITY

Consolability is the ability to move from a higher state (crying or active alert, which often involves fussing) to a lower state (quiet alert, drowsy, or sleep). Infants may console themselves at times, commonly by hand-to-mouth maneuvers or by attending (fixing attention on) something in their environment such as an interesting visual object or a sound. Faces and voices are effective stimuli for consolation. Consoling may also come from others.

Infants vary widely in both the type and amount of consolation they require. Some infants are rarely irritable and are easily consoled, either by themselves or by others. Some are frequently irritable but are able to console themselves. Others are difficult to console under any circumstances.

Because an inconsolable baby can rapidly undermine the parents' confidence in their ability to care for him, the nurse needs to help them recognize ways in which their baby attempts to console himself as well as effective means they can use to console him. The nurse should also emphasize that it is normal for some infants to be difficult to console and that this is not a reflection on their ability as parents.

As noted above, a common means of self-consoling is through hand-to-mouth movements. Many parents are uncomfortable with such movements, viewing them as a prelude to thumb or finger sucking, which is frowned upon in our society. But these movements are natural to the newborn and even to the fetus in utero, as ultrasound has often demonstrated. Reassurance may help parents accept this behavior.

Parents have commonly been conditioned to view a crying baby as a hungry baby; a bottle or breast is their first thought as they try to console their infant. They are amazed to see the baby's response to the sound of their voice as they talk to him; he may quickly become quietly alert and begin to scan the environment. Other consoling acts to which the infant may respond include the sight of a face, being rocked in a cradle or in someone's arms, having his arms held close to his body or being swaddled in a blanket, or being held to the shoulder as if to burp. Korner (1972) demonstrated the importance of position in state changes. When a crying infant was lifted and held to the shoulder with his head supported he became alert and began to scan the environment. The positions that brought the next greatest amount of visual alertness were horizontal movement and sitting up.

The nursing role, then, can be to suggest to the parents various consoling methods and to help them discover those maneuvers most useful with their infant. Additionally, when a baby has older siblings, parents sometimes need to be reminded that this infant may respond differently from previous infants. *Each infant is unique.*

Factors Affecting State

State is related to both external and internal environments. Room temperature, for example, has been shown to be related to the amount of time an infant spends in quiet sleep. In a study by Parmalee, Brueck, and Brueck (1962), newborns were found to spend 32 per cent of their day in quiet sleep at 30°C (86°F), 46 per cent at 31°C (89°F), and 55 per cent at 34°C (93°F). In a very early study Weiss (1934) found infants to be more active under minimal light than under moderate light. In the dark, background noise affected activity.

As nurses and parents might suspect, behavior when the infant is hungry is considerably different from behavior after feeding. Ashton (1973) found that postfeeding behaviors correlated with other published research related to state but that prefeeding behaviors did not correlate.

Sex differences were recognized to affect state by Korner (1972). Male infants were found to startle more frequently in all states, whereas female infants smiled reflexively more often and showed more rhythmic mouthing. Korner's findings on the effect of position on state have already been noted.

The Significance of State for Nurses

An appreciation of the concept of state is essential for nurses in both daily clinical practice and research. Perhaps the most important nursing role is to help parents recognize, and correlate their caregiving with, their infant's states. Obviously when nurses are the caregivers they must also correlate their activities with the infant's state. Nursing assessment of any infant must be within the framework of state, whether the purpose is clinical observation or research.

State-related behaviors highlight the uniqueness of individual infants. In the prenatal period, the concept of uniqueness in behavior can be introduced to the parents. The nurse may tell parents in childbirth preparation classes something like this:

> Some of you will have babies who will be easy to care for right from the start. Other babies will be more difficult. They will cry more often and will be more difficult

to quiet. Some babies have to be held. Others are squirmy, wiggly worms. Sometimes parents with more difficult babies begin to doubt themselves and think they are not good parents, particularly when they see parents who seem to be having a much easier time. Don't worry about other parents and their babies. Learn to know your baby, his likes and dislikes, his special characteristics, and you will be the best possible parents for him.

At least once during the first days after birth the nurse and both parents or the person who is to be the primary caregiver (sometimes the grandmother) should talk about the baby's individual characteristics. The nurse might begin by asking the parents what they have noticed about their baby's behavior. They may talk about the baby's crying or looking around or restlessness when he is asleep. A father may say, "Naomi really cries hard when she is hungry," to which the nurse may respond, "What seems to quiet her?"

The research of Bell and Ainsworth (1972) suggests that a mother's perception of her infant's states is important. In comparing the responses of infants whose behavior made little or no difference in determining what happened to them with infants whose behavior was met with appropriate maternal practices, the second group in general cried less, learned to express themselves in ways other than hard crying, and had more predictable rhythms and a greater tolerance of frustration. One might question whether some of these characteristics in the babies made maternal intervention easier; regardless, the infant's state seems important to the interaction.

Failure to readily recognize their infant's states is not necessarily due to parental misperception. Some infants manifest states far more indistinctly than others. Some infants move rapidly from one state to another, often skipping intermediate states. The baby may, for example, move from deep sleep (state 1) to active alert (state 5) or crying (state 6).

The concept of state should affect hospital practices; the practice of fitting babies

into institutional patterns such as rigid feeding schedules (which still exists in some hospitals) becomes obviously inappropriate. For example, it is difficult or impossible for a baby in states 1 or 2 (the sleep states) to feed well. A policy that dictates feedings at 2 AM regardless of the infant's state should be changed. Moreover, failure to appreciate the infant's state may lead the nurse to assess the baby as difficult to feed when the baby actually feeds quite well in an appropriate state for feeding.

The process of parental adaptation to their infant continues during the first weeks at home. Unfortunately for many parents, limited counsel is available during this period. Some possible strategies for changing this situation are discussed in Chapters 7 and 12.

State as a Research Question

Future research into the concept of state could answer a number of questions. Is there a relationship between differences in infant states and later development of the child? Bell, Weller, and Waldrop (1971) found an inverse relationship between intensity of behavior in the newborn period (measured by respiratory rate, tactile threshold, and reaction to interruption of sucking) and intensity of behavior in the preschool period (measured by gregariousness, communicativeness, assertiveness, participation, and low interest).

What effect does the ability of an infant to distinctly manifest state have on parent-infant interaction? It would seem difficult for the mother to interpret the needs of an infant with great variability and unpredictability of state.

Do some infants have difficulty perceiving their internal environment, just as some adults appear to (e.g., the person who cannot recognize when he is hungry)?

How much range and flexibility of state is exhibited by an infant? What is the significance of range and flexibility? What is the significance of the easy alterability of state?

Are there cross-cultural differences in the various manifestations of state?

Is there an optimum state or state pattern that will facilitate the effectiveness of stimulation?

Such questions are not merely of academic interest but, when answered, should be of value in shaping nursing practice.

PHYSICAL CHARACTERISTICS OF THE NEWBORN: NORMAL VERSUS ABNORMAL

It has been said that newborn babies are beautiful only to their parents and the nurses who care for them. To the curious stranger passing the nursery they are a rather unusual assemblage — red-faced, oddly proportioned, inclined to be easily startled. They are different in a number of ways from the baby who is just a few weeks old. The nurse's task is to recognize which of these differences is within the normal range of appearance and behavior for a newborn and which differences are indications of a pathological condition.

Babies cannot tell us, verbally, when there is something wrong with them. Yet there are few patients who communicate as dramatically through nonverbal means. Their lack of speech seems very nearly compensated for once their signal system is understood — body posture, the pitch of a cry, the character of respirations, and a multitude of other signs. Because these signals change rapidly, it is the nurse, to a very large extent, who must catch any slight change in condition so that appropriate medical attention can be given as quickly as possible. Frequently a baby may appear quite normal at 8 AM, yet be in significant distress by 2 PM. An alert nurse in the nursery can be a lifesaver in the fullest sense of the word.

It is important to develop a systematic approach to the physical assessment of the newborn. Before touching the infant, observe general characteristics as noted below.

General Characteristics

Normal
Strong flexor muscle tone

Symmetrical posture and movement

Strong cry

Edema of presenting parts

Brief tremors or twitching

Abnormal
Floppy; lack of muscle tone
Rigid

Weak, random movements
Lack of movement on one or both sides
Abnormal position or posture

Feeble cry or absence of cry
High-pitched, piercing cry

Edema of any other area

Prolonged tremors and convulsions

MUSCLE TONE

Muscle tone is assessed in relation to the gestational age of the infant (Chapter 5). The term newborn should have strong flexor muscle tone that is equal bilaterally. *Hypotonia* (lack of tone) is frequently due to hypoxia. *Asymmetric* muscle tone may be due to brain damage. The symmetry of muscle tone is assessed by extending the extremities.

When *hyperflexibility* is present, Down's syndrome is possible. The presence of a *simian crease* (a transverse crease across the palm of the hand) also occurs in many persons with Down's syndrome but occurs in other persons as well. No one physical sign in and of itself is representative of Down's syndrome.

TREMORS AND SEIZURES

Brief, spontaneous tremors are not uncommon in normal newborns. Tremors are never accompanied by any abnormal eye movements as may be seen with seizures. The movements in tremors are rhythmic and can generally be stopped by flexing the involved limb.

Seizures are more serious, and long-term prognosis is related to the underlying cause. Seizures in newborns are rarely of the generalized tonic-clonic nature characteristic of seizures in older children and adults, probably because of the immaturity of the cerebral cortex in newborns. Frequently the only signs are deviation of the eyes, repetitive blinking of the eyelids, circumoral cyanosis, and repetitive sucking or chewing movements of the mouth or drooling. Limb movements, more often of the arms, may or may not be present. Apnea can indicate seizure activity but is usually accompanied by one or more additional signs.

Distinguishing tremulousness or jitteriness from a seizure is important (Table 6–2). Because of the subtlety of these signs, careful observation and precise recording of observations is essential. To say the infant "had a seizure" is of little value. Charting should also include the duration of the seizure and the characteristics of the baby's cry and behavior before and after the seizure.

POSITION

The position of a normal term newborn follows definite patterns. When lying prone, he turns his face to one side; he flexes his legs and draws his knees up under his abdomen, raising his pelvis off the mattress (Fig. 6–1). Placed on his back, he rolls to one side or the other. When he is lying on his side, his arms and legs are flexed. This strong flexor tone of the muscles, along with symmetry, is a significant postural indicator of normality. Certain exceptions, however, do not automatically indicate abnormality. An infant born in the frank breech position with legs extended is likely to keep his legs extended during the newborn period. Other characteristics of a breech baby include abducted thighs, a flattened head, and an extended neck. An infant delivered by face presentation may appear, at first glance, to be assuming a position of opisthotonos. But this baby will have normal muscle tone, as opposed to the hypertonia of true opisthotonos.

Conditions that produce asymmetry of posture include fractures of the clavicle or humerus, injury to the brachial plexus, and asymmetry of muscle tone.

Auscultation

Because undressing the baby frequently causes him to cry and crying elevates the infant's heart rate and makes auscultation of the heart, lungs, and bowel sounds difficult, many examiners prefer to evaluate these signs before undressing the baby and proceeding with the remainder of the assessment.

Heart rate should be counted at the apex for 60 seconds. Heart rate fluctuates markedly during the transition period (Chapter 5). Following transition, the infant's state affects heart rate; the rate may fall to 100 bpm or below during periods of very deep sleep and may rise during active crying. Therefore, the infant's state should be

Table 6–2 Distinguishing Characteristics of Jitteriness and Seizure Activity

Jitteriness	Seizure Activity
Not accompanied by ocular movement	Frequently accompanied by ocular movement
Highly sensitive to stimuli	Stimuli not important in onset
Movements rhythmic, equal in rate and amplitude	Movements have fast and slow components
Flexion of affected limb can stop movement	Flexion of limb does not stop movement

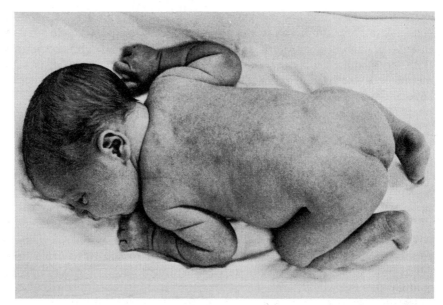

Figure 6–1. A term infant lies with his limbs flexed, pelvis raised, and knees usually drawn up under his abdomen. (Courtesy of Mead, Johnson, and Company.)

noted on the chart if state is felt to be the reason for a rate that falls outside the range of normal. Tachycardia in the resting infant is frequently an early sign of heart failure.

The apex of the heart is usually located to the left of the midclavicular line at the third or fourth intercostal space. If the

Heart

Normal
Rate:
100 to 180 bpm shortly after birth
120 to 150 bpm following transition period

Apex: left of midclavicular line at third or fourth intercostal space

Two heart sounds heard distinctly

Pulses present: femoral and dorsalis pedis

Abnormal
Tachycardia

Heart sounds on right (at right axilla)

Gallop rhythm (three sounds)

Indistinct heart sounds

Cardiomegaly
Active precordium

heart sounds indicate displacement to the right — *dextrocardia* — there may be a diaphragmatic hernia (Chapter 8), usually a surgical emergency requiring immediate attention. Dextrocardia may be unassociated with other defects or may reflect a reversal of all the organs in the body.

First and second heart sounds should be heard distinctly. In newborns, the first and second sounds are of equal intensity. When heart sounds are poorly heard, possible causes are pneumothorax (air in the pleural cavity), pneumomediastinum (air in the mediastinum, the space in the midchest between the pleura), and heart failure. Three heart sounds (having the same rhythm as the spoken word "Tennessee") constitute a *gallop* rhythm and are a sign of heart failure.

Listen for heart sounds at the right and left axillae. Heart sounds are normally not heard at the right axilla.

The presence of a murmur is not unusual in the first days following delivery and usually is related to incomplete closure of fetal structures (chapter 5). Nevertheless, any murmurs heard should be noted on the infant's record.

Cardiomegaly (cardiac enlargement) may be suspected on physical examination because of the location of heart sounds and is confirmed by chest x-ray, echocardiogram, and electrocardiogram. Infants of diabetic mothers and infants with erythroblastosis may have cardiomegaly at birth. Cardiac enlargement several days following birth may be due to heart failure.

Activity of the precordium (i.e., a visible heartbeat in the area of the chest over the heart) must be evaluated in relation to the size of the baby. The precordium may appear active in a thin, preterm baby because of the absence of subcutaneous tissue. An active precordium in an infant who is not thin suggests the possibility of certain congenital heart defects.

Cardiac assessment also includes the evaluation of *femoral* and *dorsalis pedis* pulsations. Femoral pulses are difficult to palpate in some infants. If the dorsalis pedis pulsation is present, femoral pulsation is also present. Absence of pulsation suggests the possibility of coarctation of the aorta (Chapter 8) because of diminished blood supply to the lower extremities. A bounding femoral or dorsalis pedis pulsation suggests a *patent ductus arteriosus* (Chapter 8).

Lungs

Normal
Bilateral breath sounds

Respiratory rate:
  Mean: 40 breaths/min
  Range: 30 to 60 breaths/min
Diaphragmatic and abdominal breathing

Abnormal
Rales
Rhonchi

Nasal flaring
Respiratory grunt
Retractions
Paradoxical breathing
Cyanosis
Tachypnea

There is a considerable amount of variation in the "normal" respiratory patterns of newborns. Short periods of apnea, a Cheyne-Stokes type of respiration followed by several deep breaths, and irregular respirations are not uncommon in healthy babies. Various theories have been proposed as to why this is so, but no single answer has been universally accepted.

RATE

One of the most obvious differences between the respirations of newborns and those of older children and adults is rate. The average rate is 40 breaths per minute but is often irregular. Rates of 30 to 60 breaths per minute are considered within the range of normal. This increased rate is due to the newborn's metabolic need to move much more air per minute than an adult in proportion to his body weight because of his proportionately larger area of skin surface. Because of respiratory irregularity, respiratory rate should be counted for one full minute; if irregularity is significant, the rate should be counted for two minutes and then averaged.

BREATH SOUNDS

Breath sounds should be heard bilaterally. *Rales* are *noncontinuous* sounds produced by moisture in the air passages. Fine rales, which originate in the small, distal bronchioles, may be present in the first hours after birth before all the lung fluid has been absorbed. Fine rales sound like the fizzling of a carbonated drink or the rolling of a piece of hair between your fingers near your ear. Rales are heard during inspiration and may be most apparent at the end of a deep inspiration. If rales continue, lung disease such as respiratory distress syndrome or pneumonia may be present (Chapter 8).

Rhonchi are *continuous* sounds caused by the movement of air through passages narrowed by secretions, swelling, or other obstruction. In newborns, rhonchi may indicate aspiration. Rhonchi are heard on both inspiration and expiration.

In assessing and describing respiration, specific points should always be noted. To indicate only that an infant is having "respiratory distress" is not adequate. Is *nasal flaring* present? Is there a respiratory *grunt?* Are *retractions* present? Are they intercostal (between the ribs), subcostal (at the lower margin of the ribs), or sternal (beneath the sternum)? Is there *paradoxical breathing,* i.e., a seesaw type of respiration?

What is the respiratory rate? Is the baby cyanotic? Is cyanosis subtle and localized, limited perhaps to the nailbeds, the area around the mouth, or the mucous membranes of the mouth, or is it generalized?

These signs are indications of the presence and degree of respiratory distress. "Grunting" respirations are caused by the expiration of air over a partially closed glottis. The baby closes his glottis to try to maintain increased distending pressure in the respiratory tract; it was the observation and appreciation of this physiological response of the infant by Gregory and colleagues (1971) that led to our current modes of treatment for respiratory distress (Chapter 8). Both retractions and paradoxical breathing reflect the use of accessory muscles to facilitate breathing.

Increased respiratory rate may indicate respiratory or cardiac disease. A continuous respiratory rate of more than 60 breaths per minute is often the first sign of heart disease. A chest x-ray will frequently detect the basis of the tachycardia.

Transient Tachypnea

Unexplained tachypnea may occur in both term and preterm infants. Delayed absorption of fetal lung fluid has been postulated as the etiology. Thus, the incidence of transient tachypnea is higher in infants who do not experience the "vaginal squeeze" (those born in the breech position or delivered by cesarean section) than in infants who do experience "vaginal squeeze" (those born in the vertex position). The lungs, as a result, are somewhat less flexible, but air exchange is good and blood gases are normal. The condition usually lasts from 48 to 72 hours, although it may persist through the first week.

It can be difficult to feed babies with continued rapid respirations; they aspirate stomach contents easily and must be fed with extra care and allowed frequent periods of rest. When respiratory rates are consistently faster than 60 breaths per minute, alternate routes of feeding, such as gavage, should be considered.

Bowel Sounds Heard in the Thoracic Cavity

Bowel sounds heard in the thoracic cavity may indicate diaphragmatic hernia (Chapter 8); however, it is not unusual for bowel sounds to be transmitted to the pleural cavity.

Extremities

Normal
Extended legs in baby born
   in breech presentation

Equal muscle tone bilaterally

Abnormal
Abnormal position or posture of an extremity

Unequal muscle tone
Hypotonia

Hyperflexibility
Inability to abduct thigh
Positive Ortolani's maneuver
Talipes equinovarus
Talipes calcaneovalgus
Syndactyly
Polydactyly
Simian crease

Inability to Abduct Thigh

The inability to abduct one thigh is an indication of *congenital hip dysplasia,* in which abnormal development of the hip joint occurs. Dysplasia may be partial (congenital *subluxation* of the hip), in which the head of the femur is partially dislocated from the shallow acetabulum, or complete (congenital *dislocation),* in which the head of the femur is completely dislocated from the hip. Congenital subluxation is much more common.

Early recognition and treatment of congenital hip dysplasia is important in achieving good results. Since subluxation may not result in a limitation of abduction in the first few weeks of life, every infant should be assessed using Ortolani's maneuver. With the baby lying on his back, the legs are flexed at right angles to the trunk and abducted. One thigh is then abducted, still flexed, with pressure applied in such a way that the head of the femur slips over the posterior lip of the acetabulum. A "click of exit" is felt as the femur slips posteriorly from the acetabulum; a second "click of entry" is felt when the pressure is relieved, the hip is abducted and the head of the femur consequently slips back into the acetabulum.

Other signs that may lead one to suspect hip dysplasia include shortening of the leg (Allis' sign) and asymmetry of skin folds of the buttocks; both are rare in subluxation.

Initial treatment may consist of using two diapers or a pillow covered with plastic to maintain the baby's legs in an abducted position and thereby forcing the head of the femur into the acetabulum and enlarging the socket by the constant pressure. Casts may be required. If treatment is started at birth or shortly thereafter, the hip is commonly normal by the time the baby is three months old.

TALIPES EQUINOVARUS AND TALIPES CALCANEOVALGUS

Of the several varieties of clubfoot, *talipes equinovarus,* in which the foot is turned medially and in plantar flexion with the heel elevated, accounts for approximately 95 per cent of all instances. The second most common variety is *talipes calcaneovalgus,* in which the foot deviates laterally and is dorsiflexed.

It is not difficult to recognize the presence of a clubfoot in an infant if his foot is inspected carefully. It is, however, important to differentiate true clubfoot from a foot that appears to be deformed because of the position the fetus has assumed in utero. In the latter instance, the foot can easily be positioned normally or in an overcorrected position, whereas a true clubfoot cannot.

Treatment for a true clubfoot usually begins with a cast applied before the baby leaves the hospital. Early treatment and consistent follow-up are important to achieving a good result. Exercises are frequently prescribed for a baby with a positional deformity.

SYNDACTYLY AND POLYDACTYLY

Syndactyly, fusion of the digits of the hands or feet, and *polydactyly,* extra fingers or toes, should be noted. Fingers and toes should be counted. While an extra finger or toe is hardly life threatening, the nurse's failure to notice these "small" differences and call them to the mother's attention may cause the mother to wonder how closely the nurse has attended her infant.

Skin

Normal
Milia
Mongolian spots
Toxic erythema

Abnormal
Impetigo
Hemangiomas
Cracked and peeling skin

MILIA

Milia are tiny cysts that result from the obstruction of the sebaceous glands of the face, particularly those across the bridge of the nose. They disappear without treatment.

MONGOLIAN SPOTS

Mongolian spots, sometimes called "Oriental patches," are at times mistaken for bruises. They are present in some black babies at the time of birth, usually in the area of the sacrum or buttocks. They also disappear of their own accord within a few weeks to months.

TOXIC ERYTHEMA

The most common skin disorder of infancy, toxic erythema (also known as "flea bite" rash though fleas are in no way involved) is found in 30 to 70 per cent of normal term infants. However, it is rare in premature babies. It usually occurs in the first four days of life but may appear at any time in the first two weeks. A common pattern is for the papule to appear one day, look worse on the second day, and be completely gone by the third, although it may disappear in as brief a time as two hours. Etiology is unknown and treatment is unnecessary, but the lesions must be differentiated from those of impetigo, which must be treated.

IMPETIGO

The vesicles of impetigo, a superficial skin infection usually caused by staphylococci in the newborn, are pustular, as occasionally are the vesicles of toxic erythema. In impetigo these vesicles rupture to produce thick, moist, yellow crusts, which must be soaked off before the prescribed antibiotic ointment can be applied.

HEMANGIOMAS

Hemangiomas, even when they do not pose a threat to the baby's physical well-being, are highly distressing to the baby's parents because they are so obvious. To the extent that they affect the way a mother feels about her baby and the way she treats him, they can have far-reaching significance.

A port wine stain (nevus flammeus) is a flat, purple or dark red lesion consisting of mature capillaries that is present at birth (Fig. 6–2). Those port wine hemangiomas located above the bridge of the nose tend to fade; others do not, but since they are level with the surface of the skin they can be covered with a cosmetic preparation (Covermark).

Strawberry hemangiomas (nevus vasculosus) are elevated areas consisting of immature capillaries and endothelial cells. They may be present at birth or may appear in the first two weeks following birth and continue to enlarge for six months to a year. After the first birthday they begin to be absorbed, the process of involution taking as long as 10 years (Fig. 6–3). Half to three-fourths of strawberry hemangiomas disappear by the time the child is seven years old, leaving no evi-

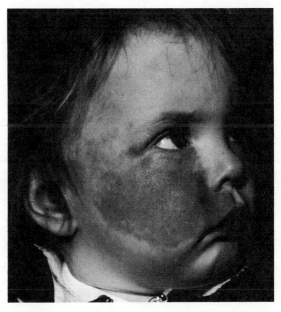

Figure 6–2. Port wine stain, present from birth, does not usually fade but can be covered with a cosmetic preparation. (From Pillsbury, Shelley, and Kligman: A Manual of Cutaneous Medicine. W. B. Saunders.)

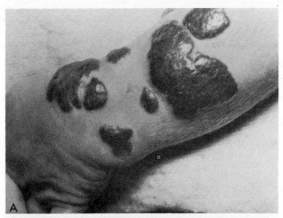

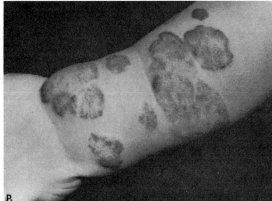

Figure 6–3. The spontaneous progressive involution of a strawberry hemangioma: *A,* age 6 weeks. *B,* age 8 months. *C,* age 2 years. (From Burgoon, Jr.: *In* Vaughan and McKay (eds.): Nelson Textbook of Pediatrics. 10th Edition. W. B. Saunders, 1975.)

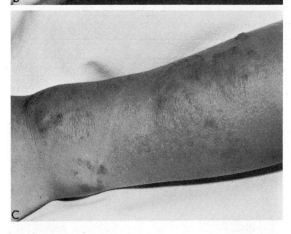

dence that they ever existed. The end result seems to be better if the hemangioma is untreated unless it interferes with normal functioning because of its location.

A third type, cavernous hemangioma, consists of dilated vascular spaces with thick walls that are lined with endothelium (Fig. 6–4). They do not regress spontaneously.

CRACKED AND PEELING SKIN

This condition is often evidence of a small-for-date baby who has experienced intrauterine malnutrition (Fig. 6–5). Postterm infants (born after 42 weeks gestation) frequently have dry, peeling skin, evidence of malnutrition from an aging placenta.

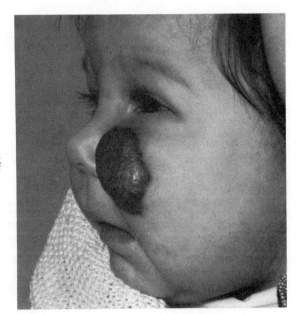

Figure 6–4. A cavernous hemangioma. (From Pillsbury, Shelley, and Kligman: A Manual of Cutaneous Medicine. W. B. Saunders.)

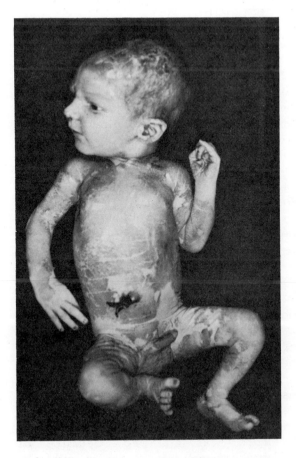

Figure 6–5. Cracked or peeling parchmentlike skin often indicates intrauterine malnutrition. (From Clifford: *In* Levine (ed.): Advances in Pediatrics, Vol. 9. Yearbook Publishers, Inc., 1957.)

Color

Normal
Red

Cyanosis of the lips, fingernails, toenails, hands, feet; cyanosis of the face in a baby born with facial or brow presentation

Jaundice after 36 to 48 hours

Harlequin sign

Abnormal
Pallor, gray color

Generalized cyanosis

Jaundice in the first 24 hours

The very red color of the newborn's skin is due to both the higher concentration of red blood cells in the vessels and the thin layer of subcutaneous fat that causes the blood vessels to be closer to the surface of the skin.

CYANOSIS

In contrast to localized cyanosis, which is due to immature peripheral circulation involving the lips, hands, and feet, and to stasis, in which the presenting parts are cyanotic, generalized cyanosis is a cause for concern. Sometimes generalized cyanosis is so slight that the baby must be compared with an infant who has obviously good respirations to detect its presence. The need for such a comparison is indicated when the baby has other symptoms of respiratory distress and the possibility of cyanosis is raised. In babies with dark skin, cyanosis can often be best observed in the mucosal lining of the mouth.

The relationship between cyanosis and crying is an important observation. The baby may be cyanotic except when he cries vigorously and thereby raises his intake of oxygen (e.g., babies with atelectasis). Or he may be cyanotic only when he cries, which can be a warning of the later, more persistent cyanosis of some types of congenital heart disease.

Cyanosis related to apnea can usually be terminated by provoking the baby to cry, by flicking either the soles of his feet or his buttocks.

Babies with bilateral choanal atresia (occlusion of the posterior nares by either bone or membrane) will be cyanotic because all infants are obligate nose breathers; they breathe through their mouths only with great difficulty. Diagnosis is made by holding a wisp of cotton in front of each naris; the air movements of respiration can then be easily observed.

Sudden cyanosis and apnea in a baby who has apparently been doing well may be related to excessive, thick mucus obstructing the upper respiratory tract. For this reason a bulb syringe should be in each baby's bed, and a suction machine with a supply of catheters should be readily available for nasal suction. Once the obstructing mucus is removed the baby becomes pink and immediately resumes respirations.

Damage to the central nervous system, either because of congenital disease or because of trauma during delivery, is another cause of cyanosis. The baby is likely to have very irregular breathing and may have some other signs of central nervous system damage — a high-pitched cry, either very rigid or very floppy muscle tone, or absence of a Moro reflex. As with babies who are cyanotic because of respiratory distress, crying and oxygen tend to improve their color.

Babies who are cyanotic because of cardiac malformations are rarely helped by oxygen and generally appear worse when they cry. At first these babies may be only briefly pale or cyanotic such as during a gavage feeding or immediately after an injection.

PALLOR

Pallor may be due to anemia, hemorrhage, hemolysis of red blood cells, or shock. Blood loss may have occurred before the cord was clamped, because of fetal/maternal transfusion, or after the cord was clamped. Sometimes when twins share a single placenta there is transfusion from one twin to the other. When there is no visible source of external hemorrhage, such as from the umbilical cord, a pale baby needs to be watched for signs of internal bleeding in vomitus or stool. Babies with intracranial damage are often pale because of shock. Gray color is also associated with infection and chloramphenicol intoxication.

JAUNDICE

About 40 to 60 per cent of term infants and even a higher per cent of premature infants are jaundiced on the second to third days of life. There is no discernible pathological reason for this such as hemolytic anemia or sepsis. This jaundice is termed *physiologic*. The following points should be noted concerning physiologic jaundice: (1) It never occurs in the first 24 hours of life. (2) It does not involve indirect bilirubin levels above 10 to 12 mg per cent. (3) It rarely lasts past the first week of life, except occasionally in breast-fed infants.

The yellow color of jaundice is due to high levels of bilirubin; the principal source of the bilirubin is the breakdown of red blood cells that normally follows birth.

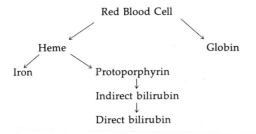

Indirect (unconjugated) bilirubin is fat soluble; it is transported in plasma bound to albumin. In the liver, fat-soluble bilirubin is conjugated mainly with glucuronic acid in a reaction in which the enzyme glucuronyl transferase is the catalyst. Once conjugated, bilirubin is water soluble; conjugated (direct) bilirubin passes into the duodenum as a component of bile and is excreted in the stool. However, in newborn infants much of the bilirubin found in the meconium is unconjugated

and can be reabsorbed from the gut. This unconjugated bilirubin contributes to an increased level of bilirubin in newborns. A normal infant produces 6 to 8 mg of bilirubin in 24 hours (more than twice the rate in an adult). The shorter life span of fetal red blood cells (90 days in comparision with the 120-day life of adult red blood cells), the higher proportion of shunt bilirubin (bilirubin from heme-containing compounds other than red blood cells, e.g., myoglobin), and, perhaps, decreased hepatic circulation contribute to this high rate of production.

As long as this bilirubin remains within the circulatory system no jaundice is visible because the red of the hemoglobin obscures the yellow of the bilirubin. But when the indirect level rises above 7 mg per cent in term infants, bilirubin moves outside the vascular space and is then visible. It often takes higher bilirubin levels to bring about visible jaundice in low birth weight babies because the capillary bed lies closer to the skin surface owing to a lack of subcutaneous fat. The red of the hemoglobin is thus reflected on the skin surface, obscuring the yellow of jaundice. Jaundice can be visualized, however, by blanching the skin with the thumb.

In 1963, Arias and co-workers reported isolated instances of neonatal jaundice associated with breast-feeding. They postulated that a steroid, pregnanediol, inhibits glucuronyl transferase activity and thus diminishes bilirubin conjugation. This concept has been questioned (Hargreaves and Piper, 1971), and at present the mechanism of breast milk jaundice is not entirely settled (Drew 1978).

Not every case of jaundice in a breast-fed infant is due to breast milk. Drew (1978) reviewed 13,102 consecutive newborns; 878 (6.7 per cent) had serum bilirubin determinations because of clinical indications of jaundice, but in only one infant (0.1 per cent) was the jaundice proved to be due to breast milk . Other feeding practices, such as delayed feeding, with concomitant weight loss, dehydration, and slowed development of intestinal flora, may be factors. Breast-fed infants may, of course, have jaundice related to other factors such as blood group incompatibility (Chapter 8).

When jaundice does appear related to breast-feeding, *temporary interruption* of breast-feeding for 24 hours will usually cause the bilirubin level to drop. Avery (1973) indicates that a single interruption may be sufficient; Guthrie (1978) suggests that if hyperbilirubinemia jaundice persists, a 12- to 24-hour period of interruption may be necessary in subsequent weeks but that there is no need to totally discontinue breast-feeding. During periods of interruption, the baby is fed formula by dropper or bottle, and the mother expresses breast milk manually or with a pump to maintain her milk supply (Chapter 9).

By definition, jaundice is considered physiologic if the bilirubin level does not exceed 12 mg/ml. Even when infants with hemolytic disease and other problems are included, only 6 per cent of infants have bilirubin levels that exceed 12.9 mg/ml (Maisels 1979). Formerly, the possibility of brain damage due to bilirubin was thought unlikely at levels below 20 mg/ml. However, it is now recognized that encephalopathy may occur at considerably lower levels but may not occur even at levels below 20 mg/ml. Pathological jaundice and its treatment, which is rarely indicated in physiologic jaundice, are discussed in Chapter 8.

Harlequin Sign

Occasionally one will glance at a baby and see one side of the infant flushed, the line of demarcation between the flushed and unflushed sides very clear. This is a very transient phenomenon and is of no known pathological significance.

Molding

Molding, the process by which the bones of the head override one another to facilitate delivery, is so natural that nurses may scarcely notice that the baby's head is asymmetrical. But the mother is often concerned and needs to know that her infant's

Head

Normal
Anterior fontanel open

Posterior fontanel may be closed

Circumference: approx. 13 to 14 inches (33 to 35.5 cm)
Craniotabes
Caput succedaneum
Cephalhematoma
Molding

Abnormal
No anterior fontanel

Sunken fontanel
Bulging fontanel
Widened fontanels and sutures

head will be normally rounded in a few days.

Fontanels

The anterior fontanel is diamond-shaped and is bounded by the frontal and parietal bones of the baby's skull. It is approximately 2.5 to 4.0 cm in width (1.0 to 1.75 inches), or about the width of two fingers. The triangular posterior fontanel is bounded by the parietal and occipital bones and is less than half the size of the anterior fontanel (0.5 to 1.0 cm or 0.2 to 0.4 inch). The posterior fontanel may be closed by birth, but the anterior fontanel should be open. While a closed fontanel is of serious concern to the physicians and nurses who care for the baby (usually being related to microcephaly), rather ironically it is the open fontanel that may distress the new mother. Hopefully she can be reassured by knowing that (1) the presence of an open fontanel helped to protect the baby's head during delivery; (2) the fontanel allowed his brain to grow before he was born and will continue to do so for the next 18 months; and (3) his brain is adequately protected by a tough membrane so there need be no fear of handling him and washing his head, which are very necessary parts of his care.

Both a bulging fontanel, which can indicate intracranial hemorrhage or infection, and a depressed fontanel, which indicates dehydration, are abnormal.

pressure is removed. The cause of craniotabes is unknown. There is no treatment; although the condition may persist for months, it eventually disappears completely.

CRANIOTABES

Craniotabes is the softening of localized areas in the cranial bones. These areas seem spongelike in that they are easily indented by the pressure of a fingertip, but they resume their shape when the

CAPUT SUCCEDANEUM

This term refers to swelling of the superficial tissues over the bone of the part of the head presenting during delivery. It is seen immediately after birth and usually is absorbed within a few days (Fig. 6–6A, C).

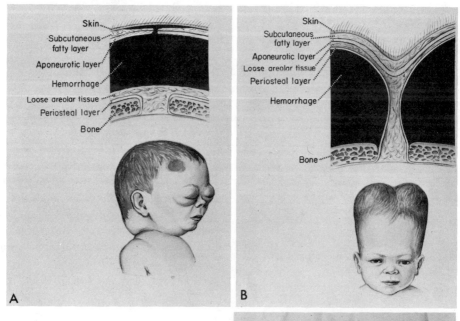

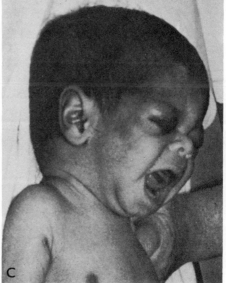

Figure 6–6. *A,* edema and hemorrhage in caput succedaneum. *B,* location of swelling in cephalhematoma; note that the swelling does not cross the suture lines. *C,* a baby with a large caput succedaneum. (Reprinted with permission of Daniel J. Pachman, MD, of the University of Illinois Pediatric Department. *A* and *C* appeared in Pediatrics, Vol. 29, 1962.)

CEPHALHEMATOMA

In a cephalhematoma blood collects between a cranial bone and the overlying periosteum (Fig. 6–6B). In contrast to caput succedaneum, it may be several weeks, even months, before it is completely absorbed. There is another difference between the two: the swelling of caput succedaneum may cross suture lines because only soft tissue is involved; a cephalhematoma is confined to one bone because it lies beneath the periosteum. This can be a help in differentiating between the two.

Treatment is not required for either condition nor is the baby in any danger (unless the hemorrhage is massive). The mother, however, may need reassurance that her baby is in no distress and does not require special handling, particularly when the baby has a cephalhematoma that may last for several weeks. The fluid is never aspirated; to do so would risk infection.

VISUAL REFLEXES

Visual reflexes are the principal means of assessing vision in newborns. Pupils should constrict in response to light (pupillary reflex); if there is no pupillary reflex by three weeks of age it is possible that the infant is blind. Newborns blink in response to bright light; therefore, eyes should be examined in subdued light.

The *red reflex* is elicited by examination with an ophthalmoscope set at "0" diopter; the pupil is viewed from a distance of 10 inches. Normally the fundus reflects a red or orange color. If the light pathway is interrupted, as in the case of opacity in the cornea, the anterior chamber, or the lens, there will be a white or a partial red reflex.

DOLL'S EYE MOVEMENTS

When the newborn's head is turned, the eyes remain in their original position. This characteristic, called *doll's eye movement*, is seen in the first 10 days of life.

Eyes

Normal
Brushfield's spots

Absence of tears

Visual reflexes present
Doll's eye movements
Strabismus
Ability to follow an object
Swelling
Subconjunctival hemorrhage

Abnormal
Brushfield's spots

Stagnant tears in eye

Large cornea
Opacity of pupil
Discharge from eyes
Hypertelorism
Prominent inner epicanthal folds

Gray-blue or brown in color, eyes may seem to be crossed at times (transient strabismus) in the newborn period because eye coordination is limited during the first month. In "normal" strabismus, movements alternate between eyes and are always convergent (i.e., toward the nose). Unilateral or divergent strabismus requires prompt medical attention.

ABILITY TO FOLLOW AN OBJECT

In the quiet alert state newborns will follow an object both vertically and horizontally. A human face is a preferred visual object; a visual stimulus combined with an auditory stimulus is more compelling than a visual stimulus alone (see Sensory Capabilities).

BRUSHFIELD'S SPOTS

Both Brushfield's spots, which are white spots scattered about the circumference of the iris, and inner epicanthal folds suggest Down's syndrome (Chapter 2). However, Brushfield's spots may also occur in normal infants.

ABSENCE OF TEARS

The lacrimal duct carries tears from the eye into the nose. The lacrimal duct may not be open at birth, and tears may normally be absent or scanty. Signs of a blocked tear duct are stagnant tears in the eye that may flow down the baby's cheek. Because mucus cannot be washed away, there may appear to be creases or a film over the eyeball. Massage over the tear-duct will frequently open the duct in a few days. If this does not occur, a lacrimal probe may be used by a physician to alleviate the problem.

HYPERTELORISM

If the distance between the inner canthi exceeds 3 cm, the term *hypertelorism* is used. Hypertelorism occurs in a number of syndromes and may be associated with congenital anomalies or mental retardation.

SWELLING

It is not unusual for swelling to develop around the eyes as a result of instillation of silver nitrate or following forceps delivery. It disappears in a few days.

SUBCONJUNCTIVAL HEMORRHAGE

Subconjunctival hemorrhage may be seen as a small patch of red or a red ring around the cornea. These hemorrhages, as well as *retinal hemorrhage,* are caused by pressure on the fetal head during delivery, which impairs venous return and leads to rupture of the capillaries. They are almost always of no significance and are absorbed in two to three weeks.

OPACITY OF PUPIL

An opaque pupil, the evidence of *congenital cataract,* is rare; it most commonly occurs in babies with rubella syndrome, galactosemia, or cytomegalic inclusion disease (Fig. 6–7).

LARGE CORNEA

A baby with an unusually large cornea is likely to have congenital glaucoma, which requires immediate treatment if the infant's vision is not to be permanently damaged (Fig. 6–8). The cornea may also be hazy or cloudy. Confirmation of the diagnosis of glaucoma is made by measuring intraocular tension. The treatment is immediate surgery.

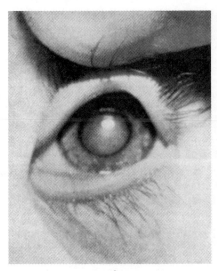

A

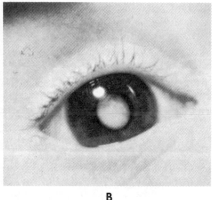

B

Figure 6–7. The opaque pupil of a congenital cataract. (*A,* from the collection of Dr. Richard Hoover, Baltimore: *In* Schaffer and Avery: Diseases of the Newborn. 3rd Edition. W. B. Saunders, 1971. *B,* from the collection of Dr. Arnall Patz, Baltimore: *In* Schaffer and Avery: Diseases of the Newborn. 4th Edition. W. B. Saunders, 1977.)

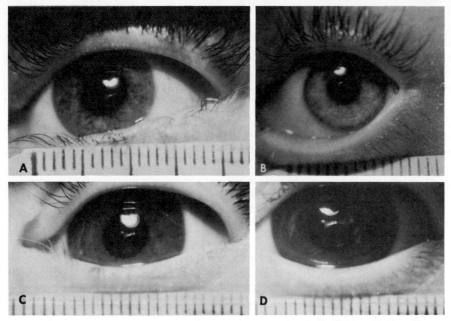

Figure 6–8. *A,* normal eyeball with cornea of normal size. *B,* small eyeball with microcornea. *C,* early glaucoma without hazing of cornea or tearing of Descemet's membrane. *D,* enlarged cornea of early glaucoma. (From the collection of Dr. Arnall Patz, Baltimore: *In* Schaffer and Avery: Diseases of the Newborn. 4th Edition. W. B. Saunders, 1977.)

CONJUNCTIVITIS

Conjunctivitis may be caused by infection of the newborn's eyes, such as that caused by *gonococci (ophthalmia neonatorum)* or *Chlamydia trachomatis* (inclusion conjunctivitis of the newborn). The inflammation may also be chemical conjunctivitis related to silver nitrate prophylaxis. Obviously it is important to distinguish the two.

Drug-related conjunctivitis occurs primarily in the first 24 hours of life; it does not last beyond the third day. Conjunctivitis due to infection appears later, commonly not until the third day and rarely in the first 24 hours. Moreover, in infection-related conjunctivitis, the initial somewhat watery discharge is followed by a thick, purulent exudate.

Once *ophthalmia neonatorum* is suspected, samples of the exudate are examined. Because the disease progresses rapidly to ocular perforation and blindness, parenteral penicillin therapy is begun as soon as the causative organism is identified as gram-positive (the group to which the gonorrhea bacteria belong). A single large dose (150,000 U aqueous penicillin) is given because peak blood level rather than total dose is the critical factor. Local treatment includes saline eyewashes and topical antibiotics. Great care is taken to protect the uninvolved eye; it may be taped shut.

Response to treatment is usually dramatic. The baby is significantly improved within 24 hours and no longer considered infective. Treatment continues, however, for two to five days. If there is no response within 24 to 48 hours, the possibility of a resistant organism is considered.

Silver nitrate prophylaxis is not effective in preventing chlamydia infections. Once infection is recognized, antibiotic therapy is begun. Prevention through prenatal screening and treatment of the mother has been suggested (Chapter 3).

Ears

Normal
Upper part of ear should be on same plane as angle of eye

Abnormal
Low set ears
Absence of response to sudden noise

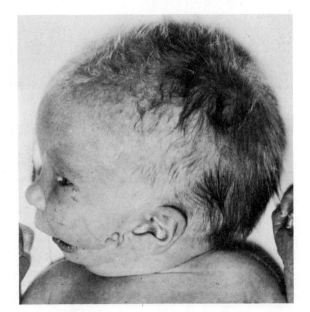

Figure 6–9. This infant has low-set malpositioned ears and extreme micrognathia. (From the files of Harriet Lane Home: *In* Schaffer and Avery: Diseases of the Newborn. 4th Edition. W. B. Saunders, 1977.)

LOW SET EARS

Low set ears are characteristic of some autosomal chromosomal abnormalities; they are also associated with some congenital renal disorders (Fig. 6–9).

ABSENCE OF RESPONSE TO SUDDEN NOISE

When a sudden noise is introduced, such as the ringing of a bell or a hand clap 12 inches from the baby's ear, he will respond with a startle or blink. Since this acoustical reflex is difficult to elicit, neither the presence nor absence of a response is considered an absolute indication of hearing or deafness.

Many infants demonstrate attention to the sound of a voice. As noted in the discussion of state, a crying infant may frequently be quieted by having someone talk to him (see also Sensory Capabilities).

THRUSH

Stimulating the baby to cry will make him open his mouth so that the inside of it can be checked for evidence of cleft palate (Fig. 6–10) and thrush (Fig. 6–11). Numerous small white and gray patches on the tongue and in the mouth are indications of thrush, an infection caused by the fungus *Monilia albicans*. The differences between thrush and the epithelial pearls found on the hard palate need to be recognized. Milk curds are also occasionally mistaken for thrush.

Babies with thrush will usually be poor eaters. Although there are many other much more serious reasons for failure to feed well — heart defects, infection, and central nervous system damage — any baby eating poorly should be given a thorough mouth examination. Babies receiving oral antibiotics are particularly

---

Mouth

Normal
Epithelial pearls

Some mucus

"Sucking blisters"

Abnormal
Thrush

Excessive, frothy mucus; "blowing bubbles"

Corners of mouth that do not move when baby cries

Cleft palate and lip

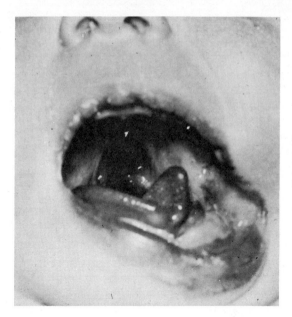

Figure 6–10. An open mouth reveals a large midline cleft in the posterior palate. (From the files of Harriet Lane Home: *In* Schaffer and Avery: Diseases of the Newborn. 4th Edition. W. B. Saunders, 1977.)

good candidates. Most healthy newborns who acquire thrush do so in the delivery process, being infected by the *Monilia* in the mother's vagina.

Treatment usually includes the administration of a nystatin solution given orally every six hours. The solution should be administered slowly and gently so that it will be widely distributed throughout the oral cavity before it is swallowed. Individual lesions are sometimes painted with a 1% solution of aqueous gentian violet. An excess amount of gentian violet should be avoided because it may be irritating if swallowed. After gentian violet has been applied, the baby should be placed face downward so that saliva containing the solution will drain outward. A paste of sodium bicarbonate can be used to remove gentian violet stains from clothing and bedding. Treatment is continued for at least three days after all visible evidence of thrush is gone to assure that the fungus itself is eradicated.

MOVEMENT ON ONE SIDE OF FACE

When there has been injury to a facial nerve either because of pressure in utero or during labor or because of the use of forceps during delivery, there will be movement on only one side of the face when the baby cries, with the mouth drawn to that side (Fig. 6–12).

EXCESSIVE MUCUS

For a day or so after birth some babies have a fairly large amount of mucus, which can usually be aspirated with a bulb syringe. Continued excessive mucus that is frothy, as if the baby were "blowing bubbles," suggests a tracheoesophageal fistula and calls for an immediate examination of the baby, whereby attempts are made to pass a catheter through his esophagus into his stomach. If the catheter curls up or will not pass, the baby must not be fed.

Jaw

Normal
Size in normal range

Abnormal
Micrognathia

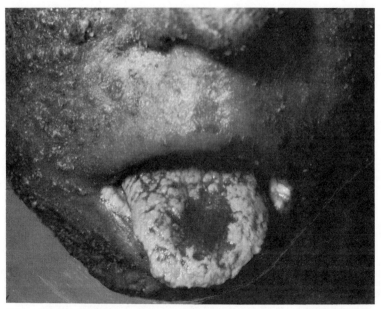

Figure 6–11. Numerous small white and gray patches on the tongue and palate are an indication of thrush. (From Pillsbury, Shelley, and Kligman: A Manual of Cutaneous Medicine. W. B. Saunders, 1961.)

MICROGNATHIA

An abnormally small jaw, micrognathia (Fig. 6–9), can cause respiratory distress, because the tongue falls back into the pharynx. This can partially be relieved by keeping the baby on his stomach so that the tongue falls forward. Sometimes the tongue is temporarily sutured in place until the jaw grows. Many babies with micrognathia have a cleft palate as well and may be more easily fed with a Breck feeder.

Chest

Normal
Circumference: 12 to 13 inches (30.5 to 33 cm)

Engorgement of breasts

Abnormal
Knot on clavicle

BREAST ENGORGEMENT

During pregnancy, maternal hormones cross the placental barrier and enter fetal circulation. When these hormones are withdrawn at birth, the breasts enlarge and may even secrete fluid resembling colostrum or milk. The enlargement lasts from several days to as long as several weeks.

Mothers should know that (1) this is perfectly normal; (2) this is not a sign of infection; and (3) the breasts should not be handled other than in routine bathing; no attempt should ever be made to express

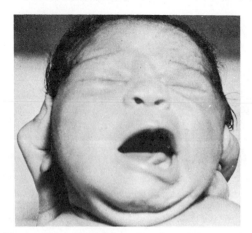

Figure 6–12. When there has been injury to the facial nerve there will be movement on only one side of the face. (From Davis and Rubin: DeLee's Obstetrics for Nurses. 18th Edition. W. B. Saunders, 1966.)

fluid from the breasts. To do so is to risk mastitis.

KNOT ON CLAVICLE

A "knot" is sometimes found on the clavicle on the third or fourth day after birth that was not evident at delivery. It indicates a fractured clavicle, which can occur in a seemingly normal delivery. The fracture heals without difficulty.

Abdomen and Back

Normal
Moderately protuberant abdomen

Bluish white umbilical cord

Granulation tissue in navel

Liver and kidneys palpable
Bowel sounds
Cutis navel

Abnormal
Scaphoid abdomen
Distended abdomen

Yellow discoloration of cord at birth

Exudate or bleeding around cord

Congenital absence of abdominal musculature
Curvature or absence of vertebrae

PALPABLE ORGANS

The abdominal muscles must be relaxed for the abdomen to be palpated. Relaxation is aided by flexing the infant's knees toward the abdomen or by holding the infant semierect with one hand while palpating the abdomen with the other. The liver is usually felt 2 to 3 cm below the right costal margin. The tip of the spleen is felt at the left costal margin; the spleen may not be palpable until the end of the first week. Kidneys are palpated by placing one hand beneath the infant's flank and the other below the costal margin and pressing them together. The tip of the left kidney and the lower half of the right kidney should be felt approximately 1 to 2 cm above the umbilicus.

BOWEL SOUNDS

Bowel sounds should be present within a few hours after birth. There is no pathological condition in 20 to 25 per cent of newborns in whom bowel sounds cannot be heard during the neonatal period.

UMBILICAL CORD

Bluish white at birth, the umbilical cord begins to dry shortly afterward and usually separates in six to eight days, the wound being healed by the time the baby is two weeks old. Yellow discoloration of the cord at birth is an indication of hemolytic disease. Exudate around the cord usually signifies infection, although the baby may have an umbilical cord infection serious enough to cause generalized sepsis without any localized sign. A weeping cord is cleaned with alcohol several times a day. Cord bleeding may be caused by inadequate tying, or it may be a symptom of a bleeding disorder.

Cutis navel describes an umbilical cord that projects beyond the skin. It looks at first glance as if the baby might have an umbilical hernia, but a hernia can be returned to the abdomen whereas the cutis navel cannot. No special treatment is required; the navel will slowly invaginate.

Granulation tissue in the naval will also spontaneously disappear; until it does, the navel should be kept clean and dry.

SCAPHOID ABDOMEN

Normally, the abdomen of a newborn is moderately distended. If it is small and scaphoid, it is very possible that the baby has a diaphragmatic hernia; part of the abdominal contents are in the thoracic cavity and the baby is likely to be dyspneic and cyanotic. Immediate surgery is essential to life.

DISTENDED ABDOMEN

An overly distended abdomen is also abnormal and may be related to several conditions. An infant with a type of tracheo-esophageal fistula in which there is an opening between trachea and stomach will become distended from the continual entry of air. Distention is also an early sign of infection. Congenital obstructions of the gastrointestinal tract and congenital megacolon are also among the conditions causing distention in newborns. It is important to know whether distention is increasing or decreasing. Marking the area of distention with a waxed pencil makes this easier to detect.

PYLORIC STENOSIS

Peristaltic waves, most prominent during or immediately after feeding and progressing from the upper left quadrant toward the pylorus, suggest pyloric stenosis. Babies with small bowel obstruction may also have visible peristaltic waves; these waves commonly move from right to left. Peristaltic waves, which are difficult to see, may be visualized by focusing a light on the baby's abdomen while he is eating.

CONGENITAL ABSENCE OF ABDOMINAL MUSCULATURE (WRINKLED ABDOMEN)

When the abdominal muscles are absent, the abdomen has a wrinkled appearance from which the term *prune-belly syndrome* is derived. The infants, 95 per cent of whom are male, may have a number of associated defects for which they must be carefully observed. These defects may include undescended testicles, intestinal malrotation, imperforate anus, dilated and tortuous ureters, hydronephrotic kidneys, and a dilated hypertrophied bladder. Prognosis is related to the degree of gastrointestinal obstruction and the extent of the renal problems.

BACK

The vertebrae should be palpated for defects in the closure of the vertebral canal *(spina bifida occulta)* and for abnormal curvature of the spine. When the meninges protrude through the bony defect, the resultant meningocele or myelomeningocele is obvious (Chapter 8).

Genitals

Normal
Vaginal bleeding

Red and swollen
Vaginal discharge
Hymenal tag
Swelling of scrotum

Abnormal
Excessive vaginal bleeding

Undescended testicles in term baby
Hypospadias; epispadias

VAGINAL DISCHARGE

A vaginal discharge of thick, white mucus is passed by all baby girls in the first week of life. Occasionally the mucus is blood tinged about the third or fourth day, staining the diaper. The cause of this "pseudomenstruation," like that of breast engorgement, is the withdrawal of maternal hormones. Excessive vaginal bleeding, however, is not normal; it may be caused by a blood coagulation defect.

A hymenal or vaginal tag may be distressing to the mother, but it will drop off in a few weeks.

SWELLING OF SCROTUM

Swelling of the scrotum is common in newborns and is especially noticeable in babies delivered in breech position. The edema disappears after a few days.

UNDESCENDED TESTICLES

Normally, testicles descend into the scrotum in the eighth month of fetal life. It is possible that a baby boy with undescended testicles is of a younger gestational age than suspected.

HYPOSPADIAS

In about one out of every 300 births, the urethra opens on the ventral surface of the penis (Fig. 6–13). This condition is termed *hypospadias.* Surgical correction is usually made by the time the boy is two years old and always before he starts school so that he will be able to urinate in the same way as the other boys in his class. These babies should *not* be circumcised, because the foreskin is used in the surgical repair.

EPISPADIAS

Epispadias (Fig. 6–13), the opening of the urethra on the dorsal aspect of the penis, is far less common than hypospadias and is also corrected by surgery.

CIRCUMCISION

Circumcision in the newborn, as suggested elsewhere (Chapter 7), is based on cultural rather than medical considerations. If circumcision is to be done, a circumcision board provides an easy method for positioning and restraining the baby. Aftercare includes applying an ointment such as Vaseline to the raw area, with frequent checks to make sure there is no bleeding.

Some babies seem uncomfortable in the first days following circumcision; others do not even seem to notice. A newly circumcised baby may not like to lie on his stomach. If the mother will be taking the baby home within a day or so after circumcision she needs to know how to care for the area until it heals completely.

Urine

Normal
Peach-colored crystals

Abnormal
Failure to void

The peach-colored crystals that can discolor the diaper of a newborn are crystals of uric acid and are not pathological at this age.

It is exceedingly important that voiding be noted on the baby's chart. Failure by the baby to void is an indication of some type of urinary tract disorder that will need to be investigated. Examples are the absence of one or both kidneys, polycystic kidneys, and various urinary tract obstructions. Dehydration is the most common cause of failure to void in newborns.

It is common for an infant not to void in the first 12 hours after birth, and he may not void until the second or third day, depending, to an extent, on his fluid intake and also on environmental temperature and the condition of his digestive and nervous systems. Failure to void within 48 hours should be reported to the physician in charge of the baby's care.

Stools

Normal
Meconium stools for 3 to 4 days; odorless, dark green to black, viscid
Transitional stools; greenish brown to yellow
Breast-fed baby: golden to mustard, from one to six in 24 hours
Bottle-fed baby: pale yellow, more formed, more frequent, and more regular than those of breast-fed baby
Darkened stools when baby is receiving iron
Faint purple when baby is receiving gentian violet for thrush
Bright green when baby is being treated under bilirubin reduction lamp

Abnormal
No stool in 48 hours
Meconium stool but no feces
Thick puttylike meconium
Small puttylike stool
Diarrhea
Blood in stool

The consistency, color, and odor of stools are all important in evaluating the baby's general condition. Because color changes can occur shortly after defecation, their evaluation has to be made immediately if it is to have meaning.

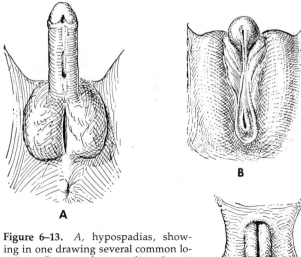

Figure 6–13. *A,* hypospadias, showing in one drawing several common locations. *B,* severe hypospadias. *C,* epispadias. (From Arey: Developmental Anatomy. 7th Edition revised, W. B. Saunders, 1974.)

Stool consistency and color vary in the first days with both age and type of feeding. The first stools are of *meconium,* an odorless viscid material that is dark green to black. Meconium stools may last from three to four days.

Meconium stools are followed by greenish brown to yellow transitional stools. In breast-fed infants, the next stools will be of a golden to mustard color. Initially, breast-fed infants may have more frequent stools than bottle-fed infants. However, in subsequent weeks some breast-fed infants may have no stool for several days and yet be perfectly normal. Breast-feeding mothers need to know this. Mothers may also interpret the soft breast-fed stool as diarrhea if they do not recognize stool characteristics.

The stools of bottle-fed babies are pale yellow in color. They tend to be more formed, are more frequent after the first days of life, and are more regular than those of breast-fed infants.

Obstruction

If no stool is passed within 48 hours there is usually an intestinal obstruction. If meconium was passed initially but then no feces are passed, the obstruction is in the ileum. Thick, puttylike meconium is the initial symptom of meconium ileus. A small, puttylike stool may be caused by stenosis or atresia somewhere in the bowel.

Diarrhea

Diarrhea is a somewhat nonspecific symptom in newborns. It may be caused by overfeeding. Some babies will have diarrhea from certain formulas that will have no effect on other infants. Gastroenteritis causes diarrhea in some babies and can spread quickly through the nursery if the baby is not quickly isolated. The degree of severity of diarrhea can be estimated by measuring the water margin around the stool if the baby has not voided in the diaper. Aside from the danger of sepsis, diarrhea is always serious in the newborn because of his extremely labile water balance (see Chapter 9).

Intestinal Bleeding

Flecks of blood in the baby's stool may come from an anal fissure. Either bright red or old blood is a sign of intestinal bleeding, as it is at any age.

Other Characteristics

CRYING

A term infant may cry vigorously for as much as two hours out of every 24. A high-pitched, shrill cry, excessive crying for which there does not seem to be a reason, and very little crying may be indications of intracranial injury or infection (also see State). A very hoarse cry suggests partial paralysis of the vocal cords.

EDEMA

Edema of the part of the infant presenting during delivery is not unusual. Some premature babies are edematous for no apparent reason. This edema is transient, making the two- to three-day-old premature infant seem dehydrated by comparison, even when fluid intake is actually adequate. Infants of diabetic mothers also may appear edematous, but their excess weight is due largely to fat rather than fluid.

Severe generalized edema at birth may be a sign of erythroblastosis, heart failure due to congenital heart disease, or electrolyte imbalance. It is not always easy to recognize this kind of edema. Pitting may or may not be present. But normally a baby should have fine wrinkles over the knuckles of his hands and feet. If these wrinkles are not evident, the area is very likely puffed with fluid.

VOMITING

Mild regurgitation is not at all unusual in the newborn and is due in part to swallowed air and in part to a "temporary inability of the cardiac sphincter to completely prevent a flow of fluid from the stomach in a reverse direction" (Craig 1969).

Vomiting is quite another matter. Occurring shortly after birth or within the first 24 hours, vomiting is likely to be caused by obstruction of the upper digestive tract or increased intracranial pressure. After the first day, vomiting may still be caused by central nervous system or gastrointestinal problems, but it can also be a sign of a multitude of other conditions including septicemia, overfeeding, pyloric stenosis, milk allergy, and adrenal insufficiency. Dark green vomitus indicates an obstruction in the gastrointestinal tract (Chapter 8).

Blood in the vomitus of a breast-fed baby, unless copious, is very possibly due to fissures in the mother's nipples. Maternal blood swallowed during delivery is also a common cause of blood appearing in the vomitus in the first two to three days of life. A laboratory test, the Abt test, is available to distinguish adult and fetal hemoglobin. The test must be performed within one to two hours after the specimen is obtained because of the chemical nature of fetal hemoglobin (Abt and Downey 1955).

Whether or not vomiting is projectile is always a significant observation. Projectile vomiting in the first week is often related to intestinal obstruction; beginning in the second week, the cause may be pyloric stenosis.

REFLEXES

Reflexes, along with other aspects of behavior that have been described in this chapter, are indications of the integrity of the infant's central nervous system. Many reflexes are unique to the first weeks and months of life; should they persist beyond the time at which they normally would be expected to disappear, central nervous system disease may be present. Major neonatal reflexes are described in Table 6–3.

A normal newborn, startled by a sudden noise or the jarring of his bed, will first abduct and extend his arms and then adduct them as if to embrace (Fig. 6–14).

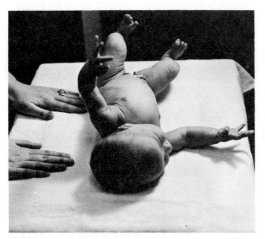

Figure 6–14. Moro response, showing symmetrical abduction and extension of the arms. (From Davis and Rubin: DeLee's Obstetrics for Nurses. 18th Edition. W. B. Saunders, 1966.)

This is the *Moro reflex,* the most commonly used of all reflexes to evaluate the neurological status of the new baby. As with asymmetry of posture, injuries to the brachial plexus, clavicle, or humerus will cause the baby to have an asymmetrical Moro reflex (Fig. 6–15). Consistent absence of the Moro reflex suggests the possibility of brain damage; there is, for example, no Moro reflex in babies with kernicterus. After the first weeks of life the Moro reflex disappears. Should it persist beyond three or four months there is some delay in the maturing of the central nervous system.

SENSORY CAPABILITIES IN THE TERM NEWBORN

Questions about the sensory capabilities of newborns were rarely raised two or more decades ago. Yet the sensory system is far more developed than motor behavior. Moreover, sensory capability is important both for parent-infant interaction and as a basis for subsequent cognitive development.

Vision

Perceptive mothers, generation after generation, have stated that their newborns looked at them. Until the late 1950s, most "scientists" disagreed. Since that time, however, the work of investigators such as Fantz, Hershenson, and colleagues, Greenman, and Brazelton have made us aware of the remarkable visual capacity that newborns possess. Although more limited than that of an older child or adult, the newborn's vision suits his needs remarkably. For example, babies see most acutely objects that are 8 to 12 inches from the eyes; this is the distance of their mother's face when the infant is at the breast or the distance to the caregiver's face when the baby is rocked in one's arms or bottle-fed. Faces, particularly eyes with their sparkle and movement, seem especially interesting to infants. The

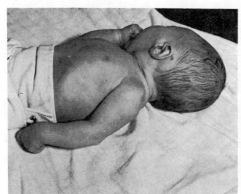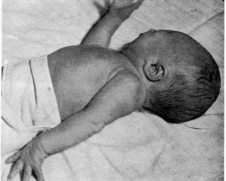

Figure 6–15. Injury to the brachial plexus is one cause of an asymmetrical Moro response. (From Behrman: *In* Vaughan, McKay, and Behrman (eds.): Nelson Textbook of Pediatrics. 11th Edition, W. B. Saunders, 1979.)

Table 6–3   Neonatal Reflexes

Reflex	Manner of Elicitation	Gestational Age when Present Consistently	Age when Disappears	Comments
Moro	A hand clap or slap on the mattress. The baby should respond with extension of the trunk and extension and abduction of the limbs, followed by flexion and adduction of the limbs (as if to embrace).	32 weeks	From 1 to 3 or 4 months	A sudden noise or motion may also elicit response. Consistent absence suggests brain damage. Absence on one side may indicate brain damage, fractured clavicle, or injury to brachial plexus.
Tonic neck	When the baby is supine and the head is turned to one side, the arm and leg the baby is facing extend while the opposite arm and leg flex in a "fencing" position.	Incomplete at birth in normal term infant; often more definite in leg than arm	During the first 6 months, although a partial response may remain until second or third year	If persistent asymmetry and a full response are easily obtained, a cerebral lesion is suggested.
Stepping	When held erect and body supported under the arms with soles flat on table top and trunk inclined forward, baby takes regular, alternating steps.	May tiptoe at 32 weeks; heel-to-toe motion at 40 weeks	6 weeks	Failure to step on several occasions suggests neurological abnormality; stepping with only one foot indicates a unilateral problem.
Neck righting	When head turned to one side, trunk will follow.	34 to 36 weeks	Continues to develop	Other righting reflexes develop as baby grows older.

Reflex	How Elicited	Gestational Age Present	Age of Disappearance	Comments
Placing	When held erect with dorsum of foot drawn against underedge of table top, foot is lifted and placed atop table.	35 weeks	6 weeks	Failure to place or unilateral placing suggests neurological abnormality, as does persistent extension or scissoring of legs.
Palmar grasp	Pressing the examiner's finger into the baby's metacarpophalangeal groove causes the baby to grasp the finger.	Finger grasp is present as early as 28 weeks, but it is approximately 36 weeks before the baby can lift himself off the mattress	4 to 6 months	
Plantar grasp	Pressure on the plantar surface of the foot causes flexion of the toes.		8 to 15 months	
Traction response	After baby grasps hands of examiner, baby pulled to sitting position; baby will flex elbows and support head.	After 36 weeks	Persists	Examiner uses other fingers to help baby grasp.
Rooting	Stroking the upper or lower lip or the side of the cheek causes the baby to turn his mouth and face toward the stimulus and open his mouth.	Fairly good by 32 weeks; complete at 34 weeks	3 to 4 months when baby awake; 7 to 8 months when baby asleep	May be difficult to elicit immediately after feeding. Utilize both rooting and sucking reflexes when putting baby to breast or offering bottle.
Sucking	Stroking the lips produces sucking.	Excellent by 34 weeks; reasonably strong at 32 weeks	12 months; diminishes at 3 to 4 months	May be difficult to elicit in recently fed baby; weak or absent in baby with brain damage.
Swallowing	Place object on back of tongue.	34 to 36 weeks	Persists	

baby's face brightens and his body becomes quiet as he gazes intently. Patterns are gazed at twice as long as plain colors (Fantz 1963). Figures with variation are preferred to plainer figures (Hershenson, Munsinger, and Kessen 1965). Red and yellow seem to be preferred colors.

Most infants not only will gaze at a stimulus but can follow it as well. Greenman (1963) studied 127 infants and found that 26 per cent followed a 4-inch red ring during the period in which they were in the delivery room. Between one-half hour and 12 hours of age, 56 per cent followed the ring, and 76 per cent followed the ring by 48 hours of age. Goren, Sarty, and Wu (1975) demonstrated that at birth a newborn will follow an ungarbled representation of the human face for 180° but will follow a scrambled representation for only 60°.

A newborn is also sensitive to light; he will not open his eyes when a bright light is shining in his face. Because eye-to-eye contact is important for parents as well as babies, the environment should be one in which the lighting is somewhat subdued.

During the first days and weeks of life, most visual stimulation occurs during caregiving activities. By three weeks, a mobile may begin to provide some visual stimulation for the baby. However, this is true only if the mobile is properly positioned. Supine infants do not normally lie so that they look above them but rather lie in the "fencing position," looking predominantly to the right and sometimes to the left. Infants see clearly between 5 and 18 inches from their face at the end of the first month. During the second month, the mobile should be at eye level and to the right of the infant, or separate mobiles should be hung to the left and right, using contrasting colors in patterns similar to a human face. An appropriately placed inexpensive mobile made from cardboard and paint or construction paper is far superior to a commercial mobile suspended directly above the baby's crib. Since a baby of this age (one to two months) cannot reach out to grab, the fragility of the cardboard mobile presents no problems.

Hearing

Infants have shown that they are able not only to attend to sound and turn their head to the sound of a voice but also that they can discriminate between highly similar speech sounds such as "ba" and "pa" as early as 24 hours after birth (DeCasper, Butterfield, and Cairns 1976).

Differences in sound frequency lead to differences in behavior. Newborns appear to be alert to and attend to female voices more readily than to male voices, probably because of the higher pitch. Many adults, male and female, automatically use a falsetto voice when talking to newborns, which in turn is rewarded by the attention of the infant.

State appears to be a factor in the behavioral response of newborns to sound frequencies; babies respond more to high frequencies when they are awake and more to low frequencies when they are drowsy or in a state of light (REM) sleep. Low frequencies have a soothing effect and also elicit gross motor activity (Eisenberg 1976). Could this differential response to the frequencies of male and female voices be a partial basis for the differential response to male and female caregivers?

Loud noises lead to startles; the absence of startles in the first days of life should lead to further evaluation of the infant's hearing.

Newborns also respond to a patterned auditory stimulus in a manner that is different from their response to a constant auditory stimulus. These differences can be demonstrated in heart and electroencephalogram changes as well as in observation of the infant's behavior, such as the initiation or cessation of crying, dilation of the pupils, and turning of the head, which characterize the response to a patterned stimulus. In addition to this response to patterned speech, Condon and Sander (1974) have shown that infants move in rhythm to speech more frequently than to disconnected vowel sounds or a tapping noise.

Since the human voice is the most readily available patterned auditory stimulus, it seems that, just as the human face is the optimum visual stimulus, the human voice is the optimum auditory stimulus. Parents who talk and sing to their babies are, therefore, providing them with important stimulation.

Taste and Smell

Research evidence indicates that newborns can discriminate not only between sweet and nonsweet substances but also between similar tastes, preferring sucrose (which is sweeter) to glucose (Engen and Lipsett 1974). This ability is present in infants as young as one day to three days of age, suggesting that it is innate rather than learned by experience, although these preferences may be altered by experience.

There is some evidence that female infants may be more responsive to sweet tastes. Nisbett and Gurwitz (1970) found that females were more responsive to a sweetened formula and increased their consumption to a significant degree when compared with males. This finding may be related to other studies that suggest a heightened oral sensitivity in females (Korner 1974).

Infants also appear to be able to discriminate between odors and to have a strong dislike for strong odors. Presenting infants with odors that adults find irritating causes babies to startle, become active, turn their heads away, and cry.

Touch

Studies with embryos show that sensitivity to touch is present long before birth. A long series of animal experiments in many species have shown the deleterious effects of lack of tactile stimulation on animal young. It should not be surprising, then, that touch is important for the human baby. The 25,000 square centimeters of skin make it by far the largest of the sense organs.

When mothers first have the opportunity to touch their babies, they move through a specific sequence of behavior. First the mother touches the baby's extremities, using only her fingertips. Within the first 10 minutes she is using the palm of her hand and is touching the baby's trunk. Still later the mother's arms enfold the baby (Rubin 1963). As with other senses (e.g., the relationship between feeding position and visual acuity) the spontaneous behavior of the mother and the needs of the infant seem amazingly well coordinated. Even when the touching sequence does not occur because of separation of mother and infant (e.g., with premature birth), the sequence at a later time is virtually identical, although the pace is considerably delayed. Klaus and colleagues (1970) found that mothers of preterm infants had not progressed to palm contact by the third visit.

Bibliography

Apt, L., Downey, W.: Melena neonatum: the swallowed blood syndrome. J Pediatr 47:6, 1955.
Arias, I., Gartner, L., Seifter, S., Furman, M.: Neonatal unconjugated hyperbilirubinemia with breast feeding and a factor in milk that inhibits glucuronide formation in utero. J Clin Invest 42:913, 1963.
Ashton, R.: The state variable in neonatal research: a review. Merrill-Palmer Q 19:3–20, 1973.
Avery, G.: Neonatal jaundice: modern trends in management. Postgrad Med 54:187, 1973.
Bell, R., Weller, G., Waldrop, M.: Newborn and preschooler: organization of behavior and relations between periods. Monogr Soc Res Child Dev 36:(1,2, serial no. 142), 1971.
Bell, S., Ainsworth: Infant crying and maternal responsiveness. Child Dev 43:1171, 1972.
Brazelton, T.: Observations of the neonate. J Am Acad Child Psychiatry 1:38–58, 1962.
Brazelton, T.B., School, M., Robey, J.: Visual responses in the newborn. Pediatrics 37:284–290, 1966.
Brazelton, T.B.: Infants and Mothers: Differences in Development. New York: Dell Publishing Co., 1969.
Brazelton, T. B.: Neonatal behavioral assessment scale. Clin Dev Med 50, 1973.
Condon, W., Sander, L.: Synchrony demonstrated between movements of the neonate and adult speech. Child Dev 45:456, 1974.
Craig, W.S.: Care of the Newly Born Infant. Baltimore: Williams & Wilkins, 1969.
DeCasper, A., Butterfield, E., Cairns, G.: The role of contingency relations in speech discrimination by newborns. Paper presented at the Fourth Biennial Conference on Human Development. Nashville, Tennessee, April, 1976.
Drew, J.: Infant feeding and jaundice. Keep Abreast J 3(1):53, 1978.
Eisenberg, R.: Auditory Competence in Early Life: The Roots of Communicative Behavior. Baltimore: University Park Press, 1976.

Engen, T., Lipsitt, L.: Ability of newborn infants to discriminate sapid substances. Dev Psychol 10:741, 1974.

Fantz, R.: Pattern vision in newborn infants. Science 140:296–297, 1963.

Goren, C., Sarty, M., Wu, P.: Visual following and pattern discrimination of face-like stimuli by newborn infants. Pediatrics 56:544–549, 1975.

Greenman, G.: Visual behavior of newborn infants. In Modern Perspectives in Child Development, A. Solnit and S. Provence (eds.). New York: Halmark, 1963.

Gregory, G., Kitterman, J., Phibbs, R. et al.: Treatment of idiopathic respiratory distress syndrome with continuous positive airway pressure. N Eng J Med 284:1333, 1971.

Guthrie, R.: Breast milk and jaundice. Keep Abreast J 3(1):49, 1978.

Hargreaves, T., Piper, R.: Breast milk jaundice. Effect of inhibitory breast milk and 3 (alpha), 20 (beta) pregnanediol on glucuronyl transferase. Arch Dis Child 46:195, 1971.

Hershenson, M., Munsinger, H., Kessen, W.: Preference for shapes of intermediate variability in the newborn human. Science 147:630–631, 1965.

Klaus, M., Kennell, J., Plumb, N. et al.: Human maternal behavior at the first contact with her young. Pediatrics 46:187, 1970.

Klaus, M., Kennell, J.: Maternal-Infant Bonding. 2nd Edition. St. Louis: C. V. Mosby, 1979.

Korner, A.: State as variable, as obstacle, and as mediator of stimulation in infant research. Merrill-Palmer Q 18:77–94, 1972.

Korner, A.: The effect of the infant's state, level of arousal, sex and ontogenetic stage on the caregiver. In The Effect of the Infant on Its Caregiver, M. Lewis and L. Rosenblum (eds.). New York: Wiley, 1974.

Maisels, J.: Annotation to text in Poland, R. and Ostrea, E.: Neonatal hyperbilirubinemia. In Care of the High Risk Neonate, M. Klaus and A. Fanaroff (eds.). Philadelphia: W. B. Saunders, 1979.

Nisbett, R., Gurwitz, S.: Weight, sex, and the eating behavior of human newborns. J Comp Physiol Psychol 73:245–253, 1970.

Parmalee, A., Brueck, K., Brueck, M.: Activity and inactivity cycles during the sleep of premature children exposed to neutral temperatures. Biol Neonat 4:317–339, 1962.

Prechtl, H.: The behavioral states of the newborn infant (a review). Brain Res 76:185–212, 1974.

Rubin, R.: Maternal touch. Nurs Outlook 11:828–831, 1963.

Weiss, L.: Differential variations in the amount of activity of newborn infants under continuous light and sound stimulation. Univ Iowa Stud Child Welfare 9:9–74, 1934.

Wolff, P.: Observations on newborn infants. Psychosom Med 21:110–118, 1959.

Wolff, P.: The causes, controls, and organization of behavior in the neonate. Psychol Issues 5:Monograph 17, 1966.

7

CARING FOR THE NEWBORN

When the first edition of *The Newborn and the Nurse* was published in 1972, the majority of infants spent much of their first days in large central nurseries. Many mothers saw their babies only briefly at feeding time, and fathers often had no opportunity to touch their infants until discharge. Siblings saw their new brothers or sisters only when they went home.

Today, a small number of infants are born at home because their parents choose this site for delivery. Other parents go to the hospital for delivery but return home within a few hours if mother and baby appear healthy. "Rooming-in," i.e., having the baby in the mother's room for large parts of the day and evening, is common. In many hospitals the father is not considered a visitor but is with the mother and baby whenever he wishes. Nurses frequently care for mother-infant pairs or families rather than just the mother or just the baby.

Although the infant's basic needs remain the same, new strategies for meeting these needs are constantly being developed. Today, nursing care for newborns includes:

1. Meeting the baby's physical needs.
2. Protecting him from environmental hazards.

3. Recognizing any signs of illness at the earliest possible stage.
4. Educating the parents.
5. Enhancing the attachment between parents and their infant (Chapter 10) and the parents' appreciation of the unique characteristics of their baby (Chapter 6).

MEETING THE PHYSICAL NEEDS OF THE NEWBORN

The Importance of Alerting the Nursery Staff

Following delivery, parents and their infant need time to become acquainted. This time is usually from 30 minutes to an hour in length and coincides with the quiet alert state of the baby (if medication has not caused undue sleepiness). As this period concludes, both mother and baby enter a stage in which rest appears to be their major need. The baby is often taken to a central nursery for assessment during this period.

Infants arrive at every hour, often when nursery personnel are intensely busy. A call from the delivery or recovery suite to the nursery means that someone must be free immediately to give the infant attention on his arrival. (Fathers may carry a healthy baby to the nursery.)

CHECKING THE BABY'S IDENTIFICATION

Some means of identification should be attached to the baby before he leaves the delivery room; identification should be rechecked in the nursery before the delivery room nurse leaves and checked against the mother's identification each time the baby is brought to his mother. Of course, it should also be checked at discharge.

THE SIGNIFICANCE OF THE NUMBER OF UMBILICAL VESSELS

The umbilical cord normally contains three vessels: a single vein (the largest of the vessels) and two arteries. In about 0.5 per cent of all deliveries (3.5 per cent of twin deliveries) there is one umbilical artery instead of two. In one-third of cases this single umbilical artery is associated with one or more congenital anomalies that are not always readily observed in the baby. The existence of a single umbilical artery must be noted on the baby's chart, and the baby should be observed with even more care than he would ordinarily be.

THE IMPORTANCE OF MATERNAL HISTORY

Since the only history a newborn has is his mother's history, the recovery room and nursery nurses need to know as much as possible about the mother and the course of her pregnancy, labor, and delivery. Although any mother can give birth to a baby who may become ill or may have a congenital defect, the chances are significantly higher for some mothers, as revealed by their history. Conditions arising during pregnancy and factors associated with labor and delivery that increase neonatal risk are discussed in previous chapters.

Recovery room and nursery nurses should also know the baby's Apgar score, as recorded at one minute and five minutes (Chapter 5), and whether the mother has had a previous child who was still-born or who had a congenital anomaly or some other illness in the newborn period. The latter is significant not only because of the genetic inheritance of some conditions but also because a mother who has already had a sick or malformed baby is likely to be overanxious about this new infant. She needs and may unconsciously demand extra reassurance. If a previous baby had a clubfoot, for example, she may check this infant's feet and legs repeatedly, asking if they seem to be all right. Nurses can better help her if they understand the reasons for her overconcern.

ADMINISTRATION OF VITAMIN K

The practice of administering 1.0 mg of water-soluble vitamin K to the baby shortly after birth has virtually eliminated hemorrhagic disease in the newborn by preventing the decrease in plasma prothrombin level that usually occurs in the neonatal period. Larger amounts of the vitamin do not carry a greater therapeutic value; in fact, they predispose the baby to hyperbilirubinemia and kernicterus. Although vitamin K has been given to the mother while in labor, this method has generally been found to be less dependable than giving the medication directly to the baby.

THE NEED FOR WARMTH

The baby's need for warmth from the moment of birth has already been discussed. Meeting this need is a nursing responsibility that can be met in several ways, depending on the baby's general condition. In the nursery or in the mother's room, the term infant who has had no difficulty during labor and delivery will probably be able to maintain body temperature with blankets. Maintaining body temperature in preterm and sick infants is discussed in Chapter 8.

Monitoring temperature In checking newborn temperature the choice lies between rectal and axillary methods. The

PROTECTION FROM ENVIRONMENTAL HAZARDS 153

initial rectal temperature taken shortly after birth enables the nurse to detect without delay the presence of an imperforate anus. Taking subsequent temperatures in the axilla eliminates the danger of perforating the rectum.

PROTECTION FROM ENVIRONMENTAL HAZARDS

Protection from Infection

Infection is one of the major hazards affecting newborns; both the prevention of infection and the early recognition of its presence, which is absolutely essential to cure, are basically nursing responsibilities.

Why are newborns more prone to infection? A complete answer to this question is not yet available. Considerations that seem to play a role are the baby's relatively poor immunity to most bacteria, a diminished capacity to produce the immunoglobulins IgG and IgM, and difficulty in localizing infection — an infection at one site quickly becomes systemic.

Moreover, there are several portals of entry that exist in the newborn but disappear shortly after birth: the vessels of the umbilical stump, circumcisions, and breaks in the skin caused by forceps delivery. In addition, delicate infant skin is easily irritated and broken down.

An increased risk of infection is inherent in certain anomalies: esophageal atresia, exstrophy of the bladder, omphalocele, congenital diaphragmatic hernia, imperforate anus with rectourinary fistula, meningomyelocele, and those anomalies that require bowel resection. Babies who receive repeated exchange transfusions or fluids or who have frequent blood sampling through the umbilical vein are at heightened risk, as are babies who must be mechanically resuscitated. In one respect infants in isolettes are protected against certain infections, but an isolette that has not been thoroughly cleaned can in itself be a reservoir of pathogenic bacteria.

Maternal factors that increase the likelihood that the baby will be infected include:

1. Rupture of membranes more than 24 hours before delivery.
2. Fever or infection in the mother during the last week of pregnancy.
3. Foul-smelling or purulent amniotic fluid.
4. Prolonged labor.
5. Excessive manipulation during labor.
6. Maternal infectious disease such as syphilis, gonorrhea, tuberculosis, residual rubella, vaccinia, polio, and salmonellosis.

PREVENTING INFECTION IN THE NURSERY

It has been said often, but it is worth repeating, that thorough hand washing with a bacteriocidal solution is an absolute essential in the prevention of nursery infection. This means scrubbing up to the elbows for two to three minutes before entering the nursery and repeated hand washing after caring for each infant. Not only must each member of the nursing staff carry out the proper techniques of hand washing but so must everyone else who enters the nursery, from cleaning personnel to aides to medical students to physicians. Mothers and fathers who are encouraged to wash their hands before they touch the baby may continue this practice after they return home.

Another source of infection is contaminated or improperly cleaned equipment. The water reservoirs in water taps, nebulizers, and equipment used in resuscitation may contribute to infection if they are not frequently and thoroughly cleaned. If it is possible, each infant confined to an incubator should be moved to a clean bed every four days, certainly weekly. The dirty incubator should be washed with an antiseptic solution and every movable part removed and cleaned separately. Just wiping or soaking with solution is not sufficient. If there are plugs of dirt or dust in corners or around screws the solution may eliminate the top layer of bacteria, but colonies of bacteria can continue to flourish beneath this layer. After the incubator or isolette is washed, it is advisable to run it in a dry condition for 24 hours to provide a further interruption of the cycle of bacterial growth.

The physical setup of the nursery can be a factor in the prevalence of infection. The ideal setup would be small, multiple nurseries of four to six infants to which no new infants are admitted until all previous babies are discharged and the nursery is thoroughly cleaned. Unfortunately such a setup is not always possible. But in every nursery each unit can be thoroughly cleaned (including the inside of drawers, shelves, walls of the cubicle) before another baby is admitted. Daily dusting of each unit with a towel dampened with an antiseptic solution is also a part of the nursing care in the control of infection. Whether the actual cleaning is done by nurses or supervised by them, there is no underestimating its importance.

Any individual with diarrhea, upper respiratory infection, or skin infection must be excluded from the nursery. Not only medical and nursing personnel but the housekeeping staff as well must observe this precaution.

There should be no visitors on the obstetrical floor during the hours when babies are with their mothers and fathers, although provision should be made for sibling visits (Chapter 10). At other times, visitors should be limited not only in terms of number at any one time but also in terms of total number. Besides providing protection from infection, strict visiting regulations — stricter than most hospitals seem willing to enforce — give the mother a chance for much needed rest, especially for the multipara who will be going home to care for other small children in addition to caring for this new infant. For the protection of both mother and baby, visitors should not sit on the mother's bed.

If the mother has symptoms of infection, such as an elevated temperature, a sore throat, or an upper respiratory infection, or has been vomiting or has diarrhea, she should not feed her baby. But neither should she be forgotten by the nursery nurse. The baby can be taken to the door of her room so that she can see him at least once during the day, and she can be given reports of his progress.

RECOGNIZING INFECTION IN THE BABY

Rarely are there dramatic signs of infection in newborns such as the sudden elevation in temperature often seen in older children. Even in sepsis severe enough to cause mortality there may never be fever; hypothermia or marked variations evidencing the infant's ability to control his temperature are often present.

Infection should be suspected when a baby is inactive and does not eat well. Jaundice, beginning after the third day, may be a sign of infection. The skin may also have a mottled appearance. Abdominal distention is a common manifestation of generalized sepsis and may be one of the first signs of infection. Temperature instability and shifts in glucose levels in blood are additional signs of sepsis, although glucose is rarely evaluated in the previously healthy term infant. A full fontanel, a high-pitched cry, and irritability usually indicate infection of the central nervous system. Babies with diarrhea need to be isolated immediately and their stools cultured. Babies who are vomiting and have changes in respiratory pattern and skin lesions need to be evaluated for infection. Most of the time these changes will first be noticed by an observant nurse who will alert the physician to the possibility of sepsis so that necessary therapy can begin as soon as possible.

Other Environmental Hazards

As important as it is to prevent infection, it is equally important that the agent used in prevention is not in itself deleterious. Boric acid was at one time widely used in newborn nurseries until evidence indicated that its use as a wet dressing or as an ointment for diaper rash could result in infant mortality rates of as high as 70 per cent.

The agents and procedures used in the laundering of infant linen and clothing can also constitute a hazard. Armstrong (1969) reported an instance in which severe illness and death in newborns was traced to a bacteriocide compound, pentachlorophenol, used in the laundry. The chemical was subsequently absorbed through the skin after the infants were repeatedly exposed to linen laundered with this compound. The babies in this particular group were in a maternity hospital for unwed mothers and thus stayed in the hospital longer than most newborns. However, their stays were probably shorter than those of tiny premature babies or babies with congenital defects. Even one such finding emphasizes how important it is that nurses know what kinds of procedures are being used in other areas of the hospital such as the laundry. Nyhan (1969) feels that only plain water should be used as a terminal rinse for infant clothing and bedding.

RECOGNITION OF ILLNESS IN THE INFANT

The assessment of variations in behavior and appearance that may indicate illness has been discussed in Chapter 6. The recognition of sepsis is described above. Continued physical and behavioral assessment is important to infant care. The condition of an infant can change rapidly. For this reason, infants in the nursery should never be left unattended, and infants rooming-in with their parents should be observed frequently for physical and behavioral characteristics as well as for parent-infant interaction. In addition, parents should be taught to recognize signs of illness in their baby.

Screening for Phenylketonuria and Hypothyroidism

Phenylketonuria (PKU) and hypothyroidism are two conditions that, if undetected, in the newborn, will lead to severe mental retardation. However, early intervention can prevent retardation.

PKU is an autosomal recessive disease (Chapter 2) in which phenylalanine, an amino acid, accumulates because of an error in metabolism. Undetected, this accumulation leads to irreversible mental retardation in affected infants. In the United States, PKU occurs approximately once in 14,000 births. Mass screening for the presence of phenylalanine in capillary blood is now required by law in most states.

Because concentrations of phenylalanine may not rise sufficiently to be detected in the first days of life, testing should be deferred until the third to sixth day or until dietary protein has been ingested for 24 to 48 hours. When mothers and infants stay in the hospital for a shorter time than usual, alternative plans for screening are necessary. A home visit for screening can provide a community health nurse an opportunity for family assessment and teaching.

If the initial screening test is negative (i.e., no phenylalanine is present) the test should be repeated within two to four weeks after birth. The most common reason for an initial negative test is an inadequate blood sample. Blood sampling is only the preliminary step in the recognition of PKU; there are other conditions in which phenylalanine is found in urine and blood. Children with these other conditions will be harmed by a low-phenylalanine diet and the use of Lofenalac, both of which are essential for children with PKU.

Dietary treatment of PKU is monitored by regular blood testing (daily during the first week, weekly until the baby is two months old, twice a month from two months to one year, and monthly after that) and urine testing (daily during the first month, twice weekly until the baby is six months old, weekly until his first birthday, and twice a month from that time on). The reason for this constant monitoring — one which parents must understand — is that although a normal dietary level of phenylalanine will cause mental retardation, a diet too low in this essential amino acid will not meet the baby's growth requirements. Phenylalanine is restricted in the diet by substituting Lofenalac for milk (with a small amount of cow's milk added to provide the phenylalanine needed for growth). Later, strained foods low in protein are added to the diet.

The routine use of mass screening for thyroid deficiency is more recent than for PKU; the same blood sample can be used. *Congenital hypothyroidism* is far more common than PKU; the incidence of thyroid dysgenesis, the most common cause of congenital hypothyroidism, is estimated at one in 6000. The etiology is unknown; rarely is more than one member of a family affected.

Without detection and treatment many affected infants die of respiratory disease or infection or survive to become mentally deficient dwarfs. If treatment (replacement therapy with thyroid hormone) is started by six weeks of life, normal development can be expected. Since it is frequently difficult to detect physical symptoms of the disease in the first weeks of life, mass screening offers the best hope for these children.

PARENT EDUCATION

Helping parents develop parenting skills has always been a primary nursing responsibility. With hospital stays for healthy mothers and infants shortened to only a few hours to one or two days, nurses who care for mothers during different phases of the childbearing cycle need to coordinate their efforts to be sure that every parent is as knowledgeable and comfortable as possible in his or her new role.

Education for parenting is addressed in many childbirth classes, but not all parents attend these classes. "Rooming-in" experiences in hospitals offer excellent opportunities for mothers and fathers to care for their babies while support persons who can answer questions are close at hand. Some parents leave too quickly to utilize rooming-in, and others may elect not to do so or, in some in-stances, may not have the chance. In some areas public health nurses make one or more home visits to every family with a new infant. Some nurses who practice in collaboration with physicians also make home visits. Nurse-midwives who deliver infants may continue to serve as resources to new parents during the first week of the baby's life. A telephone call from the hospital nursing staff to the home a few days after discharge provides an opportunity for questions from parents as well as some assessment by the nurse.

With the exception of women who are cared for throughout the childbearing cycle by a nurse-midwife or nurse practitioner, few women have a primary nurse during this period. This seems particularly true of women cared for in the private sector; the public health nurse may serve as a primary resource for some patients cared for in a public clinic, although her activity during hospitalization can be limited.

Every family needs to know where they can seek help, not just in the instance of serious illness or emergency but also for answers to day-to-day questions about matters such as diaper rash, a stuffy nose that is making feeding difficult, and crying. At each stage of the childbearing cycle nurses who care for parents will need to assess what the parents know and help them plan for their current and future learning.

Basic Information for Parents

There is a basic core of information that is important for all parents. Parents need to learn about their baby's behavior in terms of his patterns of development (including social responses) and his sensory capabilities. (Sensory capabilities have been discussed in Chapter 6.) Parents also need to learn about their baby's needs in the following areas: loving care, nutrition, safety, cleanliness, clothing and supplies, and health care. (Nutritional needs are discussed in Chapter 9.)

PATTERNS OF DEVELOPMENT

What do parents need to know about their new baby's development? Every baby develops in his own unique way, so comparisons to siblings or other children are meaningless. This is true of growth in height and weight and also of growth in motor and verbal skills. Playing with the baby, talking to him, providing interesting things for viewing, all can certainly enhance his development; nevertheless he will follow his own timetable.

Parents of newborns need to know what they can expect during the first month — from the time the baby goes home until his first checkup. The basic differences in the personality of each infant and the ways in which nurses can help parents recognize and accept their baby's unique attributes have been described in Chapter 6.

In addition to helping parents understand their infants, an overview of development in the first weeks can help parents cope with the feeling that the baby will forever consume all their time and energy. For example, although the baby may need seven to eight feedings a day during the first week, by four weeks of age he should need only five to six feedings a day. Sleep periods will become more regular, with one period that may last as long as five to six hours. The pattern of waking and sleeping will also become more predictable. A cycle in which the baby awakens when he is hungry, cries, is fed, has a period of alertness after feeding, and then becomes drowsy and sleeps will become increasingly evident.

Babies give more positive feedback to parents each week as the brief periods of alertness lengthen to six or seven minutes. The excitement the baby shows when mom, dad, or siblings come into the room, the baby's increasing ability to quiet to the sound of a familiar voice, his cooing sounds and ability to make eye contact, the decrease in crying time — all these behaviors can increase the pleasure of being a parent. By helping parents to anticipate and watch for signs of their baby's development, nurses can further the parents' appreciation of and interaction with him.

The importance of talking to the baby from the beginning can be stressed. Although many parents do this automatically, others believe that talking is silly when a baby cannot understand. Yet this early verbalization appears important in the later development of speech.

Table 7–1 summarizes major developments during the neonatal period (birth to 28 days).

LOVING CARE

Loving care for a baby means recognizing his unique needs and providing the kind of care that meets these needs. Some babies will need more holding and rocking, whereas other babies will be best served by less stimulation. One of the major concerns of parents is what to do when their baby cries. Crying is the baby's way of communicating need or distress, and parents need to respond to these cries during the early weeks and months of life. There appears to be no danger of "spoiling" during the first

Table 7–1 Development of the Newborn in the First Four Weeks

Regains birth weight by approximately 10 days of age
Has more regular respirations
Trembles and startles less frequently
Requires fewer feedings (from 7–8 to 5–6 feedings per day)
Has fewer bowel movements (vary with type of feeding)
Has fewer sleeping periods but increases the length of each sleeping period
Cries less
Has longer periods of alertness, from periods about 3 minutes long to periods 6 to 7 minutes long
Develops a more predictable sleep/wake cycle, though still disorganized
Becomes better able to focus eyes; eye-to-eye contact
Becomes excited at seeing a face
Quiets to the sound of a familiar voice
Enjoys kicking legs
Begins to make cooing noises
Makes early hand-to-mouth movements

weeks; indeed, prompt response early in life seems to lead to less subsequent crying (Chapter 6). Yet it is hard to convince parents of this. I ask parents in my childbirth education classes to respond to the statement, "It's O.K. to pick up a baby when he or she cries." I find most parents disagree or are undecided. In some classes only one or two parents will agree that it is all right to pick up the crying baby; fathers agree more frequently than mothers. A general discussion follows, and the parents are free to change their minds at any point (and some do). Parents are urged to think about this important question in the weeks that follow.

SAFETY

An understanding of safety for the baby is closely tied to an understanding of growth and development. Specific safety precautions are summarized in Table 7–2.

CLEANLINESS

For many years the only prenatal class in some hospitals was the "baby bath demonstration," usually held just for mothers (rather than for both parents). Some prenatal classes also devoted an entire evening to bathing a baby-sized doll. It was fun, but the subtle message in both of these instances was that bathing a baby involves ritual and mystique that must be mastered if one is to be a good parent. There is nothing mysterious about bathing the infant. Parents simply must keep a few points in mind.

1. It is not particularly difficult to bathe a baby.

2. Until the cord drops off and the navel heals (anywhere from one to four weeks including healing time), a sponge bath is best.

3. Even after the cord drops off a sponge bath is fine (some days a bath seems more than parents can manage).

4. As long as creases and bottoms are kept clean, a daily bath is not necessary.

5. Powders and lotions are not necessary and may irritate some babies (powder when used liberally may be inhaled by the baby).

Mother and father can sponge bathe their baby for the first time in the hospital. They will feel a lot more comfortable about bathing their baby at home after having done it in the hospital than they would from just watching an efficient nurse give a bath demonstration to a group. Of course, nursing staff should be available

Table 7–2   Safety Precautions for Newborns

Do	Don't
Consider safety in toy purchases. Be sure that toys have no small parts that can come off and be swallowed, inhaled, etc.	Never leave baby alone where he might fall, even for a moment.
Always test bath water *just before* placing baby in it (bath water can burn).	Never leave baby in or near water (tub, etc.).
Clean toxic substances from floor cabinets. Lock medicine cabinets.	Never leave baby near a portable table heater or vaporizer, wall heater, grilled floor heater, radiator, electric outlet, or connected appliance cord. Do not place crib near electric cords, lamps, or windows.
Be sure crib slats are sufficiently close together so head cannot fit between slats. Use a padded bumper on the crib. (A dresser drawer, with firm padding, is a good bed.) Avoid pillows and thin plastic covers (thin plastic can cause suffocation).	Never take baby in a car without an infant carrier placed on the seat facing backwards and secured with the seat belt.
Be sure that leadfree paint is used not only in baby's room, toys, and furniture but throughout the house.	Never leave baby in the yard in a crib or carriage while a power mower is in use (mowers can throw stones a great distance).

to support their efforts with encouragement and answers to questions.

Hospital bathtime can just as easily be in the evening as in the morning; it might vary from family to family, depending on individual needs and desires. This kind of flexibility is valuable not only during the brief hospital period but, perhaps even more important, it gives parents "permission" to be flexible and adaptive in baby care at home. Past generations of mothers (and some mothers today) felt that a daily bath before the 10 AM feeding was a binding rule. The practices of some maternity units may reinforce this kind of rigidity. Mothers should know that babies may be bathed at any time that best fits the schedule of both parents and infant. For example, nearly every baby has a "fussy" period during his first weeks — a time when he is neither hungry nor sleepy and seems at somewhat of a loss as to what he wants, probably some companionship and loving. This period varies from one baby to another in terms of the time of day but is remarkably consistent in an individual infant. In many instances this time is a good one for bathing. The following procedure is suggested for bathing the infant.

1. Gather the equipment, including the baby's clean clothes, so that you will not have to leave the baby during the bath.
2. Fill the basin, sink, or tub with water that feels comfortable to your elbow (hands accustomed to hot water used in dish washing are not as good indicators as sensitive elbow skin). If the baby is to have a tub bath, put a towel or diaper in the bottom of the tub.
3. Wash each eye from the nose outward, using a clean section of washcloth for each eye. Do not wash across the bridge of the nose; infection, if present, could be transferred.
4. Soap the baby's head with bath soap. Holding him securely, rinse his head with water. Dry with a towel. (Because of the open fontanel, many mothers are afraid to wash the baby's head, and subsequent scalp infections are not uncommon at checkup time. Therefore, this is an important part of parent education.)
5. Wash the baby's face with soap; rinse and dry.
6. Soap trunk, arms, and legs with hands; turn the baby to his abdomen to wash back. Wash genital area last. (In girls, the labia are gently separated and the genitalia cleansed from front to back. In boys, the folds of the scrotum are cleansed; the foreskin is not retracted. A Vaseline dressing covers the penis in the first 24 hours after circumcision. Soap will be irritating to the circumcision area for several days; it is best rinsed with clear water until it heals. Normally, the circumcision will be healed earlier than the umbilicus and thus prior to the baby's first tub bath.)
7. Rinse trunk, arms, and legs with washcloth and clear water, rinsing the genital area last. If the baby is having a tub bath, immerse in tub for rinsing. (Until the umbilicus heals, the baby should only have sponge baths. Immersing the baby might risk infection.)
8. Pat the baby dry. Check to be sure that creases, such as the neck folds and inguinal area, are dry and clean.
9. Clean the area around the umbilicus with alcohol until it is healed.
10. Dress the baby. Brush his hair.

ENVIRONMENTAL TEMPERATURE

Some parents (and *many* grandparents) have a tendency to keep babies too warm. An environmental temperature of 68 to 72° F is fine. At night, the temperature can be as low as 65° F.

Babies can go outdoors at any time after they return home. In summer weather, some care to protect them from sunburn is important.

CLOTHING

Just as parents may keep the environment too warm, they may also overdress the baby. Babies need no more clothing than adults. Just a diaper or a diaper and cotton shirt is sufficient if mother and father are wearing shorts. If his parents need a sweater, the baby probably does, too.

New babies need very few clothes; shirts, diapers, and two or three cotton gowns are really sufficient. Babies grow so rapidly during the first weeks and months that clothes are quickly outgrown. It makes sense to use clothing money for items of long-term value such as a good crib mattress that can be used for several years.

Plastic pants and disposable diapers with plastic coverings cannot be tolerated by some babies. When infants have a tendency to diaper rash, discontinuing use of plastic pants is the first change parents can make. Some babies will be able to wear waterproof pants during the day when diapers are changed frequently but need to avoid them at night.

Although booties, socks, and little shoes may be cute, babies are better off without foot covering. Parents should know that it is normal for a baby's hands and feet to be slightly cooler than the trunk of his body.

HEALTH CARE

Health care education for new mothers includes preventive care, the recognition of illness, and knowing what to do if the baby appears ill.

Where will the baby receive health care? From a nurse practitioner or physician? In a private office or a public clinic? Some parents have thought carefully about this aspect of baby care but others may not have. Some may need additional information about the options available to them. Many infants, even infants with high risk conditions, have no "health care home," receive few or none of their immunizations, and may be rarely if ever seen by a professional during the first year. When parents have made no plans, a referral to public health nursing can provide continuity of care. Even when parents have made a plan for continuing health care, they may not utilize that plan in the first weeks following birth. Many day-to-day questions about feeding, crying, bowel movements, rashes, and the like may seem too trivial for a call to a clinic or office yet may be a source of worry to the parents. In some hospitals, a nurse may call the mother several days after discharge to give her the opportunity to ask questions. Home visits in both the public and private sectors are available in many communities.

Preventive health care includes many areas already or subsequently described (nutrition, bottle mouth caries, safety, etc.). The importance of immunization should be emphasized; why immunization is important for *their* baby is a more significant reason for getting the baby shots than are reasons of epidemiology (e.g., the prevention of disease in the population).

How do parents recognize when their baby is ill? Every mother and father should be taught how to take their baby's temperature before they leave the hospital. They must also know that they should take the baby's temperature before calling the clinic or office if they think the baby is sick. Other clues to illness include:

1. Loss of appetite.
2. Vomiting and/or diarrhea.
3. Lack of energy (lethargy).
4. Difficult breathing.
5. Sunken eyes and/or fontanel or full fontanel.
6. Drainage from umbilical area.
7. White patches in mouth (thrush).
8. Nonspecific (looks sick).

Parents should have the telephone numbers of their health care provider and the hospital emergency room handy. A good place to put the number is on the bottom of the telephone. Families without telephones should know the location of the nearest one they can use.

Circumcision

There is evidence that circumcision was practiced in Egypt more than 7000 years ago; the oldest preserved mummies, dating from 2000 B.C., were circumcised. In the United States, from 60 to 97 per cent of newborn males are circumcised (Klauber 1973). Nevertheless, the practice of routine circumcision is debated today.

Proponents argue (1) that circumcision is a factor in the prevention of carcinoma of the penis (Speert 1953) and prostate in males and of the cervix in females, (2) that circumcision is prophylactic against a number of diseases including herpes genitalis (Taylor and Rodin 1975), (3) that hygiene is facilitated, and (4) that the absence of circumcision may make a boy feel different from his peers. Opponents argue that the studies linking cancer and the absence of circumcision are invalid for a variety of methodological reasons. Terris, Wilson, and Nelson (1973) found no significant difference in the circumcision status of marital partners of 1,148 women with histologically confirmed cases of cancer of the cervix and an equal number of women matched as controls.

In comparing the incidence of carcinoma of the penis in white male populations in temperate zones in the United States and Scandinavia, no difference was found in the rates (1/100,000) for circumcised and uncircumcised males. The incidence of cancer of the penis is higher (9/100,000) among uncircumcised males in the tropics (Gee and Ansell 1976). Ravich (1965) suggested that carcinoma of the prostate is higher in circumcised males. Studies from diverse cultures indicate that when hygiene is good carcinoma of the penis is rare; if hygiene is poor, circumcision appears to offer little protection (Grimes 1978). There is little evidence to support the belief that circumcision prevents venereal disease (Gairdner 1949); adequate studies have yet to be undertaken.

As to the ease in retracting the foreskin for purposes of hygiene in infant boys, Gairdner states that the prepuce, still developing at birth, is normally nonretractable. Of 100 newborns, only four had a fully retractable prepuce; in 54 the glans could be uncovered to reveal the external meatus, whereas even the tip of the glans could not be uncovered in the remaining 42. Separation of the prepuce from the glans usually occurs between nine months and three years. Gairdner suggests that during the years the child is incontinent the prepuce protects the glans from infection due to wet diapers.

Balanitis, infection of the foreskin, occurs only in uncircumcised males and requires staged surgical corrections. Balanitis was common among uncircumcised American soldiers stationed in desert areas during World War II because of sand under the foreskin. This may have influenced later attitudes favoring neonatal circumcision.

In 1971 the Committee on Fetus and Newborn of the American Academy of Pediatrics stated that there are no valid *medical* indications for circumcision in the neonatal period. The data were reviewed in 1975, and no basis was found for changing the statement (Committee on Fetus and Newborn 1975). Parents may, of course, have other valid reasons for wishing their sons circumcised; the religious beliefs of Jewish and Moslem families are an example. Regardless, the decision is the parents' to make.

For many parents, however, the decision to circumcise is based not on religious beliefs but on mistaken beliefs and/or lack of knowledge. For some, the first discussion of circumcision comes in answer to questions during the early stages of labor. "If it's a boy, do you want him circumcised?" In raising the question in childbirth education courses, I find some mothers do not know the meaning of the word *circumcision*. In one study, over half the women questioned did not know whether their husbands were circumcised (Terris and Oalmann 1960). In other surveys the proportion of women who did not know their husbands' circumcision status varied from 5 to 10 per cent in private practice to approximately 35 per cent in clinic populations.

Thus, if parents are to make informed decisions, a discussion of circumcision should be part of prenatal and postpartum education. Before asking parents what decision they have made, nurses should ask them if circumcision has been discussed with them and should assess their knowledge. Since circumcision should never be performed in the delivery room at birth, parents who have not discussed circumcision fully with a nurse or physician prior to labor should have the opportunity to do so in the days following delivery.

Circumcision in the delivery room at birth has been and, unfortunately, continues to be a common practice in some hospitals because it is convenient for the obstetrician. Why should this practice be abandoned? First, it is unjustified to perform a painful procedure on an infant during a time that should be devoted to allowing parents and their new infant to become acquainted. Moreover, cold stress caused by the temperature of the delivery room is a hazard. Because a neonatal anomaly or illness is a contraindication to circumcision and because these conditions may not be readily apparent in the delivery room, there is additional reason for delaying the procedure until the infant is at least 12 to 24 hours old, is stable, and has had a complete physical examination.

Few observers of circumcision doubt that the procedure causes pain. An anesthetic is rarely used, however, because it is believed that the infant will have no memory of the pain. The long-term effects of neonatal pain and stress are unknown and deserve research attention. Kirya and Werthmann (1978) suggest that a penile dorsal nerve block with 1 per cent lidocaine without epinephrine virtually abolishes circumcision pain as evidenced by the infant's quiet alert state after the initial infiltration of the medication. No complications or untoward effects of lidocaine were present in 52 infants nor were any other complications of circumcision observed. Because the infant no longer was distressed, parents were allowed to witness the circumcision.

Absolute contraindications to circumcision in the neonatal period include hypospadias (because the foreskin is needed for surgical repair), the possibility of a bleeding problem, other congenital anomalies or illness, and prematurity. If the parents of a premature infant desire circumcision, the procedure is deferred until the baby weighs at least 2500 g (5.5 lbs).

Whether or not the infant is circumcised, the need for lifelong penile hygiene must be discussed with the parents. In the uncircumcised infant, the foreskin is retracted gently, if possible, and the penis washed as part of daily hygiene. As the boy grows and becomes responsible for his own care, he is reminded about penile hygiene just as he is reminded about washing behind his ears.

For the circumcised infant, Vaseline on a gauze bandage that is changed at each diaper change may promote comfort for the first few days after circumcision. The infant may be more comfortable on his side or back while the circumcision is healing.

COMPLICATIONS OF CIRCUMCISION

In reviewing the records of 5,882 circumcised infants, Gee and Ansell (1976) found the incidence of complications to be two in 1000. The most frequent complication was hemorrhage sufficient to require physician intervention to stop the bleeding (which occurred in 59 patients — 1 per cent). Intervention included application of a sponge soaked in aqueous adrenalin, ligation of a vessel, and the use of Gelfoam as well as other methods. In only one infant (who had a Factor VIII deficiency — a type of hemophilia) was hemorrhage life-threatening; the bleeding ceased after the infant was treated with cryoprecipitate. Eight infants with hypospadias were circumcised.

Infection, diagnosed by the presence of pus and erythema, occurred in 23 patients (0.4 per cent). Local cleansing with hydrogen peroxide and 3% hexachlorophene solution was the initial treatment; four infants developed systemic symptoms and were treated with antibiotics. Infection was significantly higher ($p < .005$) following Plastibell circumcision.

Other less frequent complications included denudation of the penile shaft, edema and cyanosis following circumcision with a Plastibell that was too small (with uneventful recovery when the Plastibell was removed), and urinary retention for 34 hours after circumcision followed by spontaneous voiding.

Complications reported in other studies include urinary retention, laceration of the glans, retention of the Plastibell ring for several weeks with subsequent penile edema, and, in a rare instance, sloughing of the penis. Certainly nurses must be aware of the possibility of complications and must check each infant carefully following circumcision. When infants are circumcised on the day of discharge, parents must know whom to call if there is bleeding or pus or if the circumcision "does not look quite right" to them.

References for Parents

Reference books are helpful for some parents, and they may seek information about a choice of books. The following list is by no means inclusive. State health departments and agricultural extension services frequently have free material for parents that is well suited to particular needs. Nurses who care for childbearing families at any stage of the cycle can enhance their own practice by developing a personal library and resource file of useful materials.

Barr, E. and Monserrat, C.: *Teenage Pregnancy: A New Beginning*. Albuquerque: New Futures, 1978. Includes information about baby care as well as pregnancy and family planning. Written for teenagers.

Brazelton, T. Berry: *Infants and Mothers: Differences in Development*. New York, Dell, 1969. Follows the development of three babies, a quiet baby, an average baby, and an active baby, through the first year, emphasizing unique characteristics. For parents with high school education or beyond and professionals. Available in paperback.

Brenner, E.: *A New Baby! A New Life!* New York: McGraw-Hill, 1973. Simple, easy-to-read text and lovely drawings make this book of value for all parents. Paperback.

Caplan, Frank: *The First Twelve Months of Life*. New York, Bantam, 1978. Excellent information for parents educated beyond high school and professionals; nurses will need to adapt information for other parents. Based on research done at the Princeton Center for Infancy and Early Childhood. Available in paperback.

Child Care, J. Sutherland (ed.). Van Nuys, California: Sutherland Learning Associates, 1979. Good information; easily readable, well illustrated. Refers only to doctor as health care provider, which is unfortunate. Paperback.

Fraiberg, S.: *The Magic Years*. New York: Charles Scribner's Sons, 1968. Parent-child relationships for parents with a high school education or beyond.

Infant Development Guide. Somerville, New Jersey: Johnson & Johnson, 1978. Beautifully illustrated, comprehensive book. Shows fathers as active participants in care. Editorial advisory board includes Kathryn Barnard, Professor of Nursing at Washington School of Nursing. Hardback.

Koschnick, K.: *Having a Baby*. Syracuse, New York: New Readers Press, 1979. Written at a fourth to fifth grade reading level, this book is valuable for mothers who would be unwilling or unable to read more complex material. Includes infant as well as prenatal care. Paperback.

White, Burton: *The First Three Years of Life*. New York: Avon Books, 1975. Excellent information for parents educated beyond high school and professionals; nurses will need to adapt information for other parents. Based on research done at Harvard University. Available in paperback.

Bibliography

Armstrong, R.: Pentachlorophenol poisoning in a nursery for newborn infants. J Pediatr 75:317, 1969.
Barr, E.: Teenage Pregnancy, A New Beginning. Albuquerque: New Futures.
Brazelton, T. B.: Infants and Mothers: Differences in Development. New York: Dell, 1969.
Brenner, E.: A New Baby: A New Life: New York: McGraw-Hill, 1973.
Caplan, F.: The First Twelve Months of Life. New York, Bantam, 1978.
Child Care, J. Sutherland (ed.). Van Nuys, California: Sutherland Learning Associates, 1979.
Committee on Fetus and Newborn. Report of the ad hoc task force on circumcision. Pediatrics 56:610, 1975.
Fraiberg, S.: The Magic Years. New York: Charles Scriber's Sons, 1968.
Gairdner, D.: The fate of the foreskin: A study of circumcision. Br Med J 1433, 1949.
Gee, W., Ansell, J.: Neonatal circumcision: A ten-year overview. Pediatrics 58:824, 1976.
Grimes, D.: Routine circumcision of the newborn infant: A reappraisal. Am J Obstet Gynecol 130:125, 1978.
Infant Development Guide. Somerville, New Jersey: Johnson & Johnson, 1978.

Kirya, C., Werthmann, M.: Neonatal circumcision and penile dorsal nerve block — a painless procedure. J Pediatr 92:998, 1978.

Klauber, G.: Circumcision and phallic fallacies, or the case against routine circumcision. Conn Med 37:445, 1973.

Koschnick, K.: Having a Baby. Syracuse, New York: New Readers Press, 1979.

Nyhan, W.: Newly recognized hazard in the newborn nursery. J Pediatr 75:348, 1969.

Ravich, A.: Role of circumcision in cancer prevention. Acta Urol Jap 11:76, 1965.

Speert, H.: Circumcision of the newborn: An appraisal of its present status. Obstet Gynecol 2:164, 1953.

Taylor, P., Rodin, P.: Herpes genitalis and circumcision. Br. J. Vener Dis 51:274, 1975.

Terris, M., Oalmann, M.: Carcinoma of the cervix, an epidemiologic study. JAMA 174:1847, 1960.

Terris, M., Wilson, F., Nelson, J.: Relation of circumcision to cancer of the cervix. Am J Obstet Gynecol 117:1056, 1973.

White, B.: The First Three Years of Life. New York: Avon Books, 1975.

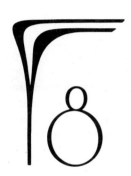

THE NEWBORN WITH SPECIAL NEEDS

When an infant is born before 38 weeks or after 42 weeks gestation, is small or large for gestational age, is ill, or has a congenital anomaly, that infant and his family have special needs in addition to those of a normal infant and family. The special needs of this infant, frequently called the high risk infant, will be addressed in this chapter. The special needs of families are discussed in Chapter 10.

Nursing Goals for Infants with Special Needs

The interest in mortality rates for high risk infants might suggest that saving lives is the primary goal in the nursing care of these patients. Although decreasing mortality does reflect improved care of mother and baby, nursing goals are far more comprehensive.

As technology has enabled us to sustain life at earlier gestational ages — first 36 weeks, then 34, now even less than 28 — there is a growing concern about the quality of life of these infants who survive the first critical weeks. Physiologically, the single most important factor in the quality of these babies' lives is an intact central nervous system. As perinatal mortality drops, this is one focus for nursing concern.

Neuronal development in the central nervous system peaks at 12 to 18 weeks gestation. Insults during this period of rapid neuronal development lead to a decreased number of neurons and to mental retardation, which is often severe. Examples of such insults are viral disease (rubella, cytomegalic inclusion disease) and radiation (Chapter 3). Nothing we know at present reverses the effects of these insults; they must be prevented.

The cerebellum reaches its peak of development in the first days after birth. If the baby fails to receive cerebellar nutrition (oxygen, glucose, maintenance of acid-base balance) in these first days, problems in cerebellar development will result in perceptual motor difficulty. As he grows older, the child may be clumsy and lacking in fine coordination, even though he may be of normal intelligence.

The cells of the brain stem and the cerebral cortex grow slowly, over a period of years, whereas the cells of the cerebellum develop during the first few days following birth. Cellular development in both cases is dependent upon continued nutritional support, but cerebellar development is obviously more critically dependent upon nutrition during the first few days of life. Without proper nutrition during this critical period, a child could be intelligent (a function mediated by the cerebral cortex) and still have perceptual motor difficulty (a function mediated by the cerebellum).

A great deal of the myelinization of the neurons also takes place following birth. Myelin is a cholesterol substance that acts as "insulation" for the neurons. Without myelinization, neuronal messages would go off in all directions. Thus, a newborn (with normally incomplete myelinization) reacts to a stimulus with his whole body. As the child grows older, his movements normally become less general and more specific, and he is able to accomplish more finely coordinated movements. When myelinization is incomplete, this fine coordination is never achieved.

Much of the care during the first hours, days, and weeks of life is aimed at protection of the central nervous system — through, for example, protection from hypoxia, hypoglycemia, and hyperbilirubinemia and adequate provision for nutritional needs and sensory stimulation.

In addition to protecting the infant from further problems, a second major goal is meeting the family's needs. We have made much progress since Dr. Martin Cooney exhibited premature babies in incubators at fairs in the United States (Fig. 8–1) and England following a demonstration of his *Kinderbrutanstalt* (child hatchery) at the Berlin Exposition of 1896. After traveling, Cooney settled down on Coney Island, where he raised more than 5000 premature infants during a 39-year period. Mothers did not participate in caring for the babies that were exhibited. (They did get free passes, however, so they could come and see them.) It is interesting to note that sometimes Cooney had difficulty persuading the mothers to take their infants back when they had matured.

Cooney's practices were reflected for many years in the custom of excluding parents from "premature nurseries," a custom that is fortunately rare today. Meeting family needs is more than allowing access. Nursing goals include the facilitation of attachment, the preservation of intact families, and the education of parents (Chapter 10).

Special Needs Based on Gestational Age

PRETERM INFANTS

Infants born prior to 38 weeks gestation are considered *preterm* infants. The word *premature* is used infrequently today because the old definition of a premature infant, i.e., an infant weighing less than 2500 g, is now inappropriate. A baby weighing less than 2500 g may be a term baby or even a postterm baby who is small for gestational age (SGA).

Preterm infants differ from term infants in a number of ways, but it is important to remember that they also differ markedly from one another. Few infants born before 24 weeks gestation survive. Infants between 24 and 30 weeks gestation (generally 500 to 1500 g in birth weight) are frequently critically ill (although not invariably) and require intensive care. Infants with a gestational age of 31 to 36 weeks, who weigh 1500 g or more if they are appropriate for gestational age (AGA), also require specialized care (Table 8–1). If the mortality of this group is compared with the mortality of severely premature infants (24 to 30 weeks gestation), there is a marked difference in prognosis.

Infants of 37 to 38 weeks gestation, sometimes referred to as "borderline prematures," frequently receive care in a nursery for term infants. Yet these infants may still have mild temperature instability and may feed slowly and become jaundiced. If delivered by cesarean section, approximately 8 per cent will develop res-

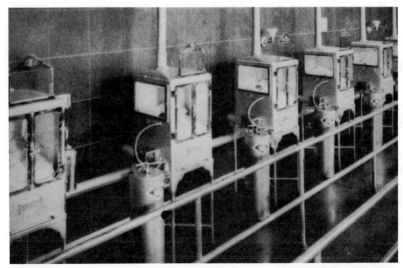

Figure 8–1. Dr. Martin Cooney's exhibit of premature infants at the Chicago World's Fair, 1933. (From Klaus and Kennell: Pediatr Clin North Am *17*:1017, 1970.)

piratory distress syndrome (RDS). Thus, they too require special attention; their needs may be overlooked if nursing observations are not thorough.

Unique Characteristics of Preterm Infants

In comparison with most parents' image of what a new baby should look like (often based on magazine pictures of six-month-old babies), the "premie" falls far short of expectations. In addition to the obvious differences in weight and proportion, the head of this born-too-early baby is large and his body is scrawny. He may also be badly bruised because of the extreme fragility of his capillaries. Such an appearance can be a disappointment to some parents in the first days after birth — a feeling they may voice or keep to them-

Table 8–1   Classification of Preterm Infants by Gestational Age

Gestational Age (weeks)	Birth Weight if AGA (g)	Approximate Percentage of all Births* (%)	Appropriate Neonatal Mortality (% of neonatal deaths)†	Special Problems/Needs
24 to 30	500 to 1500	1	26 weeks: 75 27 weeks: 50 28 weeks: 25	Highly specialized intensive care (see text)
31 to 36	1500 to 2500	6 to 7	31 weeks: 8 32 weeks: 5 36 weeks: 2	Temperature control Cannot suck and swallow before 34 weeks RDS: 12% Hyperbilirubinemia Late metabolic acidosis Hypoglycemia Hypocalcemia Anemia Susceptibility to infection
37 to 38	2500 to 3250	16	2 (1.1% at term)	Occasional temperature instability Slow feeding; tire during feeding Hyperbilirubinemia RDS: Vaginal delivery <1% Cesarean birth 8%

*Overall incidence varies from 7% in white infants to 14 to 15% in nonwhite infants.
†As care of both mothers and infants improves, these figures are changing.

selves, depending on their personalities and how comfortable they feel with the nurses and doctors who care for mother and baby.

Many of the characteristics of preterm infants form the basis for assessment of gestational age as described in Chapter 5. Preterm infants have less flexor muscle tone than infants born at term, so their extremities are frequently extended rather than flexed. The skin is thin, with visible blood vessels; even infants as old as 34 weeks gestational age have relatively little subcutaneous fat because that layer is chiefly deposited in the four weeks prior to term. Because skin is thin, insensible water loss is increased.

The lack of subcutaneous fat is important in planning care. Energy is stored in the body as glycogen and fat. Because the fat and glycogen stores of a preterm baby are practically nonexistent, they will be quickly depleted; the baby will rapidly become hypoglycemic if a source of glucose is not provided.

Thermoregulation is increasingly affected as the weight of the baby decreases; thus the ratio of surface area to body mass increases (see Thermoregulation).

The thin skin of preterm infants is easily broken in the course of everyday care through the use of tape, urine bags, and other devices that come in contact with the baby's skin. Great care must be taken to protect the baby's skin because breaks serve as portals for infection (as well as undoubtedly being uncomfortable for the baby). Small amounts of "paper tape" can be used instead. Diapers can be weighed to measure output to avoid using urine collection bags, and in many cases a specimen can be extracted from the diaper with a syringe. Solvents are available to facilitate the removal of adhesive tape.

The more premature the baby, the larger will be his head in proportion to his body because of the cephalocaudal progression of development. *Lanugo* is abundant on the body of a premature infant. Genitalia are less well developed in premature infants than in term infants. Testes do not descend until the eighth month of fetal life. The labia majora do not cover the labia minora until term approaches.

RESPIRATORY DEVELOPMENT AND FUNCTION

Of all the differences between preterm and term infants, none is more significant than the development of the respiratory tract. This is the crucial difference between viability and nonviability in a preterm infant. Prior to 26 to 28 weeks gestation, there is limited development of the alveoli (the tiny air sacs at the terminal ends of the respiratory system through which oxygen and carbon dioxide are exchanged) and the alveolar capillaries. Within the alveoli are two types of cells: Type I cells, which give structure to the alveolus, and Type II cells, which produce several compounds collectively termed *surfactant*. The most abundant of the surfactant compounds, accounting for 50 to 70 per cent of surfactant, is *lecithin*. It is the function of lecithin and the other surfactant compounds to prevent the collapse of the alveoli on expiration. When surfactant production is inadequate, respiratory distress syndrome (RDS) results.

Preterm infants also differ from term infants in their breathing; respirations are more irregular in preterm infants, with periodic apnea. Both the relative weakness of the respiratory muscles and the decreased rigidity of the thoracic cage lead to hypoventilation, which results in the retention of carbon dioxide and subsequent acidosis. The treatment of respiratory distress in preterm infants is directed toward the correction of these problems.

Respiratory complications may also arise because of the weak cough and gag reflexes of preterm babies, which increase the possibility of aspiration.

GASTROINTESTINAL DEVELOPMENT AND FUNCTION

Gastrointestinal motility is decreased in preterm infants; stools may be infrequent, with abdominal distention. Glycerin suppositories will usually stimulate defecation. For a small preterm infant, a small piece of a suppository is shaped in the nurse's warm hands before insertion.

The sucking and swallowing reflexes of the baby born before 34 weeks gestation are not sufficiently coordinated to allow direct feeding from breast or bottle; alternate feeding methods are necessary. In addition, the immature digestive system of the preterm baby makes certain dietary adjustments necessary. Not only must the types of carbohydrate, fat, and protein given be adapted to the special needs of the preterm baby, but factors such as renal solute load must be considered (Chapter 9).

Liver Development and Function

The liver of a preterm infant is relatively less mature than that of a term infant; this increases the likelihood of hyperbilirubinemia. Great care must be taken when drugs that must be excreted through the liver are administered.

When the liver is immature there is a decreased ability to conjugate bilirubin (i.e., convert indirect bilirubin to direct bilirubin). This is one factor in the increased incidence of hyperbilirubinemia in preterm infants. Another factor that may be equally or more significant is the decreased number of Y and Z carrier proteins in the liver cells, to which bilirubin must bind in the conjugation process. If the level of protein is low (as when blood volume is decreased) or if other substances are competing for binding sites (when the baby is acidotic or receiving certain drugs), there is a danger of kernicterus even when total bilirubin levels may not be excessively high because of the higher level of unconjugated bilirubin free to enter brain cells.

An increased susceptibility to bruising in preterm infants, which leads to increased red blood cell destruction, and delayed feeding, which may allow reabsorption of bilirubin from the bowel, also increase the risk of hyperbilirubinemia. In addition, any condition that leads to lower levels of albumin in the infant, such as decreased blood volume, decreases the number of available sites for bilirubin to bind to albumin and thus allows greater circulation of unconjugated bilirubin.

For all these reasons, serum bilirubin is monitored closely in preterm infants. The treatment of hyperbilirubinemia is discussed later in this chapter.

Cardiovascular Development and Function

The transition from fetal to adult circulation, described in Chapter 5, is sensitive to the increased level of oxygen in the baby's circulatory system following his initial respiration. When oxygen levels are low, fetal circulation may persist; particularly frequent in the small preterm infant is a persistent patent (open) ductus arteriosus (PDA) or an intermittent PDA. A distinct murmur caused by the rush of blood through the PDA can be heard on auscultation and should be assessed along with vital signs. If the ductus arteriosus remains open, the baby's condition will usually deteriorate.

Renal Development and Function

Because of a reduced glomerular filtration rate, preterm infants are more likely to retain fluid and to excrete drugs poorly than term infants. Moreover, when blood pressure is low, kidney perfusion and, therefore, urinary output will be diminished. When body water is low, however, the kidneys are not able to concentrate urine to conserve water, so the baby may become easily dehydrated.

Within the renal tubules themselves both reduced absorption and reduced secretion may occur. Reduced absorption of glucose and amino acids means that glucose and protein may be spilled into the urine at lower serum levels than in more mature infants or older children. Metabolic acidosis is more likely because of the decreased ability to retain bicarbonate. Reduced secretion in the tubules, like reduced glomerular filtration rate, limits drug clearance. The doses of medication given to preterm infants are very small, but they may accumulate in the body nevertheless.

In the infants with a gestational age of less than 29 to 30 weeks, abnormal fluid retention with pedal edema and, later, more generalized edema may occur. Pulmonary congestion may follow. Furosemide (Lasix) (1 mg/kg of body weight) is the preferred treatment, along with some restriction of fluids (see Chapter 9).

IMMUNOLOGICAL COMPETENCE

Immunological competence refers to the ability of an organism to resist infection. Immunological competence involves cellular factors such as white blood cells, factors that enhance the ability of white blood cells to destroy bacteria, and immunoglobulins such as IgG, IgM, and IgA. For a variety of reasons white blood cells are less effective in their action in the preterm infant. Moreover, the amount of immunoglobulin IgG available, which crosses the placenta and provides the newborn with immunity against certain infections to which his mother is immune (e.g., diphtheria, measles, tetanus), is limited because transplacental passage occurs primarily in the third trimester. IgA, the primary immunoglobulin of colostrum, is not available to the baby who does not receive breast milk (many preterm babies do not).

THERMOREGULATION

The basic need for warmth at birth and the basic mechanisms of heat loss have been described in Chapter 5. For healthy term infants, normal room temperature and light clothing and blankets usually provide sufficient warmth following the transition period. When infants are preterm, small for gestational age, or ill, thermoreg-

ulation requires meticulous care based on an understanding of both neonatal physiology and the principles of physics.

Temperature assessment in the newborn Axillary temperature should be used to assess infant warmth. Besides the potential damage to the rectal mucosa and the vagal stimulation that the frequent taking of rectal temperatures may cause, skin temperature varies more rapidly than core temperature and gives an earlier indication of hypothermia or hyperthermia, thus allowing earlier intervention to correct the cause. Axillary temperature is approximately 0.3° C (0.5° F) higher than skin temperature.

When the baby's temperature is unstable, axillary assessment may need to be as frequent as every 15 minutes. As infants recover, temperature as well as other vital signs may be monitored every two to four hours.

Thermoneutral environment A thermoneutral environment is one in which the infant's metabolism is at a minimum and his thermoregulation is achieved by nonevaporative methods (Bligh and Johnson 1973). An environment that maintains the infant's abdominal skin temperature at 36.5° C (97.8° F) is considered a thermoneutral environment. The temperature range of a thermoneutral environment varies with the gestational age, the chronological age, and the weight of the baby and the relative humidity of the environment. Table 8–2 combines age and weight to calculate thermoneutral environmental temperatures.

Providing a thermoneutral environment The incubator and the radiant warmer are the two principal means of providing a thermoneutral environment for the infant.

INCUBATOR   The *incubator* uses the principle of convection to provide heat — currents of warm air surround the infant. Most incubators currently available are single-walled. Room temperature affects incubator wall temperature; if the incuba-

Table 8–2 Thermoneutral Environmental Temperatures*

Age and Weight	Starting Temperature (°C)	Temperature Range (°C)
0–6 hours		
Under 1200 gm	35.0	34.0–35.4
1200–1500 gm	34.1	33.9–34.4
1501–2500 gm	33.4	32.8–33.8
Over 2500 gm (and >36 weeks)†	32.9	32.0–33.8
6–12 hours		
Under 1200 gm	35.0	34.0–35.4
1200–1500 gm	34.0	33.5–34.4
1501–2500 gm	33.1	32.2–33.8
Over 2500 gm (and >36 weeks)†	32.8	31.4–33.8
12–24 hours		
Under 1200 gm	34.0	34.0–35.4
1200–1500 gm	33.8	33.3–34.3
1501–2500 gm	32.8	31.8–33.8
Over 2500 gm (and >36 weeks)†	32.4	31.0–33.7
24–36 hours		
Under 1200 gm	34.0	34.0–35.0
1200–1500 gm	33.6	33.1–34.2
1501–2500 gm	32.6	31.6–33.6
Over 2500 gm (and >36 weeks)†	32.1	30.7–33.5
36–48 hours		
Under 1200 gm	34.0	34.0–35.0
1200–1500 gm	33.5	33.0–34.1
1501–2500 gm	32.5	31.4–33.5
Over 2500 gm (and >36 weeks)†	31.9	30.5–33.3
48–72 hours		
Under 1200 gm	34.0	34.0–35.0
1200–1500 gm	33.5	33.0–34.0
1501–2500 gm	32.3	31.2–33.4
Over 2500 gm (and >36 weeks)†	31.7	30.1–33.2
72–96 hours		
Under 1200 gm	34.0	34.0–35.0
1200–1500 gm	33.5	33.0–34.0
1501–2500 gm	32.2	31.1–33.2
Over 2500 gm (and >36 weeks)†	31.3	29.8–32.8
4–12 days		
Under 1500 gm	33.5	33.0–34.0
1501–2500 gm	32.1	31.0–33.2
Over 2500 gm (and >36 weeks)†		
4–5 days	31.0	29.5–32.6
5–6 days	30.9	29.4–32.3
6–8 days	30.6	29.0–32.2
8–10 days	30.3	29.0–31.8
10–12 days	30.1	29.0–31.4
12–14 days		
Under 1500 gm	33.5	32.6–34.0
1501–2500 gm	32.1	31.0–33.2
Over 2500 gm (and >36 weeks)†	29.8	29.0–30.8
2–3 weeks		
Under 1500 gm	33.1	32.2–34.0
1501–2500 gm	31.7	30.5–33.0
3–4 weeks		
Under 1500 gm	32.6	31.6–33.6
1501–2500 gm	31.4	30.0–32.7
4–5 weeks		
Under 1500 gm	32.0	31.2–33.0
1501–2500 gm	30.9	29.5–32.2
5–6 weeks		
Under 1500 gm	31.4	30.6–32.3
1501–2500 gm	30.4	29.0–31.8

*Adapted from Scopes and Ahmed: Arch Dis Child 47:417, 1966 *In* Klaus and Fanaroff: Care of the High-Risk Neonate. 2nd Edition. W. B. Saunders, 1979, p. 102. Scopes had the walls of the incubator 1 to 2° warmer than the ambient air temperatures.

Generally speaking, the smaller infants in each weight group will require a temperature in the higher portion of the temperature range. Within each time range, the younger the infant, the higher the temperature required.

†Gestational age.

tor wall is cool, the baby will suffer radiant heat loss. A plastic shield can be placed between the baby and the wall of the incubator to conserve heat. The baby will then radiate heat to the wall of the shield, which is the same temperature as the air within the incubator, rather than to the cooler wall of the incubator. One or two oxygen hoods placed over the baby can serve as a shield. Very tiny infants who have great difficulty maintaining temperature may be placed on a K-pad covered with a blanket.

When the infant is in an incubator, the incubator temperature should be recorded along with the baby's temperature (some means of distinguishing the two, such as circling the incubator temperature, is necessary). Incubator temperature (or the set point of the servomechanism on the radiant warmer) will indicate the degree of warmth needed to maintain the baby's temperature at the desired level, which is important because the baby's axillary temperature may vary little, particularly when an Infant Servo-Control (ISC) monitor is used. A continuing rise in incubator temperature indicates a drop in the baby's temperature; the reverse is also true.

Incubator temperature may be controlled by an ISC monitor or by manually adjusting the temperature. When an ISC sensor probe is used, it is securely taped to the infant's abdomen or back in the area of the liver (because of the liver's high metabolic activity). The probe should be on the infant's back when he is lying on his abdomen and vice versa. The sensor probe is set at 37° C (98.6° F). If no probe is used, incubator temperature should be set to maintain a thermoneutral environment (see Table 8–2).

A major disadvantage of an incubator, particularly when an infant is ill and needs frequent attention, is the change in environmental temperature each time the doors are opened. If the doors must remain open for a period of time (e.g., when starting an IV), some additional means of providing warmth will be necessary. Examples include using a radiant warmer, placing a 40-watt bulb in a gooseneck lamp approximately 18 inches from the baby, wrapping the extremities, and covering the head with a cap (Fig. 8–2), and/or using a K-pad. Frequent assessment of skin temperature (at the axilla) is essential to prevent either chilling or overheating.

One major advantage of an incubator is the lower level of insensible water loss in comparison with the baby under a radiant warmer.

RADIANT WARMER   An overhead radiant warmer provides radiant heat through infrared heat rays that are absorbed by the skin and warm the peripheral blood; heat is transferred to deep structures by conduction and the circulation of peripheral blood. Whereas some warmers produce continuous heat and can be controlled only manually, others offer the option of Infant Servo-Control (ISC), just as some incubators do.

Some nurses place great reliance on radiant warmers with manual control. The potential problems with these warmers, however, are serious. Hyperthermia and even burns may occur when output is high. Low output may produce heat insufficient to prevent hypothermia. Unless the baby can be observed constantly, a skin temperature sensor (ISC) must be used in conjunction with the radiant warmer. The skin sensor should be covered with gauze or a folded piece of tape to insulate the sensor from the heat of the warmer, which can interfere with its proper functioning. There must be nothing else between the baby and the warmer. Even bending over the baby to give care may interpose the caregiver's head and shoulders between

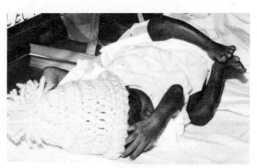

Figure 8–2. A hat, easily made by the family or made from stockinet, will decrease heat loss.

the probe and the warmer and thus interfere with its function. Care in placing the baby in the bed beneath the warmer is important; not all of his bed will be warmed by the rays. The baby may be on his abdomen, side, or back, but the sensor probe must always be uppermost, never beneath the baby.

Most radiant warmers have alarm systems that give auditory and visual signals when the temperature is outside the present range of 36° to 37° C (96.8 to 98.6° F). It is easy to turn off the alarm and forget to turn it on again, a potentially serious error.

Radiant warmers offer the advantage of easy access to the baby for caregiving. In addition, a barrier between parents and baby is removed. The importance of early touching of the baby by his parents is widely recognized (Chapter 10). Yet many parents are hesitant to reach into the "box" (incubator). They seem less reluctant to hold the baby's hand or stroke him in an open bed.

There are also disadvantages to care in an open bed with a radiant warmer. Infection control may be more difficult. There is sometimes a tendency to touch the baby without the proper preliminary hand washing. This can be overcome with proper teaching. A major disadvantage, especially for the small preterm baby, is an increase in insensible water loss (Chapter 9), which can lead to dehydration. A number of studies have shown marked increases in insensible water loss from both radiant warmers and phototherapy (Wu and Hodgman 1974; Yek, Vidyasagar, and Pildes 1975; Jones, Rochefort, and Baum 1976; Oh et al. 1976). Wu and Hodgman found that insensible water loss increased from 50 to 190 per cent, depending on the size of the infant and the type of warmer. The greatest losses were seen in infants weighing less than 1500 g.

Heat production There are three basic mechanisms of heat production in humans: shivering thermogenesis, nonshivering thermogenesis, and voluntary muscle activity. Nonshivering thermo-genesis is the principal means of heat production in the newborn.

Nonshivering thermogenesis occurs when norepinephrine stimulates the metabolism of brown fat. Brown fat, which accounts for 2 to 6 per cent of the body weight in newborns, contains fat vacuoles, mitochondria, and an abundant blood and sympathetic nerve supply. Most brown fat is found between the scapulae at the base of the neck, surrounding the kidneys and adrenal glands, and in the mediastinum. Oxygen is required to metabolize brown fat for energy.

High risk infants may be compromised in heat production in one or more of the following ways:

1. Because brown fat accumulates more rapidly in the third trimester, preterm infants have decreased amounts of brown fat, as do infants who are small for gestational age.

2. Norepinephrine (noradrenalin) release may be decreased in preterm infants (Stern 1965).

3. Because oxygen is required for the metabolism of brown fat, infants who have been or who are hypoxic will have a diminished capacity for heat production. Infants with decreased perfusion will also be limited in their ability to transport oxygen to the necessary areas of heat production.

4. Reduced caloric intake decreases the number of calories available for thermogenesis.

Heat conservation Newborns do make some attempts to conserve heat. A term newborn may assume a flexed position, which diminishes exposed surface area. Preterm infants, however, have difficulty conserving heat by changing body posture. Peripheral vasoconstriction is a second mechanism of heat conservation.

Heat loss Not only is heat production limited in high risk newborns, but heat loss is increased. Two major factors in infant heat loss are the ratio of skin surface to body mass and the lack of subcutaneous fat. Both of these factors become increasingly important as the baby's weight decreases. In addition, the normal position of a preterm infant (extension rather than flexion) allows for greater heat loss. The transfusion of blood that has not been warmed and the feeding of formula directly from the refrigerator may be sources of chilling, also contributing to heat loss. (Although most formulas used in nurseries today are stored at room temperature and need no warming, breast milk and some special formulas are refrigerated). The basic mechanisms of heat loss are summarized in Table 8–3, along with nursing intervention to prevent heat loss.

Cold stress   A change of as little as 2° C (3.6° F) from a thermoneutral environment can produce profound changes in an infant. Increased production of norepinephrine along with peripheral vasoconstric-

tion leads to the cycle shown in Figure 8–3 and ultimately to brain damage from hypoxia or death if intervention does not occur. Note that, once begun, the cycle is self-sustaining. Pulmonary vasoconstriction can cause hypoxia directly as less blood circulates through the lung or by increasing pulmonary artery pressure, thereby shunting blood from the pulmonary (right heart) circulation to the systemic (left heart) circulation through the foramen ovale and ductus arteriosus (which may remain patent or may reopen when PaO_2 is low). Pulmonary vasoconstriction can also cause hypoxia through an effect on the alveolar cells of the infant's lungs, thereby reducing surfactant production and initiating or exacerbating respiratory distress syndrome (RDS).

In addition to direct respiratory effects, the loss of heat indirectly requires an

Table 8–3   Heat Loss in Newborns

Type of Heat Loss	Mechanism	Conditions Contributing to Heat Loss	Nursing Intervention
Conduction	Conduction to surfaces that skin touches	Cool temperature of contact surfaces Thermal conductivity of material of contact surfaces	Avoid placing infant on cold surfaces (e.g., scales, x-ray plates, examining tables); pad with a warm diaper or blanket
Evaporation	1. Insensible evaporation from skin	Insensible evaporation accounts for 25% of heat loss	Maintain relative humidity of 50 to 80%
	2. Evaporation of moisture on skin (e.g., amniotic fluid, bath water)	Increased skin permeability leads to insensible water loss and thus evaporative heat loss	Keep skin dry Do not bathe baby unless temperature is stable
	3. Evaporation from the mucosa of respiratory tract	Tachypnea increases rate of heat loss from respiratory tract	Bathe and dry only small area at a time Warm any soaks or solutions applied to skin; keep warm
Convection	1. Air moving over the skin	Exposure to currents of air, including oxygen that has not been warmed and humidified	Avoid currents of air moving across skin
	2. Warm air expired during respiration 3. Conduction of heat to skin surface	Thermal sensors on face and forehead are sensitive to cold even when rest of body is warm	Warm and humidify oxygen When infant must leave nursery (e.g., for surgery) transport in prewarmed incubator
Radiation	Transfer from infant's skin to surrounding environment	Difference between skin temperature and environment (e.g., walls of single-walled incubator) Total radiating surface of infant; the smaller the infant the greater the surface area in relation to weight and thus the greater his loss Large surface area of infant's head exacerbates loss	Raise incubator air temperature to 36°C Clothe infant when possible Keep infant's bed away from outside walls and out of drafts Use a heat shield in incubator Swaddle Put on cap or bonnet (nearly doubles insulating effect of infant's own tissues)

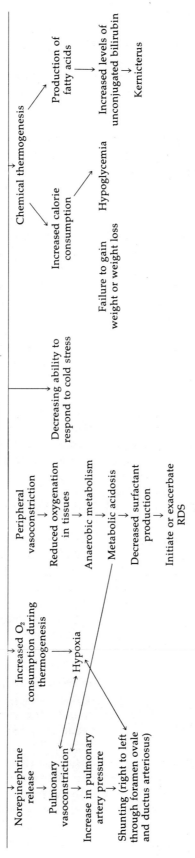

Figure 8–3. The cold stress cycle.

increase in calories that may be difficult to supply; because of increased fatty acids and H_2 ions that bind to albumin and decrease binding sites, this increase in calories may lead to increased levels of unconjugated bilirubin and kernicterus (see Hyperbilirubinemia).

SIGNS OF COLD STRESS   Clinical signs that an infant is experiencing cold stress are summarized in Table 8–4. Many of these signs are general in that they may result from problems other than cold stress. Bright red skin color is due to the effect of low temperature on oxyhemoglobin dissociation, i.e., oxygen remains bound to hemoglobin. *Sclerema* is a hardening of the skin seen in babies with sepsis and those who are moribund as well as infants with cold stress.

WARMING A COLD-STRESSED INFANT   It is far better to prevent cold stress than to treat it. Once the baby is cold, warming should occur slowly. Klaus and Fanaroff (1979) suggest that air temperature should be about 1.5° C (2.5° F) warmer than abdominal skin temperature, because oxygen consumption is minimal at this temperature gradient. A rapid increase in body temperature may produce apnea (Perlstein, Edwards, and Sutherland, 1970). During the rewarming period careful attention must be given to correcting the other problems produced by cold stress such as metabolic acidosis and hypoglycemia. Axillary temperature should be checked every 15 minutes during the rewarming period and the

Table 8–4 Signs of Cold Stress

Failure to feed well
Lethargy
Slow, shallow, irregular respirations
Bradycardia
Bright red or rosy skin color, cyanosis, or pallor
Poor cry
Edema (especially of face and extremities)
Sclerema
Oliguria
Diminished or absent reflexes
Hypoglycemia
Metabolic acidosis
Hyperkalemia

environmental temperature adjusted accordingly until skin temperature reaches 36.5° C (97.8° F).

Hyperthermia   When an infant's skin temperature exceeds 36.5° C (97.8° F), metabolic activity and thus oxygen and glucose consumption increase as when he is cold. Excessive environmental temperature is a major cause of hyperthermia. When either the incubator or the radiant warmer is controlled manually, hyperthermia can result. The use of phototherapy lights or extra lighting for procedures, or sun shining on an incubator may produce overheating if a servomechanism is not utilized. If the servosensor probe is not taped securely to the skin or if it becomes detached, the warming unit may continue to produce heat.

Other causes of hyperthermia include dehydration and problems in central nervous system functioning resulting from injury or drugs. Infection may cause hyperthermia, but changes in body temperature during infection are much more variable in infants than in older children and adults. Hypothermia may also be a response to sepsis.

POSTTERM INFANTS

From four to nine infants in every 100 are born following pregnancies of 300 days or longer (more than 42 weeks). The reason for delay in the onset of labor is not clearly understood.

Although many of these infants appear healthy and normal, others have characteristics that have come to be associated with postmaturity. Some of these characteristics appear to be related to a decreased ability of the aging placenta to nourish the baby. Loss of subcutaneous tissue is apparent; hypoglycemia may be more common and is related to this loss of tissue. Muscles may appear wasted. The baby is long and thin with dry, cracking skin. Vernix may be absent; skin cord and membranes may have a green-yellow staining. The likelihood of birth asphyxia and meconium aspiration increases.

Mortality rates increase after 42 weeks gestation. For this reason, some obstetricians choose elective induction in mothers with prolonged pregnancy.

Following birth, early oral feeding and/or intravenous gluocse is started to avoid hypoglycemia. Glucose levels should be monitored. If the infant requires resuscitation, care is planned as for any infant with respiratory difficulty.

INFANTS WHO ARE SMALL FOR GESTATIONAL AGE

Infants whose weight is less than the tenth percentile for their gestational age are called *small for gestational age* (SGA); other terms include *intrauterine growth retarded* (IUGR) and *light-for-date.*

About one-third of all babies weighing less than 2500 g are term infants who are SGA. Preterm and postterm infants may also be SGA. Inadequate weight gain in the mother, intrauterine infection, maternal smoking or heroin addiction, any condition that compromises placental functioning, and chromosomal abnormalities are some of the major causes of failure of the fetus to gain adequate weight (Chapter 3). A woman who has already delivered an SGA infant is more likely to have a subsequent low birth weight infant than a woman who has not. Thus, the relationship between birth weight and gestational age is an important aspect of maternal history in every pregnancy.

Table 8–5 summarizes some problems common to many SGA babies and the nursing interventions appropriate to those problems. If the infant is both preterm and SGA, the problems of prematurity will be added to those of growth retardation. Because SGA infants have a higher incidence of birth asphyxia, which requires immediate attention at delivery, recognizing intrauterine growth retardation prior to delivery is important. Assessment of fundal height and biparietal diameter during pregnancy aids in the identification of babies who may be SGA.

Hypoglycemia and thermoregulation are both related to a lack of tissue and involve decreased carbohydrate stores and a decreased amount of brown fat for thermogenesis. The reason for polycythemia is unknown; it may be related to intrauterine hypoxia. These problems are most critical in the first three to four days of life; it is then that babies need specialized care.

INFANTS WHO ARE LARGE FOR GESTATIONAL AGE

Preterm, term, or postterm infants may be large for gestational age (LGA). A major problem of the preterm baby who is LGA

Table 8–5 Nursing Interventions for Common Problems of SGA Infants

Problem	Intervention
Birth asphyxia	Recognition of intrauterine growth retardation prior to delivery
Meconium aspiration	Preparation for resuscitation at delivery
Aspiration pneumonia	Careful observation postdelivery for signs of
Pneumothorax	respiratory distress
Pneumomediastinum	
Pulmonary hemorrhage	
Hypoglycemia	Blood sugar concentrations monitored
	Intravenous glucose if necessary
Hypocalcemia	Serum calcium monitored
	Supplemental calcium if necessary
Difficulties in thermal regulation	Careful attention to thermoneutral environment
Polycythemia	Assessment of hematocrit
	Exchange transfusion may be required
Increased incidence of congenital malformations	Careful assessment to detect anomalies not readily apparent

is that his immaturity and the problems associated with it are not readily recognized because of his size. He may, for example, have RDS or a hyperbilirubinemia level that might be expected for his gestational age but is not usually associated with a baby of his size. His sucking reflex is appropriate to his age rather than his size, his ability to maintain his temperature in an open bed may be poor, and his muscle tone may be diminished (again appropriate to age but not size); for all these reasons he may be falsely regarded as ill.

For reasons that are unknown, infants with transposition of the great vessels tend to be LGA.

Infants of diabetic mothers (IDM), particularly diabetic mothers whose disease has not been in good control during the last trimester of pregnancy, are typically LGA. When delivered at 37 weeks, they may weigh 9 or 10 lbs. (About 10 per cent of the infants of Class D through F diabetic mothers are SGA and resemble infants with placental insufficiency.) The increased size of the large IDM is due to fat (and not to edema as once believed) through a process described in the discussion of glucose metabolism. Characteristically, the large IDM baby is sleek and plethoric, lying quietly, moving very little, and crying infrequently. Not only the baby but also the cord and placenta are oversized.

With very careful control of the mother's diabetes, especially in the last weeks of pregnancy, some mothers with diabetes can deliver babies who do not have this classic appearance and who have decreased neonatal mortality as well. Although fetal and neonatal death rates are still higher for all IDMs (except those of Class A diabetic mothers) than for infants of nondiabetic mothers, neonatal mortality of IDMs has decreased from 40 to 10 per cent.

The IDM needs careful nursing observation in the first hours and days of life. Major potential problems are hypoglycemia, hypocalcemia, hyperbilirubinemia, and respiratory distress. The incidence of

congenital anomalies is also higher in these babies.

About 50 per cent of IDMs may become *hypoglycemic* in the first six hours after birth, probably because of the following sequence. Diabetic mothers whose disease is not well controlled are hyperglycemic. The excess sugar, like other nutrients in maternal blood, crosses the placental barrier, causing hyperglycemia in the infant as well. To metabolize this excess sugar, the islets of Langerhans in the fetal pancreas hypertrophy to secrete increased amounts of insulin. The sugar is converted to glycogen and stored as excess fat, hence the large size of the baby. When the baby is born, he is removed from the source of his sugar but his pancreas continues to work for several hours and thus he becomes hypoglycemic. The more closely the mother's blood sugar can be kept within normal limits during her pregnancy, the less likely her baby is to develop hypoglycemia following delivery. The higher the maternal blood sugar, the greater the infant's problem may be.

Most IDMs will have a transient hypoglycemia, lasting from one to four hours, after which the blood sugar level will begin to rise. In a few infants the hypoglycemia will be prolonged and severe.

Blood sugar levels must be closely monitored (at least hourly). Waiting for clinical signs of hypoglycemia to appear (tremors, apnea, cyanosis, limpness, failure to feel well, convulsions) would seem to violate standards of good care. Treatment for hypoglycemia is a constant, slow infusion of 10 to 15 per cent glucose. (Rapid infusion of 25 to 50 per cent glucose is contraindicated because insulin production is increased as a response, with a subsequent drop in blood sugar.)

An increased incidence of *hypocalcemia* has been reported in IDMs; tremors are the most obvious clinical signs. *Hyperbilirubinemia* at 48 to 72 hours occurs more frequently in IDMs than in normal infants of comparable weight or gestational age.

The incidence of RDS is also increased in babies of Class A through C diabetic mothers. Apparently, high levels of insulin produced by the baby interfere with the synthesis of lecithin, which is necessary for lung maturation. In the Class D, E, or F diabetic mother, in whom the intrauterine environment is even less favorable, the stress resulting from poor blood supply to the uterus may lead to increased

production of steroids and thus acceleration of lung maturation.

Because IDMs have more fatty tissue than most babies in the nursery, their temperature must be monitored carefully; they may become hyperthermic if a servocontrol is not used (see Thermoregulation).

Special Needs Based on Respiration Disorders

Respiratory difficulty in a newborn may be due to one or more factors. Respiratory tract problems, central nervous system disorders, metabolic disruptions, acute blood loss, and a variety of congenital abnormalities as varied as diaphragmatic hernia and congenital heart disease may all result in respiratory difficulty (Table 8–6).

RESPIRATORY DISTRESS SYNDROME

The most common of all respiratory tract diseases in newborns both in the United States and throughout the world is respiratory distress syndrome (RDS), also called hyaline membrane disease (HMD). RDS occurs in approximately 0.5 to 1.0 per cent of all deliveries and in approximately 10 per cent of all preterm deliveries. In a hospital delivering 400 infants a month, from two to four infants each month could be expected to have respiratory distress syndrome. The incidence will most likely be higher, of course, in major medical centers to which large numbers of high risk mothers are referred in premature labor.

The Physiology of RDS

The lungs develop more slowly in the fetus than many other organ systems. The alveoli, the tiny air sacs at the terminal ends of the respiratory system through

which oxygen and carbon dioxide are exchanged, are not developed until 26 to 28 weeks gestational age. Alveolar capillaries, necessary for gas exchange between the alveoli and blood, develop at 28 weeks.

Lining the alveoli are Type I and Type II cells. A fatty soaplike substance called *surfactant* (actually a collective name given to several compounds) is produced in the Type II cells and enables the alveoli to remain open during exhalation when the amount of air pressure in the lungs is

Table 8–6 Sources of Respiratory Distress in Newborns*

Pulmonary
  Respiratory distress syndrome (RDS)
  Transient tachypnea
  Meconium aspiration
  Pneumothorax
  Pulmonary infection, hemorrhage
  Wilson-Mikity syndrome
Extrapulmonary
  Central nervous system
    Hemorrhage
    Drugs (including those administered to mother during labor/delivery)
    Edema
  Cardiovascular
    Congenital heart disease
    Persistent fetal circulation
    Blood loss
    Hyperviscosity
  Metabolic
    Metabolic acidosis
    Hypoglycemia
    Hypothermia

*Adapted, in part, from Klaus and Fanaroff: Care of the High-Risk Neonate. 2nd Edition. W. B. Saunders, 1979.

decreased. Lecithin is the most abundant of the compounds, accounting for 50 to 70 per cent of surfactant. Lecithin production begins at about the twenty-second to the twenty-fourth week of gestation. (The assessment of the presence of lecithin and another compound, sphingomyelin, in the fetus has been described in Chapter 4.)

The production of surfactant is impaired in RDS. When the baby exhales, the alveoli collapse. Lung compliance is decreased, i.e., the lung becomes "stiff," and the work of breathing is increased. In addition, there is diminished gas exchange: oxygen cannot be effectively delivered to the blood stream nor can carbon dioxide be removed for exhalation. As Po_2 (partial pressure of oxygen in the blood stream) decreases, pulmonary vasoconstriction occurs, further compromising oxygenation.

The baby works hard to compensate for the physiological problems associated with RDS. The *audible grunt*, which is a distinct symptom, results from the baby's attempt to keep the alveoli from collapsing. The glottis closes to prolong expiration and thus allow a better diffusion of the inspired oxygen across the alveolar membrane. Marked *retractions* (intercostal, suprasternal, substernal, and sternal) demonstrate intense respiratory effort to overcome lung stiffness. *Tachypnea* (a respiratory rate greater than 60 breaths per minute) is an attempt to move air in and out more rapidly. When these efforts are unsuccessful, cyanosis results from lack of oxygen; respiratory acidosis and subsequently metabolic acidosis occur.

The aim of nursing care is to prevent deterioration of the baby's respiratory effort by early and appropriate intervention until he is able to produce lecithin at a rate sufficient to prevent alveolar collapse. Such care includes provision of a thermoneutral environment, maintenance of adequate respiration, therapy to combat acidosis, and provision of fluids and nutrition (Chapter 9). The baby must be closely observed and carefully cared for by nurses throughout this critical period.

Maintenance of Respiration

Although neither oxygen nor assisted ventilation is a cure for RDS, these treatments may enable the baby to survive until he is able to begin surfactant production on his own. The amount of oxygen given to the baby (the FIO_2 or fraction of inspired oxygen) is dependent upon the arterial oxygen concentration (PaO_2) of the baby. If the PaO_2 is greater than 90 to 100, there is a risk of retrolental fibroplasia and/or pulmonary oxygen toxicity. At Pao_2 levels of less than 50, pulmonary blood vessels constrict, further hindering gas exchange in the alveoli. Brain damage may occur at PaO_2 levels below 40. The level of FIO_2 necessary to maintain PaO_2 levels between 50 and 90 will vary not only from baby to baby but from hour to hour in the same baby. Thus, the assessment of oxygenation in the baby, and not merely in the baby's environment, is critical.

Assessment of Oxygenation

Adequate oxygenation in an infant may be assessed by (1) observing the color of the trunk, face, and mucous membranes of the mouth, (2) determining the PaO_2 in blood samples, or (3) monitoring PaO_2 continuously via catheter or transcutaneous monitor.

Color is the least valuable means of assessment and should be relied on only for short periods (e.g., during transport) when other means of assessment may not be available. Oxygen is provided at a level that just prevents visible cyanosis of the mucous membranes of the mouth. Cyanosis of the extremities is not a useful guide in newborns because acrocyanosis is not unusual in otherwise healthy infants.

Blood may be obtained from an umbilical artery catheter, the right radial artery, or a heel capillary that has been sufficiently warmed to "arterialize" the specimen (i.e., wrapping the baby's foot in a warm diaper for five minutes to increase the blood flow).

The right radial artery rather than the

left is chosen because blood circulates there before reaching the ductus arteriosus; a right-to-left shunt of blood through the ductus arteriosus will affect the PaO_2 in the left radial artery but not the right. PaO_2 in the right radial artery is essentially the same as PaO_2 in the carotid arteries supplying the brain.

When the right radial artery is used for intermittent assessment, pressure is applied for five minutes or until the bleeding stops (whichever is longer) after withdrawing the needle to prevent bleeding. An indwelling radial artery catheter may be inserted in the right radial artery for frequent determinations; this is most commonly done when it is difficult or impossible to perform umbilical artery catheterization.

Capillary blood is of limited value in assessing oxygenation in sick newborns; it is impossible to assess the extent to which this blood is arterialized. Lower values of Po_2 are usually accepted when capillary blood is used (35 to 45 mm Hg), but since one is not really sure what is being measured, this is potentially dangerous. Levels of pH and Pco_2 should not vary in capillary and arterial blood. The amount of blood withdrawn for blood gas determinations should be recorded and the record frequently assessed. In a small baby it is possible to significantly compromise blood volume with the withdrawal of frequent blood specimens.

A third means of assessment in increasing use in intensive care nurseries is continuous measurement of oxygenation, by either intravascular oxygen electrode or transcutaneous oxygen monitor. The transcutaneous oxygen monitor is most widely used.

Transcutaneous oxygen ($tcPo_2$) is oxygen that has diffused from the arterial capillaries near the surface of the skin to the skin surface. Because preterm infants have so little fatty and subcutaneous tissue, $tcPo_2$ measurements and arterial oxygen measurements (PaO_2) have been found to correlate well (Martin and Okken, 1979). The advantage of transcutaneous monitoring is its ability to monitor oxygenation continuously in a noninvasive manner. This is particularly helpful to nurses when they care for infants with respiratory problems. The effects of position change, suctioning, chest bag ventilation, physical therapy, and many other aspects of care can be quickly assessed and care modified for the needs of each baby.

One valuable insight that has come from the use of transcutaneous monitoring is that there is continuing variation in oxygenation as measured by $tcPo_2$ (Fig. 8-4), although these changes are usually within the range of 50 to 90 mm Hg. When the administration of care causes a marked change (either increase or decrease) in tc Po_2 on the print-out, indicating the reason for the change by writing on the strip aids in the overall assessment of the infant's condition.

When a baby has diminished peripheral blood flow because of severe hypotension, $tcPo_2$ is believed to correlate with PaO_2 less closely.

The electrode attached to the baby's

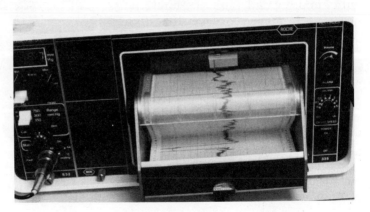

Figure 8-4. A transcutaneous monitor. Note the fluctuation in $tcPo_2$.

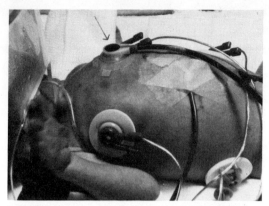

Figure 8–5. The transcutaneous electrode is identified by the arrow. Note the erythematous area lateral to the electrode where the electrode was previously placed.

skin is heated (Fig. 8–5); the proper temperature of the electrode is very important. If the temperature is too low, Po_2 may be underestimated; if the temperature is too high, the baby's thin skin may be burned. As further protection against burns, the electrode is repositioned every four hours. Even with frequent repositioning, a reddened area may appear beneath the electrode, but it will usually disappear within a few hours. This information needs to be shared with parents.

Assessment of $tcPo_2$ obviously is an adjunct to blood sampling, since Pco_2 and pH are not measured. However, the transcutaneous monitoring of Pco_2 is now being evaluated.

Oxygen Therapy

Oxygen given to a baby (or to any patient) must be administered in combination with humidity and warmth. Humidity is necessary to prevent oxygen from drying out the respiratory mucosa. This leads to mucosal crusting, which impedes the normal function of the respiratory cilia and not only makes suctioning the baby difficult but also increases the chance of airway obstruction. Moreover, the crusted mucus provides a medium for bacterial growth.

The need for humidity is one reason warmth is so important. Warm air holds more moisture than cold air. To give warm, moist oxygen to the baby, the gas must be heated to 38.3 to 38.8° C (101 to 102° F) at the oxygen source. Cooling occurs in the tubing that carries the oxygen to the baby; as a consequence, condensation occurs and water is seen in the tubing. Cold air robs the body of water and is an additional source of chilling. Condensed water in the tube must be frequently emptied; this is particularly important when oxygen is given in conjunction with airway pressure, because water will affect the diameter of the tubing and thus the pressure, flow, and tidal volume of the oxygen.

Currently, the most common means of delivering oxygen to babies with respiratory distress are the head hood, continuous positive airway pressure (CPAP), and mechanical ventilation with end expiratory pressure.

OXYGEN BY HOOD

If the baby simply needs to breathe air with a higher concentration of oxygen, a level of fraction of inspired oxygen (Fio_2) of from 80 to 90 per cent can be achieved with a head hood (Fig. 8–6). The hood does not correct CO_2 levels nor does it

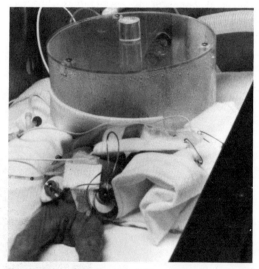

Figure 8–6. A baby receiving oxygen via hood. Note the condensation within the hood caused by the warm, moist oxygen. The opening of the hood around the baby's neck is partially covered to help maintain oxygen concentration.

assist ventilation in any way. Oxygen concentrations in the hood should be checked and charted every 30 minutes with an instrument specifically designed for that purpose. Temperature within the hood should also be monitored every 30 minutes; this area can become quite warm (note the condensation on the hood in Fig. 8–5). Constant observation of the baby's respiratory efforts is essential.

CONTINUOUS POSITIVE AIRWAY
PRESSURE

Because the basic problem in RDS is the tendency of the alveoli to collapse on expiration, it is logical that some form of therapy that prevents this collapse would be of value. This is the principle of continuous positive airway pressure (CPAP). Positive pressure on both inspiration and expiration prevents alveolar collapse and enables oxygen to diffuse into the bloodstream. CPAP has no effect on the elimination of carbon dioxide. If Pco_2 levels are high (as determined by blood gas measurement), periodic bag and mask ventilation may eliminate excess carbon dioxide.

CPAP may be administered through nasal prongs (Fig. 8–7) or by endotracheal tube. In either case the baby continues to

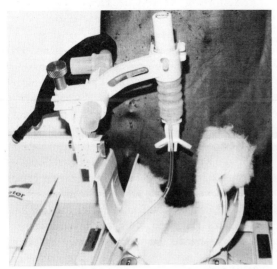

Figure 8–7. One method of delivering nasal CPAP. The baby's head is cradled in sheepskin.

breathe by himself. His respirations are less labored, however, because he is not working against collapsed alveoli.

CPAP is ordered according to pressure (usually from 1 to 10 mm Hg) and FiO_2 level. As already noted, the baby's respiratory effectiveness is closely monitored through blood gas values. If nasal CPAP is used, the prongs must be adjusted so that they do not lie on the baby's lip; the tender skin beneath can easily necrose. As with an older patient receiving oxygen, mouth care with lemon and glycerin is helpful. A newborn's secretions are acidic and should be wiped from his cheeks and neck.

Babies on both CPAP and ventilation should be turned every one to two hours and suctioned at regular intervals; the frequency of suctioning is related to the amount of mucus present.

MECHANICAL VENTILATION WITH END
EXPIRATORY PRESSURE

If the baby is unable to breathe by himself, if PaO_2 is less than 50 when FiO_2 is 100 per cent, or if respiratory acidosis is severe, a mechanical ventilator may assist him. Unlike oxygen by hood and CPAP, mechanical ventilation controls the level of carbon dioxide as well as that of oxygen. Ventilators are either pressure-cycled, volume-cycled, or time-cycled (Table 8–7). The time-cycled ventilator is frequently used in the care of newborns.

There are three possible breathing patterns on most mechanical ventilators used with newborns: assist, assist-control, and control (Fig. 8–8). On *assist* the baby initiates every breath himself. The *assist-control* pattern, or intermittent mandatory ventilation (IMV), allows the baby to initiate his own breathing as often as he is able; if he stops breathing the ventilator will give him a programmed number of breaths per minute. On the *control* setting, the baby has no role in his own respiration; the ventilator breathes for him. *Positive end expiratory pressure* (PEEP) is frequently used in connection with ventilators. PEEP serves the same function

Table 8–7   Classification of Continuous Mechanical Ventilators

Type of Ventilator	Characteristics	Examples
Pressure-cycled	Terminates inspiration when predetermined pressure is reached Volume and time interval may vary	
Volume-cycled	Fixed volume of air with each respiratory cycle Pressure and time interval may vary	Bourns LS 104 Cavitron Siemens-Elema Starling Pump Vickers
Time-cycled	Both inspiratory and expiratory durations may be adjusted Volume and pressure may vary Commonly used in care of infants	Baby Bird Bourns–BP 200 Veriflo

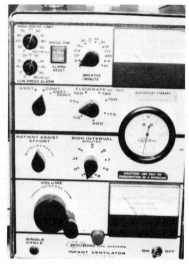

Figure 8–8. A ventilator can be adjusted to meet the specific needs of each baby.

as CPAP; it prevents alveolar collapse on expiration by maintaining positive pressure in the airway.

The infant assisted by a ventilator has an endotracheal tube that is either oral (most frequent) or nasal. Caring for this infant requires nursing skill and continual attention; if the baby is acutely ill a nurse for each baby or one nurse for every two babies is required.

Nursing care for infants on ventilators is summarized in Table 8–8. Changes in management are based on both blood gases and the nurse's clinical observations. Clinical evidence that the baby is doing well includes improved color (pink mucous membranes as well as skin), im-

proved muscle tone, and heart rate and rhythm within normal limits (absence of either tachycardia or bradycardia). When the endotracheal tube is properly placed, breath sounds are bilateral and chest movement is symmetrical. If breath sounds are heard more clearly on one side, the endotracheal tube may be in a main stem bronchus or a pneumothorax may have occurred. If breath sounds are heard over the stomach, the tube may be in the esophagus. Abdominal distention may also indicate esophageal placement, but abdominal distention may also occur with the endotracheal tube in the trachea. For this reason, an indwelling gastric tube is frequently placed when the baby has an endotracheal tube.

Suctioning of mucus from the endotracheal tube is essential; the frequency of suctioning varies with the amount of mucus. Careful sterile technique, including a sterile glove on the hand that holds the catheter, is essential. Preoxygenation of the baby for approximately two minutes with a bag and oxygen at the same FiO_2 the baby is receiving (or a slightly higher concentration) will prevent a rapid drop in Po_2 during the procedure. Sterile saline (0.2 ml) may be placed in the tube prior to suctioning to help liquify secretions. A sterile suction catheter should be used and replaced after each suctioning. Suction should be applied only on the withdrawal of the catheter. The catheter should be put down quickly (remember that the baby receives no oxygen while the suction cather is in the tube) and withdrawn quickly with a slight rotation of the catheter. The entire process from entry to withdrawal should take no more than five to 10 seconds; after 15 seconds apnea and bradycardia may begin. The transcutaneous monitor is helpful during suctioning because $tcPo_2$ can be continually assessed.

Curran and Kachoyeanos (1979) have questioned the value of suctioning in relation to the apparent stress to the baby. Although their study raises some important issues that deserve further nursing research, three points must be made about their procedure: (1) suctioning was of the nasopharynx, which would be highly stressful to anyone; (2) the infants were not oxygenated prior to or following the procedure; and (3) there was no evaluation of blood gas levels reported prior to or following the procedure. In addition, their sample included only six infants; there were no control infants.

Both position change and chest percussion are aids in preventing the accumulation of secretions. Although several meth-

Table 8–8   Caring for an Infant on a Ventilator

Assessment	Comments/Care
Baby	
Blood gases	
Appearance: color, symmetrical movement of chest, abdominal distention	Insert gastric tube to compress stomach
Auscultation: heart rate and rhythm bilateral; equal breath sounds	
Behavior: active with good muscle tone vs lethargic with poor muscle tone	
Secretions: amount, character (thick, blood-tinged, yellow, etc.)	Suction prn Change position every 1 to 2 hours to promote drainage of secretions
Pressure: blanching of gums (oral tube) blanching of nares (nasal tube)	Chest percussion
Signs of occluded tube or extubation: color change, absence of breath sounds or chest movement, apnea, bradycardia, poor muscle tone	If extubated, support with bag and mask ventilation until new tube can be inserted An occluded tube must be removed and a new tube reinserted
Signs of pneumothorax	
Ventilator	
FiO_2 Heart rate End expiratory pressure Peak pressure	Information should be recorded on chart
Alarm on (not all systems have alarms or alarm switches)	
Tubing connected properly	
Oxygen warm	Cold oxygen can chill infant very quickly
Condensed water in tubing	Observe tubing and empty at frequent intervals (water in tubing decreases diameter of tube, increases resistance and pressure in system, and decreases tidal volume)
Sterility of all respiratory equipment	Change sterile tubing and attachments every 24 hours; use only sterile distilled water in the system; perform all procedures, including intubation and suction, under sterile conditions

ods of chest physiotherapy (CPT) are utilized (a hand, a padded nipple, an electric toothbrush with a nipple attached), the electric toothbrush is a gentle method and seems more appropriate for small preterm infants who are easily fatigued (Fig. 8–9). Curran and Kachoyeanos found color, breath sounds, and Po_2 and Pco_2 (24-hour means) to be higher in babies receiving CPT by electric toothbrush, but their small sample size makes it impossible to draw any conclusions. Meier (1979) suggests that CPT is appropriate for those infants with atelectasis, such as infants with RDS, but not for infants who have respiratory symptoms for other reasons (e.g., apnea of prematurity or heart failure). Infants may, of course, have RDS in combination with these other problems; x-ray will indicate the presence of atelectasis. The unanswered question is, will CPT, by preventing the accumulation of secretions, prevent secondary atelectasis?

Meier also suggested that positioning the infant for postural drainage for one minute in each of the positions used for CPT, without using CPT, is effective in aeration. Research to confirm this impression is also essential.

Muscle paralysis for infants on ventilators Some infants, especially larger infants, appear to "fight" mechanical ventilation yet are unable to breathe adequately without assistance. Pancuron-

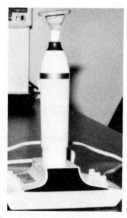

Figure 8–9. An electric toothbrush adapted with a nipple for chest physiotherapy.

ium bromide (Pavulon) or curare may be used to paralyze muscles and allow improved oxygenation and gas exchange. Curare relaxes not only the pulmonary vascular bed but also blood vessels in other parts of the body and thus may cause hypotension and may decrease perfusion. Pavulon does not decrease pulmonary vascular resistance and may actually increase resistance. Careful observation of infants receiving these drugs is obviously essential.

When the infant's condition worsens A marked worsening of the baby's condition may be due to occlusion of the endotracheal tube, extubation, a pneumothorax, a leak in the system, or general deterioration of the baby.

If the endotracheal tube is occluded (e.g., by mucus) or has become dislodged, absence of chest movement and/or breath sounds, color change, apnea, bradycardia, and diminished muscle tone may be evident. Until a new tube can be inserted, the baby's ventilation is supported by bag and mask ventilation.

Weaning from mechanical ventilation It is not particularly difficult to initiate mechanical ventilation for a baby. It is often far more difficult to wean that baby from the ventilator. Weaning involves reductions in rate, end expiratory pressure, and oxygen concentration. The weaning is monitored by blood gas determinations; oxygen and/or pressure is reduced and values are checked within 30 minutes to see if the baby is able to tolerate the lower levels. Careful nursing observations are equally important (see Table 8–18). Weaning frequently involves a transition from assisted ventilation to CPAP and then to the head hood.

Endotracheal tubes should not be left in place once the baby is "disconnected" from mechanical ventilation. A baby can no more breathe through an endotracheal tube without assistance than we could breathe through a straw. The resistance of the tube makes adequate air exchange impossible.

Another consideration during weaning

is the way in which oxygen concentration is decreased. A very rapid drop will cause reflex constriction of the pulmonary arteries with a subsequent decrease in blood flow to the lungs, cyanosis, and other signs of respiratory distress. This behavior is sometimes termed the *flip-flop phenomenon*.

HAZARDS OF OXYGEN THERAPY

The two chief hazards of oxygen therapy, as noted previously, are retrolental fibroplasia and pulmonary oxygen toxicity (bronchopulmonary dysplasia). Pneumothorax, pneumopericardium, and/or pneumomediastinum may occur when oxygen is given under pressure (CPAP or ventilation).

Prior to 1940 *retrolental fibroplasia* was virtually unknown. By 1950 it had become the largest single cause of blindness in children in the United States, greater than all other causes combined. The fact that almost all the cases occurred in the better-equipped medical centers while the condition was virtually unknown in small towns and rural areas was a mystery until 1953, when it was shown that high oxygen concentrations were to blame. (The large centers with the newest equipment were able to deliver oxygen much more efficiently.)

As oxygen was monitored more closely the incidence of retrolental fibroplasia dropped. If arterial oxygen is not closely monitored, there may be a resurgence of retrolental fibroplasia as we save more and more infants of earlier gestational age through the use of high concentrations of oxygen.

The basis of retrolental fibroplasia is in the development of the blood supply system of the retina. No retinal vessels are present until the fourth month of gestation; vascularization of the retina is not complete until after the eighth month. A baby born at 30 weeks gestation, for example, has no blood vessels in much of his retina (Fig. 8–10). It is the incompletely vascularized retina that is susceptible to oxygen damage. Once the vessels are completely developed, they are not damaged by oxygen.

Since newborn puppies and kittens also have incomplete retinal vascularization, it is relatively easy to demonstrate on them the sequence of events when oxygen is given. The initial effect is the immediate and almost total constriction of retinal vessels. This can happen within five minutes after oxygen is given at concentrations of 70 to 80 per cent. It has been suggested that a careful examination of the fundus is one means of determining the level of oxygen concentration to be used, the presence of vasoconstriction indicating an immediate need to lower oxygen concentration. (This is rarely done, however.)

After about 10 minutes of sustained oxygen, the arterioles and capillaries reopen and remain dilated for the next sev-

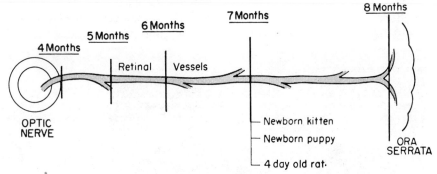

GESTATIONAL AGE OF FETUS

Figure 8–10. Schematic drawing showing the chronology of the development of the blood supply of the retina in the human fetus. (From Patz: Pediatrics *19*:508, 1957.)

cral hours. New blood vessels appear in the retina. Leakage of fluid and blood from these newly formed vessels and invasion by fibroblasts eventually lead to retinal detachment in the weeks that follow.

A second or cicatricial stage, during which the retrolental membrane is formed, occurs several weeks later. The extent of damage done in the second stage depends on the severity of the first stage and is related to (1) the concentration of oxygen, (2) the length of time during which oxygen is administered, and (3) the degree of immaturity of the eye. There is no cure for a fully developed case of retrolental fibroplasia (Fig. 8–11).

It is believed that by keeping PaO_2 levels within the supposedly safe limits of 50 to 90 mm Hg the danger of retrolental fibroplasia can be minimized. The danger cannot be totally eliminated because, for some babies, there appears to be a danger at any oxygen level above that of room air. It is important to recognize that arterial levels in the baby can suddenly change without a change in oxygen concentration if the baby's ability to ventilate improves.

All preterm infants who have received oxygen therapy should have an eye examination at discharge and again at three to six months following discharge by a person experienced in recognizing retrolental fibroplasia.

Bronchopulmonary dysplasia (BPD), also termed pulmonary oxygen toxicity (POT), is a second condition that may occur in newborns exposed to high concentrations of oxygen. It has been recognized even more recently than retrolental fibroplasia; it was first described by Northway and his associates in 1967.

Pulmonary oxygen toxicity appears to be related to (1) the concentration of oxygen, (2) the length of time during which oxygen is given, (3) the use of a positive pressure respirator, and (4) an endotracheal tube that disrupts normal ciliary function in the respiratory tract. Even when these four factors are constant, some infants appear more susceptible to bronchopulmonary dysplasia than others.

Infants with bronchopulmonary dysplasia may require oxygen for a number of weeks with very slow weaning. Not only does the baby need special care but his family will need a great deal of support to keep them from becoming discouraged.

Pneumothorax A third complication is not related to oxygen per se but is often caused by the pressures of ventilation (either manual or mechanical). This is pneumothorax (air in the thoracic cavity). Related conditions that may or may not also appear are pneumomediastinum (air in the mediastinum) and pneumopericardium (air in the pericardial sac). A pneumothorax may also occur spontaneously. It is estimated that some degree of pneumothorax is present in approximately 7 per cent of all babies, but it is not always symptomatic.

The cause of pneumothorax is rupture of the alveoli from pressures that are too high, with the subsequent escape of air into the pleural space. As more and more air escapes, breathing becomes more and more difficult. Nurses need to be alert for signs of possible pneumothorax, which often appears as *sudden* respiratory distress. Listening through a stethoscope for air exchange on both sides of the chest should be routine when pulse and respiration are checked.

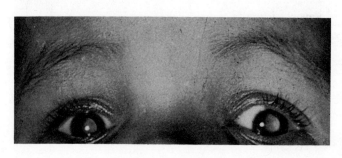

Figure 8–11. Terminal stage of retrolental fibroplasia. The child is totally blind. (From Patz: Pediatrics *19*:508, 1957.)

Kuhns (1975) has described the use of a high-intensity transilluminating light to detect pneumothorax and pneumomediastinum. After the overhead lights in the nursery are turned out, a high-intensity transilluminating light is placed against the baby's chest, first superior and then inferior to the nipple on both sides. "If an area around the sternum appears translucent, or if either side of the chest transilluminates more than the other, several other spots at varying distances from the sternum on either side are transilluminated" (Kuhns: 356). It would seem very useful for nurses to become familiar with rapid, noninvasive means of observation (Fig. 8–12).

Needle aspiration of air and/or placement of a chest tube is the treatment for pneumothorax. Transillumination is also used to guide the needle and tube placement.

RESPIRATORY DISEASE OTHER THAN RDS

Not all infants with respiratory distress have respiratory distress *syndrome*. Other respiratory problems include transient tachypnea of the newborn (Chapter 7), meconium aspiration syndrome, apnea of prematurity, pneumothorax, pulmonary infection or hemorrhage, and Wilson-Mikity syndrome. The treatment and nursing care of respiratory diseases other than RDS are the same as for RDS (as well as other general supportive measures).

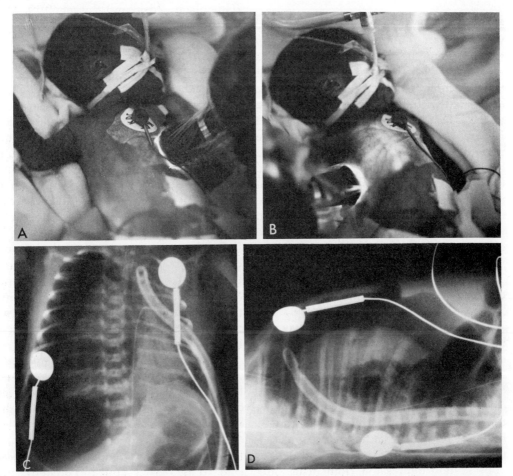

Figure 8–12. Transillumination to detect pneumothorax. *A,* corona of light around the thorax; no pneumothorax indicated. *B,* entire thoracic cage transilluminates; suggests large pneumothorax. *C* and *D,* chest x-ray showing massive right pneumothorax. (From Kuhns: Pediatrics 56:355, 1975. Copyright American Academy of Pediatrics, 1975.)

Meconium Aspiration Syndrome

The presence of meconium in the amniotic fluid suggests some degree of neonatal asphyxia. When an infant is delivered through thick meconium the vocal cords should be visualized through a laryngoscope; if meconium is present it is suctioned through an endotracheal tube before the baby is stimulated to breathe. Ting and Brady (1975) have shown this procedure to markedly reduce mortality and morbidity. Carson et al. (1976) have suggested suctioning the nasopharnyx and oropharnyx as soon as the head is delivered, prior to the delivery of the chest.

Apnea of Prematurity

Nearly all infants born at less than 30 weeks gestation and a signficant proportion of infants born at less than 32 weeks gestation will have periods of apnea that last for more than 20 seconds and are associated with bradycardia and a change in the infant's color and tone. Avery and Fletcher (1974) distinguish apnea from the periodic breathing that is characteristic of healthy preterm infants. *Periodic breathing* (1) follows a cyclic pattern; periods of regular breathing for 10 to 15 seconds are followed by periods of no breathing for 10 to 15 seconds; and (2) does not involve changes in color, tone, or heart rate.

Causes of Apnea of Prematurity

A single specific cause of apnea has not been identified. Immaturity of the various components of respiratory regulation in the central nervous system is a major factor. Important contributing factors include hypoxia, environmental temperature outside the thermoneutral range, hypo- or hypercapnia, hypoglycemia, hypocalcemia, anemia, sepsis, central nervous system depression from drugs, increased vagal tone, intracranial hemorrhage, and heart failure. Because many of these variables can be recognized

and corrected, understanding the relationship between these factors and apnea is necessary for nursing practice.

Hypoxia and hypoxemia may occur in preterm infants because of airway congestion, poor positioning, or tiring in a baby with RDS. When respiratory centers are depressed by hypoxia, response to an elevation in $PaCO_2$ or a decrease in pH is compromised, and the likelihood of apnea is increased.

Airway obstruction is prevented by close observation, gentle suctioning of the nose and oropharnyx when secretions accumulate, or suction through an endotracheal tube.

When the baby is supine, a rolled diaper beneath the shoulders aids in maintaining the slight hyperextension that facilitates respiration. Two studies (Hutchison, Ross, and Russell 1979; Martin et al. 1979) have shown that when the baby was placed in a prone position respiration improved. Hutchison's group measured a number of respiration components in preterm infants, finding significant differences in several indicators including tidal volume, minute volume, and the total work of breathing when infants were in a prone position. Martin's group found that when infants were placed in a prone position PaO_2 rose by a mean 15 per cent in preterm infants and 25 per cent in five infants with residual cardiopulmonary disease. In addition to the rise in PaO_2, there was a decrease in the amount of time the infants exhibited asynchronous chest wall movements, from 90 per cent in a supine position to 28 per cent in a prone position. These studies indicate that position deserves careful attention in both nursing practice and research.

The effect of *environmental temperature* on oxygen requirements has been noted in several chapters. A *decrease* in environmental temperature, even when slight, leads to increased oxygen consumption and can result in apnea. A sudden *increase* in environmental temperature can also lead to increased apnea (Perlstein, Edwards, and Sutherland 1970). Consider the infant under the radiant warmer. The servocontrol becomes detached and the warmer stays on continuously, even for a brief period. Aside from the very real danger of burning (see Thermoregulation), hyperthermia is inevitable and apnea a possibility.

Hypoglycemia, hypocalcemia, and/or sepsis may cause apnea, probably by depressing the respiratory centers in the brain. These conditions are discussed individually. If apnea is due to metabolic causes, treating the underlying cause will usually result in decreased apneic episodes.

though the baby's breathing is satisfactory. However, any malfunction must be quickly corrected lest nurses ignore the monitor when the baby is truly apneic.

When apnea occurs, careful assessment of accompanying behavior is important. Is apnea accompanied by significant bradycardia (heart rate below 100 bpm within 30 seconds after the onset of apnea)? Is there a color change or a change in muscle tone? Are other factors present (summarized in Table 8–9) that could account for the increasing apnea?

IMPLICATIONS FOR NURSING CARE

As noted in the discussion of cardiac and respiratory monitors, the respiratory monitor is frequently set to allow a 10- or 15-second delay so that normal periodic breathing will not constantly trigger the monitor. If the baby appears to be breathing normally, the monitor itself needs to be checked. A loose connection may cause the monitor to sound the alarm even

PLANNING CARE FOR THE INFANT WITH APNEA

All infants who might be expected to develop apnea (including all infants under 1800 g) should have continuous monitoring of both cardiac and respiratory status. Bradycardia may not accompany apnea (nursing records should indicate the presence of bradycardia). A variety of preventive measures are summarized in Table

Table 8–9 Assessment and Intervention in Factors Related to Apnea

Factor	Assessment	Intervention
Immaturity of central nervous system	Continuous monitoring of respiratory and cardiac rates	Tactile stimulation
	Evaluation of other possible causes of apnea	Based on identified cause Assisted ventilation
Variation in thermo-neutral environment	Frequent assessment of axillary temperature	Use of servomechanism to maintain thermoneutral environment (36.5° C [97.6° F] temperature in baby)
Hypoxia	Continuous assessment of oxygen levels: transcutaneous and/or arterial	Positioning for maximum oxygenation
	Evaluation of causes of hypoxia: airway congestion, poor positioning, tiring from respiratory efforts, patent ductus arteriosus (PDA)	Correction of underlying causes: suction Assisted ventilation Medical or surgical closure of PDA
Hypoglycemia	Dextrostix to quickly assess blood sugar level	Administration of glucose
Hypocalcemia	Assessment of serum calcium levels	Administration of calcium
Anemia	Record blood withdrawn for laboratory evaluation Assessment of hemoglobin and hematocrit	Replacement of blood
Sepsis	Apnea may be early symptom of sepsis; assess other parameters	Treatment of sepsis, including supportive treatment and antibiotics
Central nervous system drug depression	Note drugs given to mother in labor	

8–10. The value of a pulsating waterbed is documented (Korner et al. 1975), as are the effects of CPAP (Kattwinkel et al. 1975).

Theophylline has been shown by several investigators to reduce the incidence of apnea (Kuzemko and Paala 1973; Shannon et al. 1975; Uauy et al. 1975). The mechanism seems to be increased respiratory center output (Gerhardt, McCarthy, and Bancalari 1979), which supports the theory that apnea of prematurity is due to an immature respiratory center which is responsible for decreased respiratory drive. One of two regimens is usually utilized in the prescription of theophylline: a loading dose of 5 mg/kg followed by a maintenance dose of 1 mg/kg/dose at intervals of four to eight hours (Klaus and Fanaroff 1979) or 2 mg/kg every six hours (Gerhardt, McCarthy, and Bancalari 1979). Heart rate is assessed and charted immediately before administering a dose because increased heart rate may be an early sign of theophylline toxicity. (Aminophylline is not given in our nursery when heart rate exceeds 180 bpm without physician consultation in relation to that particular dose.)

Prompt intervention by rubbing the infant's back and other methods of generalized cutaneous stimulation will be effective in 80 to 90 per cent of apneic episodes. Painful stimuli are not necessary. If the infant does not respond quickly to cutaneous stimulation, bag and mask resuscitation may be necessary. The resuscitation bag and infant face mask should be available at the baby's bed and should already be connected to an oxygen source. The nurse should need only to turn the oxygen on. Avoid using high concentrations of oxygen. If the infant is currently receiving oxygen, he can be resuscitated using the same concentration. If the baby is breathing room air, it may be possible to resuscitate with room air or, if not, at concentrations no greater than 30 to 40 per cent oxygen. Nurses need to be continually aware of the hazards as well as the benefits of oxygen therapy.

When a baby is having constantly recurring apnea, a careful evaluation to determine the possible causes is essential.

Pulmonary Hemorrhage

Pulmonary hemorrhage most frequently occurs in infants who are already ill. Blood-stained fluid appears in the trachea, preceded or accompanied by apnea, bradycardia, and peripheral vasoconstriction.

Table 8–10   Apnea of Prematurity: Nursing Approach

Need	Method
Assessment	
Continuous apnea monitoring of preterm infants, particularly infants below 1800 g, until no apnea for 3 to 7 days (recommendations vary)	Apnea monitor
Prevention	
Treatment of underlying causes	See text and Table 8–9
Proper positioning	Head slightly extended; roll under shoulders
Infant stimulation	Cutaneous, vestibular, proprioceptive (see sensory stimulation), including pulsating water bed
Nasal CPAP at low (2 to 4 cm) pressures	Oxygen may be needed to maintain Po_2 at 50 to 60 mm Hg
Theophylline (oral or IV)	See text
Treatment (of specific episode)	
Stimulation	Diffuse cutaneous stimulation (e.g., rubbing entire back) is superior to painful stimuli; will be sufficient to end most episodes
Bag and mask ventilation if response to stimulation is not prompt	Use oxygen concentration in which infant has previously been kept; may be room air or no more than 30 to 40 per cent

The fluid is usually not whole blood but primarily edema fluid that forms because of increased pressure in the pulmonary capillaries. Prevention of birth asphyxia, a predisposing factor, and prompt recognition and adequate treatment of other predisposing factors (Cole et al. 1973), which include hypothermia, Rh incompatibility, and congenital heart disease, are probably decreasing the incidence of pulmonary hemorrhage. Treatment includes mechanical ventilation and blood transfusion, with excellent supportive care.

Wilson-Mikity Syndrome

Wilson-Mikity syndrome is a respiratory condition of infants who generally weigh less than 1500 g. Symptoms usually begin after the first week of life in infants who may have had very mild respiratory symptoms initially. Etiology is unclear. Early signs are mild cyanosis, periodic apnea, and tachypnea. Symptoms become increasingly severe, reaching maximum severity about four to eight weeks after onset and may remain for weeks and even months, although most infants survive.

The care of babies with Wilson-Mikity syndrome is similar to that of infants with bronchopulmonary dysplasia. Because this is a long-term condition, parents are going to need emotional support over a period of weeks and months. There will be times when they will despair of their baby's recovery. Primary nurses on each shift who give the baby consistent care and also know the parents well can be important in maintaining parental attachment during hospitalization.

Special Needs Based on Other Problems

Intraventricular Hemorrhage

Intraventricular hemorrhage (IVH) occurs in 40 to 60 per cent of small preterm infants, probably because of hypoxia, which damages the walls of fragile blood vessels and also causes congestion in cerebral veins. Many of these infants will subsequently develop hydrocephalus (if they survive the initial insult) as the flow of cerebral spinal fluid is obstructed. A tense fontanel may be the initial sign of IVH; the diagnosis is confirmed by a lumbar puncture in which the spinal fluid is bloody. Continued nursing assessment includes daily measurement of head size to detect possible hydrocephalus. Computerized tomography is an additional assessment tool. Daily lumbar punctures have been used to reduce intracranial pressure and prevent the deleterious effects of hydrocephalus (Goldstein, Chaplin, and Maitland 1976; Papile et al. 1978). A shunting procedure for hydrocephalus may be necessary.

PROBLEMS OF ACID-BASE BALANCE

Acid-base balance is evaluated by determining gas levels of pH and Pco_2 and by calculating HCO_3. Sites for blood gas determinations have been previously described. The infant should be quiet and in a constant oxygen concentration for at least 10 minutes prior to the drawing of the blood specimen. If the baby has been crying or oxygen concentration has varied (e.g., if the hood or nasal prongs have been removed to weigh the baby), arterial gases will not correctly reflect the baby's response to the prescribed concentration of oxygen. When the blood sample is withdrawn from an indwelling line (umbilical or arterial) the blood withdrawn to clear the line must be replaced because of the infant's low blood volume. A careful record is kept of blood withdrawn for specimens for the same reason. Transfusion may be necessary.

Acidosis

When the pH falls below 7.3, the baby is considered acidotic. A mild acidosis (7.2) is not uncommon immediately following birth, even in newborns who are healthy, but this acidosis is generally resolved within the first 30 to 60 minutes of life as carbon dioxide levels drop to normal limits. Our concern here is with severe acidosis.

When the infant becomes acidotic, pulmonary vascular resistance increases, thereby decreasing the flow of blood to the lungs and subsequently leading to further increases in carbon dioxide levels. Acidosis also compromises myocardial contractility and adversely affects cell metabolism.

RESPIRATORY ACIDOSIS

It has previously been noted that infants with respiratory distress have difficulty not only in oxygenating but in getting rid of carbon dioxide, resulting in *respiratory acidosis.* Unlike the adult or older child who usually responds to respiratory acidosis by increasing acid excretion through the kidneys, the immature kidney of the preterm infant has a marked incapacity to excrete acid. Thus, preterm infants do not develop compensatory metabolic alkalosis.

Normal levels of Pco_2 in newborns are between 30 and 40 mm Hg; a Pco_2 level of over 45 mm Hg is considered to indicate respiratory acidosis. Acidosis that is purely respiratory in origin requires respiratory treatment; if CO_2 increase is mild, bag and mask ventilation may correct a transient problem. If the problem is more severe or persistent, assisted ventilation (CPAP or ventilator) may be necessary.

Sodium bicarbonate ($NaHCO_3$) is not used in the treatment of *respiratory* acidosis. Consider:

$$NaHCO_3 \rightarrow Na + H_2O + CO_2$$

The administration of sodium bicarbonate requires adequate ventilation to remove carbon dioxide from the lungs.

METABOLIC ACIDOSIS

When the baby is unable to inspire adequate oxygen to meet his metabolic needs, anaerobic metabolism results, with the production of lactic acid. In metabolic acidosis, HCO_3 is decreased. The HCO_3 level is not directly measured but is calculated from values that are directly measured. Bicarbonate levels in adults in acid-base balance are approximately 24 mEq/liter. However, newborns are less able to conserve bicarbonate than adults; bicarbonate levels may be somewhat lower (20 to 21 mEq/liter in term infants and as low as 18 to 20 mEq/liter in preterm infants).

For practical purposes, the *base deficit* is calculated; one method utilizes a Siggaard-Andersen nomogram (Fig. 8–13) in this manner: after the pH and Pco_2 are determined, connect the two values with a straight line. Find the point at which this line intersects with hemoglobin concentration. The base deficit (negative number) or base excess (positive number) is read at this point. If the base deficit is 6 or more and the pH is less than 7.3, metabolic acidosis exists. The treatment for metabolic acidosis is the administration of alkali in the form of sodium bicarbonate.

Hemoglobin is important in the calculation because tissue perfusion is compromised when hemoglobin is low. If Pco_2 is 60 and pH is 3.0, base deficit is 14 with a hemoglobin of 10 but 20 with a hemoglobin of 20. The lower hemoglobin value indicates inadequate perfusion, which is corrected by administration of blood products.

In an emergency, such as severe asphyxia, when blood gas values are not available, an initial dose of 2 to 3 mEq/kg sodium bicarbonate is given, the smaller dose for infants under 2000 g.

Once blood gas values are available, base deficit can be calculated in the manner described. Once base deficit is known, a common method of calculating bicarbonate dosage is:

baby's weight in kilograms × base deficit
× 0.3 = mEq bicarbonate

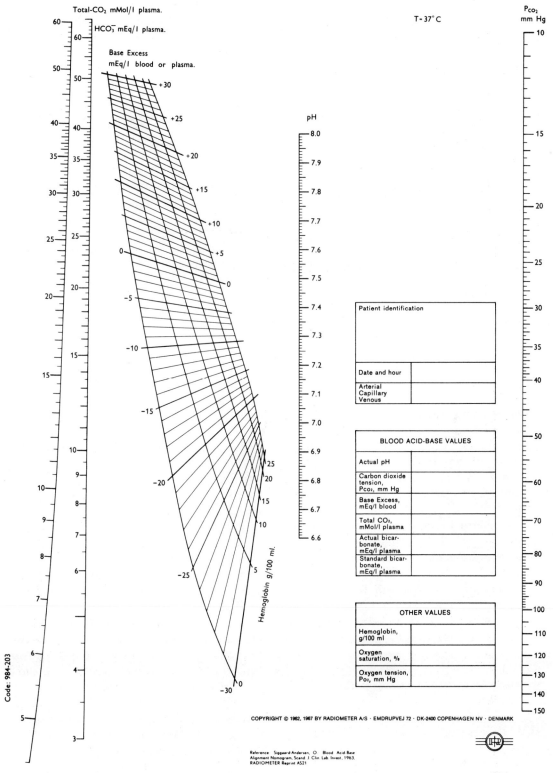

Figure 8–13. Siggaard-Andersen alignment nomogram. (Copyright © 1962 by Radiometer A/S.)

For example: a 1300 g baby (1.3 kg) is determined to have a base deficit of 6.

$$1.3 \text{ kg} \times 6 \times 0.3 = 2.34 \text{ mEq bicarbonate}$$

Note that if the base deficit doubles, the dosage doubles.

$$1.3 \text{ kg} \times 12 \times 0.3 = 4.68 \text{ mEq bicarbonate}$$

Any formula is, of course, only a rule of thumb; careful evaluation of the baby's behavior and appearance is also essential.

In administering $NaHCO_3$, several guidelines are important.

1. Dilute the prepared dose with equal parts water for injection to lower the osmolality. Sodium bicarbonate solutions are hypertonic; rapid injection of hypertonic solutions causes water to move into the plasma from the extravascular space, increasing plasma volume, venous pressure, and cerebrospinal fluid pressure. The pressures can lead to intracranial hemorrhage with resultant neurological deficit or death.

2. Infuse slowly (1 mEq/min) to avoid tissue damage as well as changes in osmolality.

3. Be aware of the total dosage given; under all but the most unusual circumstances 24-hour dosage should not exceed 8 mEq/kg. Again, the concern is osmolality.

4. Ventilate the baby, if the baby is not breathing well, by bag and mask or other means of assisted ventilation, so that the carbon dioxide that results from the dehydration of $NaHCO_3$ will be eliminated. Otherwise Pco_2 will rise, Po_2 will fall, and the net result will be worsening rather than an improvement.

MIXED METABOLIC AND RESPIRATORY ACIDOSIS

When acidosis is purely respiratory, the HCO_3 will be normal and the CO_2 increased. The reverse is true for metabolic acidosis; HCO_3 is decreased and CO_2 is normal. Both respiratory and metabolic acidosis can exist concurrently. Both alkali therapy and excellent ventilation will be required to restore pH to normal limits. Reevaluation of blood gases approximately five minutes after treatment will serve as a guide to further treatment.

Alkalosis

Alkalosis is seen far less frequently in newborns than acidosis. *Respiratory alkalosis* may occur when an infant is hyperventilated by a mechanical ventilator. CO_2 is low because too much is expired. Treatment is an adjustment of ventilator settings.

Metabolic alkalosis may occur when the body loses acid, as in the persistent vomiting that can accompany an obstruction in the gastrointestinal tract such as pyloric stenosis. Treatment is usually not of the alkalosis per se; measures to inhibit vomiting (NPO) and correct fluid and electrolyte deficits usually restore blood pH.

PROBLEMS OF BLOOD VOLUME AND PERFUSION

Blood volume in the term newborn averages approximately 85 ml/kg, with slightly higher values (89 to 105 ml/kg) in preterm infants. Thus, the total blood volume of a 3000 g infant will little more than fill an 8 oz glass, and the blood volume of an infant weighing 1000 g is approximately 3 oz. The baby does not have to lose much blood to become hypovolemic. Hypovolemia, in turn, is the chief cause of hypotension and is also important as a cause of anemia.

Hypovolemia may result from a variety of circumstances. Many are self-explanatory (Table 8–11); some require further comment. Fetal-maternal bleeds may be spontaneous; some amnioceneses are followed by fetal-maternal bleeding. When there is cord compression during the second stage of labor blood may be pooled in the placenta, and the fetus will have relatively decreased blood volume. If hypovolemia is due to a shift of plasma from the intravascular spaces, hematocrit

Table 8–11   Causes of Hypotension in Newborns

Hypovolemia	
Prenatal factors	Fetal-maternal bleed
	Twin-to-twin transfusion
Intrapartal factors	Rupture of umbilical cord
	Placenta previa
	Abruptio placentae
	Umbilical cord compression (second stage of labor)
	Accidental incision of placenta or cord during cesarean birth
Neonatal factors	Hemorrhage
	Shift of fluid from intravascular space (e.g., large cephalhematoma, edema)
Iatrogenic factors	Excessive blood removal for laboratory tests
	Rapid clamping of umbilical cord
Medications given to mother	
Beta-adrenergic blocking agents	Vasodilan, ritodrine
Antihypertensive agents	Aldomet, Apresoline
Increased intrathoracic pressure	Pneumothorax
	Pneumomediastinum
Septic shock	

will be higher than normal (normal is 55 to 65 per cent in term infants, slightly lower in preterm infants).

Because of the infant's small blood volume, blood for laboratory tests can decrease circulating volume quickly. In the 1000 g infant, 10 ml represents 10 per cent of total volume. A "blood out" record should be kept at the bedside and all specimens recorded. Techniques that use only small amounts of blood for laboratory tests are essential.

If the mother is given drugs that will affect infant blood pressure, that information must be on the infant's record so that nurses can be particularly watchful of hypertension. The drugs listed in Table 8–11 lower blood pressure by dilating the vascular bed. Pneumothorax and/or pneumomediastinum may occur spontaneously or may be secondary to assisted ventilation.

Blood pressure is most commonly measured in infants with the Doppler ultrasound technique. The sensor is placed over an artery (most commonly the brachial or the popliteal artery). In small preterm infants, blood pressure is best measured in the leg because of the relation of the size of the cuff to the limb. In many term infants, the arm is a better choice. If the infant is crying when the cuff is applied, soothing him before checking the pressure will result in a more accurate reading. Mean blood pressures are summarized in Table 8–12.

Haddock (1980) suggests the following general guidelines as criteria for hypotension.

1. A systolic blood pressure of less than 55 in term infants.

2. A systolic blood pressure of less than 50 in large preterm infants.

Table 8–12   Mean Blood Pressures*

Weight (g)	Systolic (mm Hg)	Diastolic (mm Hg)
1000 to 2000	49 to 53	26 to 31
2000 to 3000	57 to 64	32 to 37
≥3000	65 to 70	39 to 44

*Adapted from Kitterman, Phibbs, and Tooley: Pediatrics 44:959, 1969.

3. A systolic blood pressure of less than 40 in small preterm infants.

Hypotension is treated with volume expansion; common solutions include blood, frozen plasma, Plasmanate, and albumin. Initial doses are 10 to 20 ml/kg of body weight; if blood pressure does not stabilize in an appropriate range additional doses may be required.

HYPERBILIRUBINEMIA

Hyperbilirubinemia in infancy is a result of either overproduction of bilirubin or interference with bilirubin metabolism and excretion. The production and metabolism of bilirubin was discussed in Chapter 6; the reasons for an increased susceptibility to hyperbilirubinemia in preterm infants was discussed previously in this chapter. Table 8–13 summarizes a number of other causes of hyperbilirubinemia.

Hemolytic Anemia

Hemolytic anemia is most commonly due to Rh_d or ABO incompatibility (Chapter 3). Although the incidence of Rh_d incompatibility has markedly decreased since the introduction of anti-D immunoglobulin (Rho-GAM), hemolytic anemia continues to occur.

RH$_d$ INCOMPATIBILITY

As soon as the baby is delivered, blood is Rh typed and a Coombs' test for the presence of antibodies is done. The Coombs' test is given in addition to the type test because a baby with negative type blood who has a great many antibodies may type positive. If the Coombs' test is negative, there are no antibodies present and the baby should have no difficulty from Rh_d incompatibility. If the Coombs' test is positive, indicating that the infant's erythrocytes are coated with antibodies, further blood studies are done (hemoglobin, hematocrit, indirect bilirubin level,

reticulocyte count). Even with a positive Coombs' test, about 45 per cent of D positive babies born of D negative mothers do not require exchange transfusions. Phototherapy may be used when babies seem to be only mildly affected, with frequent checks of indirect bilirubin level and other blood studies.

In contrast to those D positive babies who do not appear to be in serious danger, other D positive babies are obviously in distress at birth. They are pale and edematous and have enlarged livers and spleens; blood studies show marked anemia, which can lead to heart failure and metabolic acidosis. These babies will nearly always have their blood exchanged shortly after birth. A third group of infants may not appear in such immediate danger but because of subsequent anemia and hyperbilirubinemia will also need treatment.

OTHER BLOOD GROUP INCOMPATIBILITIES

About 10 to 20 per cent of babies with ABO incompatibility have hyperbilirubinemia to the extent that they require exchange transfusion. Group O blood, cross-matched against maternal serum, is used.

In less than 5 per cent of all infants with hemolytic anemia, a blood factor other than Rh_d, A, or B is involved. E, C, and the Kell (K) factors may be responsible for severe hemolytic disease and even for hydrops fetalis. The Coombs' test is positive. Very careful cross-matching with maternal serum is necessary so that the blood used for transfusion will not contain the antigen responsible for maternal sensitization.

Other Causes of Hyperbilirubinemia

Several causes of hyperbilirubinemia occur rarely; several are related to genetic defects (e.g., Crigler-Najjar). For a more complete discussion see Maisels (1975) and Poland and Ostrea (1979). Several conditions mentioned in Table 8–13 are sufficiently common that nurses should be particularly alert for the possibility of increased bilirubin levels in infants in which they exist.

When there is blood in any extravascular space, the breakdown of the RBC may elevate serum bilirubin. Maternal blood swallowed during delivery, as well as fetal hemorrhage, contributes to the supply of extravascular blood.

In polycythemia, the number of RBCs is large, so that increased RBC destruction is possible. If the passage of meconium is delayed by intestinal obstruction, the meconium is in the intestine longer and more bilirubin is deconjugated and reabsorbed into the system.

Albumin binds to acceptor proteins. A lack of binding sites, either because serum proteins or total blood volume is limited or because other substances (e.g., hydrogen ions in acidosis, certain drugs) have utilized the sites, results in high levels of unconjugated (indirect) bilirubin. When the ductus venosus remains open and much of the circulating blood is shunted past the liver where conjugation occurs, less bilirubin is conjugated. A patent ductus venosus (like a patent ductus arteriosus) is most common in preterm infants and hypoxic term infants.

The reason for increased levels of bilirubin in many instances is unclear.

Treating Hyperbilirubinemia

Infants with hyperbilirubinemia will generally receive phototherapy and may receive an exchange transfusion.

PHOTOTHERAPY

None of us can doubt that the careful observations of nurses contribute to the care of individual patients every day. What we do fail to recognize is that the careful observations of nurses can lead to new and important developments in patient care that will have far-reaching effects. It was such an observation that led to the use of phototherapy as a tool in the treatment of hyperbilirubinemia.

The incident occurred at the General Hospital in Rochford, Essex, England. The sister (nurse) in charge of the premature nursery, whose name unfortunately is not recorded in the published report, noted that jaundice faded after babies had been in direct sunlight for a short time. Cremer, Perryman, and Richards (1958) then began to place naked babies in direct sunlight for 15 to 20 minutes, withdrawing them for a similar period before exposing them again. During exposure the babies' eyes were protected with a plastic shield. It was discovered that jaundice quickly disappeared from the exposed areas, but re-

Table 8–13 Some Causes of Neonatal Hyperbilirubinemia

Overproduction of Bilirubin	Problems in Bilirubin Clearance (Metabolism and/or Excretion)	Problems of Overproduction and Clearance (Mixed)
Destruction of red blood cells	Decreased bilirubin uptake	Prenatal infection
Physiological destruction of fetal red blood cells	Competition for binding sites	TORCH diseases (Chapter 3)
Hemolytic anemia from blood group incompatibility	Low serum albumin	Hepatitis
Hemolysis from medications (e.g., vitamin K)	Persistent ductus venosus Hypovolemia	
Extravascular red blood cells (bruising, petechiae, cephalhematoma, etc.)	Defects in bilirubin conjugation Crigler-Najjar syndrome	Neonatal sepsis
Polycythemia	Hypothyroidism	
Intestinal obstruction	Human milk factors	
	Impaired bilirubin transport	Infants of diabetic mothers
	Specific genetic conditions	Galactosemia
	Obstructed flow of bile	Oxytocin and diazepam given to mother during labor

mained in the shaded areas. The initial test group included 13 infants, weighing from 3 lb 3 oz to 5 lb 14 oz, whose levels of indirect bilirubin ranged from 10 to 25 mg per cent. After two to four hours of exposure the bilirubin levels dropped 2 to 12 mg per cent in 11 of the babies; there was no change in one infant, and indirect bilirubin rose 2 mg per cent in one infant. In general, the higher the initial serum bilirubin level and the longer the exposure time, the greater the fall. Cremer and his associates next devised a source of artificial light that was tested with nine jaundiced premature infants and was also found to be effective in reducing serum bilirubin levels. Subsequent studies have supported his findings.

Light causes bilirubin to break down into water-soluble products that are rapidly excreted in the bile and, to a lesser extent, in the urine. Because of the mode of excretion, the stools of a baby who has been under the light are brown or dark green; the urine may be a dark golden brown.

Blue light is more effective than white light in causing bilirubin breakdown. However, it is difficult to detect changes in the baby's color, particularly cyanosis, under blue lights. They must be turned off frequently for observation of the baby. The baby will appear "strange" to his parents under blue lights. Even the effects of white lights are frightening and should be carefully explained. Lights should be turned off and the infant's eyes uncovered when the parents visit him. If parents remain throughout the day, phototherapy must continue, of course, but can be interrupted for brief periods of interaction.

Following are specific considerations in the care of infants receiving phototherapy.

1. Because photodegradation of bilirubin takes place in the skin, the baby should be fully undressed while under the lights.

2. As stated in the discussion of thermoregulation, bilirubin lights increase environmental temperature; axillary temperature should be assessed frequently.

3. Fluid intake should be increased because of increased insensible water loss, which may be increased by as much as 300 per cent in the preterm baby (and approximately 40 per cent in the term baby). The baby should be weighed twice a day and fluid intake further increased if weight loss exceeds 2 per cent of body weight.

4. Both of the baby's eyes should be shielded completely. There are no data concerning eye damage to humans, but some retinal damage has been produced in experimental animals.

5. Skin color is not an adequate guide to serum bilirubin levels; bilirubin level in the blood must be measured often.

6. Babies under the bilirubin light may have a rash from ultraviolet radiation. There should always be a Plexiglas shield between the baby and the light to filter out this radiation.

7. Light emission from the bilirubin light may decay over time. Specific instructions for various types of lights are contained in instruction manuals and should be reviewed periodically.

Concern about the potential dangers of phototherapy in human infants is unanswered at this time. Some studies in vitro and in animals suggest varying kinds of damage on a cellular level that may (or may not) be important in humans. Prophylactic phototherapy, to prevent the initial rise in serum bilirubin, is not currently recommended. However, the dangers of hyperbilirubinemia are well known; exchange transfusion, the only other treatment modality currently available, also involves some risk.

EXCHANGE TRANSFUSION

A second method of treatment for hyperbilirubinemia is exchange transfusion. When bilirubin levels are rising rapidly, exchange transfusion is generally preferred to phototherapy.

Blood for exchange may be O negative that has been cross-matched against maternal serum. If it is indicated before delivery that an immediate exchange will be necessary, blood should be ready. If there is time following delivery to type the baby's blood before exchange, negative blood of the baby's type that has been cross-matched against maternal serum is used. A sample of maternal serum should be saved for future exchanges. Obtaining additional maternal blood is not a serious problem when the mother is in the same hospital as the baby. But as the transfer of very sick infants from smaller community hospitals to intensive care units of major medical centers becomes increasingly more common, the nurses at the involved hospitals must make sure that maternal blood accompanies any baby with hemolytic anemia.

Why are D positive babies given negative blood? If D positive blood is used, the antibodies already present in the infant's circulatory system will destroy the new erythrocytes, just as they are destroying his own cells; nothing will have been accomplished by exchanging one set of positive cells for another.

In addition to proper type, blood for exchange must be the freshest available, never more than three to four days old. Older blood is more likely to undergo hemolysis, the exact process that exchange transfusion is attempting to prevent. Heparinized blood is always fresh since it must be discarded if it is not used within 24 hours after being collected. Babies who receive heparinized blood must be watched for bleeding following transfusion; 0.4 mg protamine sulfate for each milligram of heparin in the donor unit is given intravenously following an exchange with heparinized blood. Blood that has had acid citrate dextrose (ACD) added as an anticoagulant can lower blood calcium levels. Because of this, calcium gluconate is given through the exchange catheter after each 100 ml of blood is exchanged. Calcium levels are checked one to two hours postexchange; further treatment may be necessary.

Hypoglycemia is also a potential problem; heparinized blood, in particular, contains very little glucose. Therefore, glucose levels are assessed during and after exchange transfusions.

The danger that the baby will become chilled during any procedure has already been discussed. In addition to the measures normally used to keep the infant warm, the blood for exchange should be warmed. An easy and safe way to do this is to place the blood in a basin of water warmed to, but not exceeding, 37° C (98.6° F). Overheating the blood can damage erythrocytes and can also increase the level of free serum potassium.

The amount of blood that will be used is figured at 85 ml × the weight of the baby in kilograms × 2 (85 ml per kilogram is the assumed blood volume of the newborn). An amount equal to twice the blood volume is used because research indicates that this quantity will assure 85 to 90 per cent effective replacement of circulating erythrocytes.

During the exchange itself there must be one person—doctor or nurse—who can devote full attention to the baby by monitoring pulse and respiration, observing the infant's color and general condition, checking glucose levels, and suctioning him if necessary. The amount of blood injected and withdrawn and the venous pressure must also be accurately recorded.

After the exchange is completed, the baby is observed closely both for his general condition and for signs of hemorrhage from the exchange site.

INFECTION IN THE NEWBORN

Neonatal septicemia is acute infection in which the baby appears ill and a culture of his blood demonstrates the causative organism. About one baby in every 1000 to 2000 live term births and one in every 230 to 250 live preterm births has neonatal sepsis. With the exception of group B (β-hemolytic) streptococcal infections, septicemia is more common in male infants. This may be because factors regulating the synthesis of immunoglobulins are located on the X chromosome. Other acute infections in newborns are gonorrheal conjunctivitis, urinary tract infections (which may lead to sepsis), meningitis, infectious diarrhea, and monilia (thrush).

A number of infections, several of which are acquired transplacentally, may affect the baby's long-range development but are not always obvious in the immediate newborn period. The most common causes of chronic infection are the organisms that are collectively known as the TORCH group (Chapter 3).

Factors That Predispose Newborns to Infection

The nature of defense mechanisms in all newborns, individual injuries or anomalies, maternal factors, and the nature of the hospital experience — all these factors predispose infants to infection (Chapter 7).

Once acquired, an infection in newborns quickly becomes systemic. The reason for this rapid invasion, multiplication, and dissemination of bacteria is the inability of newborns (both term and preterm) to concentrate leukocytes (white blood cells) at the site of an infection, the reduced capacity of those leukocytes for phagocytosis (ingestion of bacteria), and an impaired bacteriocidal capacity. Limitations in complement activation also limit response to infection.

Although the fetus acquires several types of antibodies transplacentally, there are limits to the spectrum of immunity conferred for several reasons.

1. Only IgG crosses the placenta. IgA and IgM, which contain specific antibodies for gram-negative organisms, are not acquired by the baby. IgA is present in breast milk (Chapter 9); IgM must be produced by the fetus/newborn.

2. The mother may lack antibodies to some antigens; if so, the fetus will also lack these antibodies.

3. The shorter the gestation period the more limited the transplacental transfer of antibodies, resulting in a decreased ability of preterm infants to fight infection.

When Sepsis is Suspected

Interventions to prevent infection and clinical signs of infection have been dis-

cussed in Chapter 7. When sepsis is suspected, specific laboratory studies are initiated. Table 8–14 summarizes both clinical and laboratory evidence of neonatal septicemia. Symptoms of sepsis are very general and can apply to many other conditions as well as sepsis. The nursing observation that the baby behaves very differently from previously is probably a key to early recognition. This means that the baby's behavior as well as appearance must be precisely communicated from one nurse to another. Primary nursing, with one nurse having responsibility for an individual baby from the time of admission, is helpful in this regard.

Normal white blood cell count in newborns varies from 6000 to 25,000 and also changes from day to day, so a single value is of little help in recognizing sepsis. Any marked and sudden change (either increase or decrease) suggests sepsis. The level of band cells, a form of immature white blood cell, may be abnormally elevated or decreased. Band cell count in the first weeks of life normally averages from 5.5 to 9 per cent, the higher values occurring at birth.

Platelet counts decrease in septic in-

Table 8–14   Signs of Neonatal Sepsis

Clinical Signs
  Subtle indications of behavioral change ("not doing as well as previously")
  Apnea
  Any change in respiratory status
  Inability to maintain body temperature
  Jaundice or mottled skin
  Abdominal distention
  Vomiting and/or failure to feed well
  Decreased blood pressure
  Pustules or furuncles on skin (staphylococcus)
  Lethargy
  Irritability
  Bleeding
Laboratory screening
  Glucose intolerance (hypoglycemia and/or hyperglycemia)
  Changing blood counts
  Hyperbilirubinemia
  Metabolic acidosis
Specific evaluation for sepsis (septic workup)
  Complete blood count
  Blood culture
  Urine culture (suprapubic aspiration)
  Spinal fluid culture
  Culture of any skin lesion or drainage

fants; platelet counts normally exceed 80,000 to 100,000, although in preterm infants they may be as low as 60,000 in the first three days.

Blood cultures are drawn from a peripheral vein after disinfection of the skin with iodine. Umbilical vessels should not be used to obtain blood for culture because the outer several millimeters may be contaminated by bacteria. Urine for culture is obtained by suprapubic aspiration because it is less dangerous than catheterization and more reliable than a clean catch specimen. Cerebrospinal fluid is aspirated via lumbar puncture. Any skin lesion should also be cultured.

Causative Organisms

The types of organisms most often responsible for neonatal sepsis change from time to time. Currently, group B (β-hemolytic) streptococci are the chief source of infection in most nurseries in the United States. Since these organisms are part of the normal vaginal flora of many women, fetal infection is difficult to prevent. However, only a small percentage of mothers with group B β-strep will infect their infants.

E. coli, once the leading cause of neonatal sepsis, remains a major source of infection in nurseries. Other significant organisms are *Klebsiella, Staphylococcus aureus,* and *Pseudomonas.* Table 8–15 indicates major sources of the organisms that cause neonatal sepsis.

Nursing Intervention

Good nursing care, with emphasis on careful hand washing, should effectively isolate every infant in the nursery. Babies with sepsis may be isolated in separate rooms as well but never where they cannot be closely observed, for they are usually very sick. A septic baby in a normal term nursery should be transferred to a high risk nursery to protect other healthy infants as well as to assure him the special care he needs.

In addition to the supportive treatment that all sick newborns need, babies with sepsis receive parenteral antibiotics. Because drugs are excreted more slowly by the immature kidney of newborns, blood levels of antibiotics remain high for a longer period of time than in older children and adults. Dosage is calculated on the basis of body weight. Antibiotics

Table 8–15   Organisms that Cause Neonatal Sepsis*

Organism	Source	Form of Sepsis	Comments
Group B (β-hemolytic) streptococcus (gram-positive)	Mother: vaginal flora	Septicemia within first 12 hours of life with 50% mortality	Leading cause of neonatal sepsis
	Environment: nursery personnel and infected infants	Meningitis at 2 to 12 weeks of life with 20 to 40% mortality	
E. coli (gram-negative)	Mother (initial case in nursery) Hands of nursery personnel in subsequent cases	Diarrhea Septicemia Meningitis	Leading cause of neonatal sepsis until recently
Aerobacter (gram-negative) Klebsiella (gram-negative)	Intubation Surgery	Pneumonia Septicemia Meningitis	
Staphylococcus (gram-positive)	Nursery personnel (particularly hands) Other infants	Septicemia (Phage I group) Skin infection — scalded skin syndrome (Phage II group)	
Pseudomonas (gram-negative)	Respiratory equipment Bottles of distilled water, etc. Sink traps	Septicemia Pneumonia Meningitis	Difficult to treat

*From Moore: Realities in Childbearing. W. B. Saunders, 1978, p. 579.

commonly used in the care of newborns are listed in Table 8–16.

Four antibiotics have been found to be highly toxic to newborns: the sulfa drugs, tetracycline, chloramphenicol, and potassium penicillin. The sulfas compete with bilirubin for albumin-binding sites and can thus cause kernicterus and death at levels of serum bilirubin that would generally be considered safe. Tetracycline inhibits the linear growth of infants because it is deposited in the growing epiphyses. It also causes permanent yellow-green staining of the enamel of the baby teeth (as does the ingestion of tetracycline by the mother during late pregnancy). Chloramphenicol, because it is poorly excreted by newborns, can lead to sudden collapse and death (known as the gray syndrome). Potassium penicillin can cause heart block in infants.

CONGENITAL HEART DEFECTS

Although the compilation of truly accurate statistics is difficult, it is suspected that one out of every 130 liveborn babies will have a significant congenital heart defect. In a medium-sized hospital where 30 to 35 babies are delivered each week, this means that on the average one baby each month will have a cardiac malformation. Approximately 10 per cent of all congenital defects involve the heart. Congenital heart defects are second only to prematurity as the leading cause of death in referral centers in the first month of life. Approximately one-third of all infants with congenital heart disease die within a week after birth.

Many symptoms of congenital heart defects are vague in the first days of life because certain structures of fetal circulation, such as the patent foramen ovale or ductus arteriosus, may help the baby to compensate (Chapter 5). Since hospital stays of apparently normal mothers and babies are often limited to four or five days, clear-cut symptoms may not appear until after discharge. Of course, it is better if the defect can be found before this, so nursing observations are extremely important.

Congenital heart defects are usually divided, for obvious reasons, into two groups based on the presence or absence of cyanosis. Here we will consider some of the most common defects in categories based on the anatomical changes involved: shunts, blocks, underdevelopment, and complex defects.

Table 8–16   Antibiotics Frequently Given to Neonates with Sepsis

Drug	Dosage	Route	Expiration after Mixing	Comments
Ampicillin	50–200 mg/kg/day (q 8–12 hours)*	IV or IM	1 hour	Effective against certain gram-negative organisms along with kanamycin Initial drug used
Carbenicillin	200–400 mg/kg/day (q 6–8 hours)*	IV only	72 hours	Used for *Pseudomonas* in newborn Alters platelet function
Gentamycin	3–7.5 mg/kg/day (q 8–12 hours)*	IM	Indefinite	Effective against staph and resistant gram-negative organisms; potential ototoxicity and nephrotoxicity
Kanamycin	15 mg/kg/day (q 8–12 hours)*	IM	Indefinite	Effective against gram-negative organisms except *Pseudomonas* Not used for more than 12 days; potential ototoxicity and nephrotoxicity
Nafcillin	100–200 mg/kg/day (q 6–8 hours)*	IV or IM	48 hours	Nephrotoxic; watch for hematuria
Penicillin G.	50,000–200,000 U/kg/day (q 8–12 hours)*	IV or IM	72 hours	Effective against gram-positive organisms

*Less frequent intervals in preterm infants

Etiology

Congenital cardiac disease may be genetic in origin or it may be related to intrauterine infection (particularly rubella) or to other factors in the intrauterine environment such as drugs and nutrition. Nora (1968) found that 34 per cent of 417 patients with cardiac anomalies had relatives with cardiac anomalies in comparison with 9 per cent in a matched control group. When there is a genetic predisposition, the same lesion is usually found in siblings. In most instances, however, the risk of recurrence is not considered sufficiently high to warrant the avoidance of future childbearing.

Because most heart development occurs between the second and eighth weeks of embryological life (Chapter 1), this is the period when teratogens will have their chief effect.

Shunts

Shunts are "leaks" or openings where no postnatal openings should be. There are three types of shunts: atrial septal defects, ventricular septal defects, and patent ductus arteriosus. *Atrial septal defects* are virtually never discovered in newborns and are seldom a problem in children of preschool age.

The most frequently occurring of all congenital heart defects, the *ventricular septal defect* (VSD) is rarely symptomatic in the newborn period because the normally high pressure in the blood vessels of the lung prevents shunting from the left side of the heart to the right side through the defect. As pulmonary pressure drops between two weeks and three months, blood is shunted from the left to the right side of the heart through the VSD. The lungs are flooded and signs of congestive heart failure develop. Banding of the pulmonary arteries is a palliative procedure to keep blood from flooding the lungs. When the baby grows to weigh over 20 lbs, the septal defect is repaired and the band is removed.

It is important to understand why symptoms are delayed, because parents often feel that a diagnosis was missed or that their baby was not carefully examined at birth, when in fact it was not possible to recognize the defect at that time.

The third type of shunt, *patent ductus arteriosus,* is a result of an opening between the aorta and the pulmonary artery which is normal in fetal life but which normally closes functionally at birth (illustrated in Chapter 1). If the patent ductus arteriosus (PDA) is small in term infants, there are usually no symptoms during infancy and early childhood. If the shunt is large the baby may develop congestive heart failure toward the end of the first week as the pulmonary vascular bed dilates, pulmonary vascular resistance decreases, and the lungs are flooded with blood.

A PDA is more likely to be present in preterm infants than in term infants because there is less muscle in the ductus and because preterm infants with respiratory distress frequently have hypoxia and acidosis, which cause the ductus arteriosus to remain open. In addition, because there is decreased pulmonary vascular resistance in preterm infants and because cardiac output is already high, heart failure may occur rapidly.

A *murmur* may be present in conjunction with a PDA but it may be intermittent. If the baby is on a ventilator, it may be necessary to disconnect him briefly to auscultate heart sounds. A *widened pulse pressure* is common, as are *bounding femoral and posterior pedis pulses.*

Treatment of heart failure is initially with digitalis and diuretics. Indomethacin, a drug that inhibits prostaglandin synthesis, has been used to bring about medical closure of the PDA (Gersony 1977; Moss 1979). The dosage should not exceed 0.2 mg/kg of body weight times three doses. Long-term effects of indomethacin are not known at this time: one potential short-term danger is renal shutdown. Therefore, urine output must be carefully measured in infants receiving indomethacin therapy. Bleeding and problems of bilirubin metabolism, as well as compromised renal function, are contraindications.

Indomethacin therapy is most successful during the first 10 days of life and in infants who are not extremely premature. When medical closure is unsuccessful, surgical ligation may be necessary. Some physicians consider surgical ligation the treatment of choice.

Persistent fetal circulation is a syndrome in which right-to-left shunting occurs through both the foramen ovale and the ductus arteriosus. Pulmonary vascular resistance is high, pulmonary artery pressure is high, and thus the right-to-left shunt. The structure of the heart is normal; there is no evidence of congenital heart disease. The baby is usually critically ill, generally requiring 100 per cent FiO_2 and assisted ventilation.

Tolazoline (Priscoline) has been given to infants with persistent fetal circulation to avoid right-to-left shunting through the foramen ovale. The initial dose is 1 to 2 mg/kg of body weight, followed by either continuous infusion (1 to 2 mg/kg/hour) or intermittent doses. Hypotension is a possible side effect, so blood pressure must be closely monitored. Skin flushing is sometimes seen following administration of the drug.

Heart Blocks

There are also three varieties of congenital heart blocks: aortic valvular stenosis, pulmonary valvular stenosis, and coarctation of the aorta.

Aortic valvular stenosis is relatively rare, and unless it is severe it will usually not be detected in newborns but rather will be found at some later time during routine physical examination. The prognosis is good for children with mild to moderate stenosis but rather poor for those babies who develop respiratory distress, tachycardia, and pallor in the first few weeks of life. Although these babies are initially treated with digitalis and oxygen, prompt surgery (aortic valvulotomy) is necessary to save their lives. The surgery itself carries a high risk at the present time.

Complete obstruction of the aortic valve (*aortic atresia*) is always fatal, generally by the time the baby is four to five days old. These babies also have an underdeveloped left heart and ascending aorta, the combination known as *hypoplastic left heart syndrome*.

Pulmonary valvular stenosis is also rare in newborns, occurring most often in the infants of mothers who had rubella in early pregnancy. In combination with other defects, pulmonary stenosis may be an asset in that it reduces excess blood flow to the lungs, just as banding of the pulmonary artery does artificially, and thus protects the baby from congestive heart failure.

Atresia of the pulmonary artery carries a very high risk; untreated patients die within two weeks to two months after birth and mortality is very high following transarterial valvulotomy.

Coarctation of the aorta usually occurs in combination with other defects, thus the term *coarctation syndrome*. This syndrome is the most common malformation causing cardiac failure during the newborn period. Often the baby shows no symptoms during the few days he is in the hospital. But the absence of femoral pulses, which should be routinely checked, gives the clue. If the defect is not discovered before the baby goes home, the classic triad of rapid breathing, feeding difficulty (due to rapid breathing), and tachycardia may follow. On the other hand, many children will have no symptoms and the coarctation will be discovered only on routine examination. As with patent ductus, treatment during infancy is aimed at eliminating congestive failure, with surgery ideally postponed until the baby is at least five years old. Surgery is performed in the newborn period only when heart failure has not responded to medical treatment. To a large extent the success of surgery depends on the nature of the related cardiac anomalies in the coarctation syndrome.

Underdevelopment

Either the right or left ventricle may be hypoplastic (underdeveloped). Infants with hypoplastic left ventricle have systemic circulation only through a patent ductus arteriosus. As the ductus narrows, systemic circulation is increasingly impaired. Death commonly occurs in the first week of life. Because blood flow to the lungs is increased, the baby is usually not cyanotic.

In contrast, very little blood flows to the lungs in infants with hypoplastic right heart. When this anomaly is associated with tricuspid atresia and a ventricular septal defect, the baby will be cyanotic, but some pulmonary and systemic circulation is possible. This baby may do very well during the neonatal period. When pulmonary atresia accompanies hypoplastic right ventricle, pulmonary blood flow depends on the ductus arteriosus and the baby is seriously ill. Surgery linking a systemic artery to a pulmonary artery has been performed, but the risk of death is high.

Complex Malformations

The most common of the complex heart anomalies are transposition of the great vessels and tetralogy of Fallot.

Cyanosis is the outstanding sign of *transposition of the great vessels,* although even with this defect the cyanosis may not be severe in the first days until the ductus arteriosus closes and eliminates the mixing of blood from the two sides of the heart. After it closes, the baby has two separate circulatory systems. The aorta arises from the right ventricle rather than from the left; blood is circulated through the body and returned to the right atrium. This blood never gets to the lungs to be oxygenated. The pulmonary artery carries blood from the left ventricle to the lungs where it is oxygenated and returned to the left atrium. Intercommunication must be established between the two circuits or the baby will die in a few days. Treatment is the creation of an atrial septal defect that allows the blood to mix. This is commonly done through the use of a balloon cardiac catheter; an inflated balloon is drawn through the foramen ovale to enlarge the opening (Fig. 8–14). Further corrective surgery may be done when the child is older.

The four defects that comprise *tetralogy of Fallot* are (1) pulmonary stenosis (occasionally pulmonary atresia), (2) right ventricular hypertrophy, (3) ventricular septal defect, and (4) overriding aorta, which receives blood directly from both right and left ventricles.

Although tetralogy is considered a cyanotic heart disease, even here cyanosis is relatively rare during the time the baby spends in the newborn nursery, even when the pulmonary stenosis is severe. Only half of the newborns with tetralogy will have a murmur, the murmur being due to the ejection of blood through the narrowed pulmonary valve. Lack of this murmur is considered a serious sign; death from anoxia will occur in a few weeks unless high risk surgery can increase pulmonary blood flow. If the baby is having cyanotic attacks during the new-

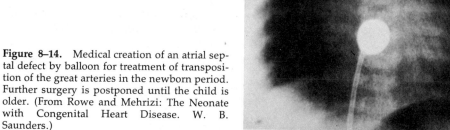

Figure 8–14. Medical creation of an atrial septal defect by balloon for treatment of transposition of the great arteries in the newborn period. Further surgery is postponed until the child is older. (From Rowe and Mehrizi: The Neonate with Congenital Heart Disease. W. B. Saunders.)

born period an anastomosis between the aorta and the pulmonary artery (an artificial patent ductus) may be palliative until the child is older and better able to withstand open heart surgery. Anastomosis of the left pulmonary artery to the descending aorta is called a Pott's procedure, and anastomosis of the right pulmonary artery to the ascending aorta is called a Waterston procedure.

Obviously, not every cardiac malformation has been mentioned here; for descriptions of rare anomalies the reader is referred to pediatric cardiology texts.

Diagnosis of Heart Defects

Once a heart defect is suspected diagnosis is made on the basis of (1) clinical signs that have been observed and recorded, (2) x-ray, (3) electrocardiography, (4) echocardiography, and (5) cardiac catheterization.

The clinical signs associated with individual defects have been mentioned. The role of x-ray in evaluating heart size and some outstanding anatomical changes seems obvious. It is very important that the baby be comfortably at rest and not crying when chest films are taken if they are to be detailed enough to be of any real value. If the baby is to go to the x-ray department for films he should be transported in a heated bed and should spend as little time as possible outside it. A nurse should both go with him and remain with him throughout the entire procedure, wearing a protective apron to shield her from radiation while the pictures are being taken. A bottle of water or a pacifier will help to soothe the baby and keep him from crying. A bulb syringe for suctioning and a hand-operated bag resuscitator should accompany the baby; infants at times become apneic in x-ray departments and other areas of the hospital away from the nursery, and equipment for resuscitation is not always immediately available. Mouth-to-mouth resuscitation can be used in acute emergency, of course, but there is always a risk of introducing pathogens into the respiratory

tract of an already sick baby. It is much easier to be prepared.

Electrocardiograms of newborns differ from those of children from age two through adulthood, and those of premature infants often vary from the EKGs of term babies. The problems involved in the interpretation of newborn EKGs are beyond the scope of this book. As with babies who are to be x-rayed, the infant should be warm and comfortable so that he will lie quietly during the procedure.

Echocardiography is a noninvasive technique that uses ultrasound to diagnose congenital heart disease. Information available in an echocardiogram includes the size and location of chambers in the heart and the great vessels. The motion of valves can also be seen. Some conditions, such as hypoplastic left ventricle, can be diagnosed with great accuracy; others can only be suspected. In many instances cardiac disease can be differentiated from respiratory disease. Echocardiography is proving extremely valuable because it eliminates the need for cardiac catheterization in some infants.

Cardiac catheterization presents somewhat different problems in the newborn period from those encountered in other periods. Although the mortality rate in newborns is in the neighborhood of 5 per cent, a large proportion of the babies who die have inoperable defects and would have died under any circumstances. Nevertheless, catheterization is a hazardous procedure in the newborn period for several reasons.

1. The hazards of chilling the baby during the procedure are greatest in newborns.

2. The baby is often in very serious condition before the catheterization — he may be cyanotic or acidotic or in congestive heart failure.

3. Needle punctures and even traction on small vessels can cause thrombosis and can impair circulation.

4. Catheterization in newborns is often combined with angiography so that an accurate anatomical diagnosis can be made, thereby necessarily increasing the risk.

5. Full exploration of the heart, rather than just right-heart catheterization, may be necessary.

Measures that minimize the risk include:

1. Early detection of the possibility of a heart defect before the baby is critically ill.

2. Avoidance of premedication and anesthesia; local anesthesia and a cutdown are used. The umbilical artery is sometimes used in the first days of life.

3. Treatment of acidosis.

4. Treatment of serious arrhythmias by electrical conversion.

5. The use of a minimum of contrast material.

Once the baby returns from catheterization there must be careful monitoring of temperature (which often drops during the procedure), apical pulse, respiration, and acid-base balance and fluid intake. The cutdown site should be checked for bleeding and the color and pulsation in the limb in which the cutdown was done should be observed. Thrombosis is a particular danger in tiny newborn vessels. If there is no pulse four hours after the study has been completed, arterial thrombosis has usually occurred. Fortunately, collateral blood supply usually prevents gangrene, but occasionally surgery will be necessary.

Congestive Heart Failure

It takes very little time for a baby to progress from the first sign of heart failure to complete vascular collapse. It becomes a major nursing responsibility, then, to spot that first sign — not an easy thing to do because the symptoms are so often vague. The instinctive feeling that "something is not quite right about this baby" may be the first indication.

Tachypnea is often the initial symptom. Respiratory rates, after the first two hours, of more than 45 breaths per minute in a term baby or 60 breaths per minute in a premature baby are usually abnormal if the baby is at rest when the observation is made. In term babies respirations are often not counted as a routine measure; perhaps they should be. But because they rarely are, *failure of the baby to feed well* may be the first sign noticed by the nurse. The baby is breathing so rapidly he cannot suck; he forsakes eating to continue breathing, or he may attempt to do both and choke or vomit, possibly aspirating his food and further compounding the problem. There are many other possible reasons for tachypnea in the newborn and not all of them are of serious consequence (see Transient Tachypnea, Chapter 6). Yet any baby who breathes rapidly needs extra watching.

Another sign of possible congestive heart failure is *tachycardia*. A heart rate of more than 150 beats per minute is unusual in a healthy baby who is not crying.

Edema, if present (and often it is not), is more likely to be found about the face; the baby looks "puffy." The ankle edema seen in adults with congestive heart failure is not present in a recumbent baby.

Older babies (past the newborn period) perspire excessively in congestive heart failure. Although it is rare for a newborn to perspire for any reason, the occasional occurrence of *perspiration* can be a valuable clue in helping to diagnose possible heart failure.

The liver in healthy newborns is felt 1 to 2 cm below the right costal margin; the edge feels "sharp." In heart failure the liver is 3 cm or more below the costal margin and the edge is less sharp. The heart may also be enlarged.

Dyspnea may be due to cardiac disease; retractions in heart failure are more likely to be lateral than substernal because the enlarged heart restricts movement of the sternum.

Once congestive heart failure is suspected, treatment is begun as early as possible. The principal agent in treatment is digoxin. Digitalizing doses for newborns are: .05 to .07 mg/kg of body weight orally or .04 to .05 mg/kg of body weight IM for term infants, and .03 mg/kg of body weight orally for premature infants. One-half of the total dose is administered immediately, the remaining half divided into two doses to be administered in the

next 12 to 18 hours. The average maintenance dose for newborns is .01 mg per kg.
Toxicity to digitalis is revealed by rate and
rhythm changes on EKG. Both term and
preterm infants have an intolerance for
digitalis preparations and must be carefully monitored.

Furosemide (Lasix) is the diuretic most
commonly used in infants; the dosage is 1
mg/kg/day intravenously (2 to 3 mg/kg/day
orally). Careful records of urine output are
kept by weighing diapers (weigh dry and
again following voiding). Serum electrolytes must be carefully evaluated when
diuretics are used (Chapter 9). Oxygen is
used to relieve cyanosis and dyspnea.

Additional Nursing Responsibilities

In addition to careful assessment that
leads to the recognition of the infant with
congenital heart disease and to changes in
his condition, nurses must help parents
learn to care for their infant at home and,
in many instances, to cope with a chronic
problem, offering appropriate protection
but avoiding overprotection, a very fine
and often difficult distinction.

Parents want and need answers about
the nature of their infant's problem — the
prognosis and timetable if surgery is contemplated, for example. They also need
help in day-to-day planning. Feeding
problems are discussed in Chapter 9. If
the baby is to receive digoxin following
discharge, whoever is to give the digoxin
must have instruction and practice while
the baby is in the hospital. Jackson (1979)
suggests the following guidelines for
parents (which I have modified slightly).

1. Give the prescribed dosage without
variation.
2. If one dose is missed, do not be
concerned; do not double or increase the
next dose to compensate. If two or more
consecutive doses are missed, notify
physician, clinic, or nurse.
3. Give doses ar regular intervals as
prescribed (usually every 12 hours).
4. Give doses one hour before or two
hours after feedings (this facilitates passage into the bloodstream and avoids

loss in case of vomiting during feedings).
If dose is vomited within 15 minutes
after it is administered and most appears
lost, repeat dose. If more than 15 minutes
has elapsed, or you feel little has been
lost, do not repeat dose.
5. Notify physician, clinic, or nurse at
the first sign of any illness including
colds or flu. (Loss of appetite, vomiting,
and diarrhea are all signs of illness.)
6. Store digoxin in a safe place; if it is
accidentally taken by anyone, bring the
victim to an emergency room immediately. Bring the digoxin bottle with you.

These guidelines may seem simple, but
Jackson found that many parents who
were giving their infants digoxin did not
know these basic principles. In addition,
many were unsure of how to measure the
dosage, particularly if the original dosage
was changed. Parents need opportunities
for supervised practice in the administration of digoxin not only during initial
hospitalization but whenever the dosage
is changed.

THE NEWBORN REQUIRING SURGERY

Some of the more common conditions that
require or benefit from immediate surgical
correction are: (1) anomalies of the gastrointestinal tract (tracheoesophageal fistula,
diaphragmatic hernia, intestinal obstruction, imperforate anus, and omphalocele),
(2) skull fracture, (3) bilateral choanal atresia, (4) meningocele and encephalocele,
(5) certain congenital heart defects, and (6)
certain disorders of the genitourinary tract
(patent urachus, obstructions).

Preoperative Care of Newborns

Preoperative care of newborns involves
attention to the basic principles of stabilization: thermoregulation; provision of
glucose, fluids, and electrolytes; maintenance of acid-base balance; and specific
care directed toward the special needs of
the individual baby.

Perhaps the most difficult task is explaining to parents that their new baby has a defect that needs emergency surgery. Although the doctor will undoubtedly make the initial explanation, it is not very long before the father and perhaps a grandmother appear at the nursery door to see the baby and ask many of the same questions again, because they need to hear the answer again. And they need to see for themselves, so they can try to understand what is happening.

Some Special Problems Related to Surgery in Newborns

Major areas of difficulty for newborns who need surgery include anesthesia, hyperbilirubinemia, and maintenance of adequate warmth during surgery.

Anesthesia is complicated by the limited pulmonary reserve of the baby, by the fact that his rapid respiratory rate must be maintained even during deep anesthesia, and by his sensitivity to relaxant drugs.

Physiologic jaundice may be intensified by the stress of surgery or by conditions related to the surgery such as sepsis, the initial condition for which the baby is being treated, dehydration, or the anesthesia. On the other hand, adequate hydration, antibiotics, and good general supportive care may bring about a significant fall in bilirubin level without other treatment.

KEEPING THE BABY WARM DURING SURGERY

One of the biggest hazards to a newborn in a modern, air-conditioned operating room is chilling. Even a healthy term newborn lying on the table for an hour or more, without undergoing a surgical procedure, could experience difficulties because of chilling that might be fatal or, at the least, damaging. For an infant who is sick enough to require an emergency operation and who, in addition, is often of low birth weight, this chilling is a significant danger. Exposure of internal organs

during surgery, such as the bowel, hastens the fall of the baby's temperature.

How can heat be conserved in the operating room ?

1. From the standpoint of the baby, an operating room temperature of 29.4°C (85° F) with a relative humidity of approximately 50 per cent is ideal, yet this degree of warmth will probably be unacceptable to many surgeons. An overbed warmer that uses radiant heat keeps the operative area warm, but this too may make the surgical team uncomfortable. If such a warmer is used the distance between the baby and the warmer in relation to the temperature of the warmer is important; hyperthermia is no more desirable than hypothermia.

2. The baby should be transported to the operating room (as well as to the x-ray room or any other area of the hospital) in a heated, covered incubator. The bed should be plugged in once he reaches the operating room, and he should stay in it until the surgeons are scrubbed (Figure 8–15).

3. Wrapping the baby's arms and legs in a protective covering, such as the sheet wadding used to line plaster casts, not only reduces heat loss but helps protect his extremities against injury during surgery and also partially immobilizes him. His head should also be covered because a baby loses heat through his bare scalp. All of this can be done while the baby is in his warm bed.

4. During the surgical procedure itself, the baby must be kept warm without being burned or overheated, and his temperature, both rectal and axillary, must be monitored and recorded.

5. Nonvolatile liquids should be used for skin preparation, since evaporation leads to cooling.

6. Only the area required for operation should be uncovered.

7. Blood for transfusion should be warmed to body temperature (37° C or 98.6° F).

8. A warmed incubator should be ready to receive the baby immediately following surgery and should be used to transport him to the nursery.

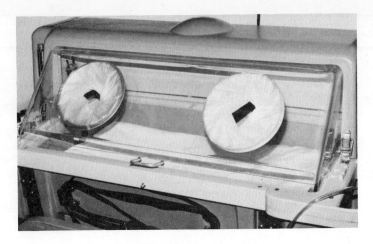

Figure 8–15. A transport incubator should be used if the infant is transported from one area to another within a hospital as well as between hospitals.

The Baby with a Tracheoesophageal Fistula

The signs indicating that a baby has a tracheoesophageal fistula vary somewhat with the type of anatomical anomaly involved (Fig. 8–16). In the most common type of anomaly (*A*), the esophagus ends in a blind pouch (a catheter cannot be passed through it), accounting for the almost immediate vomiting of any fluid taken orally. The trachea is connected to the stomach by a short fistula; thus the stomach becomes quickly distended as air enters with each breath. Gastric secretions can enter the tracheobronchial tree through the fistula. When the baby is not being fed there is drooling and frequent bubbly mucus — the classic symptom. Spotting this excess mucus before the baby is fed for the first time contributes to the successful care of these babies.

In *B*, air does not enter the stomach nor can gastric juice reach the trachea and lungs, but milk and saliva do overflow the esophagus into the respiratory tract.

The fistula in *C* is often not suspected in the newborn period because the esophagus does lead to the stomach and the baby can take his feedings. However, there is a fistula, although it may be as small as a pinpoint, and its presence is suspected as the baby grows older and has repeated pneumonitis.

Fortunately, the fistulas in *D* and *E* are rare. Because the upper esophagus is connected to the trachea any feeding taken orally will be carried directly to the lungs; the baby will cough and become cyanotic, "drowning" in the fluid.

Maternal polyhydramnios is a diagnostic clue available even before the baby is examined. Polyhydramnios often means that obstruction exists somewhere along

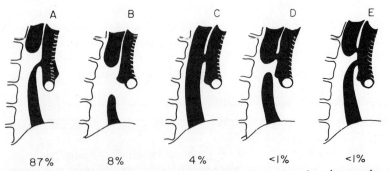

A	B	C	D	E
87%	8%	4%	<1%	<1%

Figure 8–16. The most common forms of esophageal atresia and tracheoesophageal fistula, in order of frequency. (From Vaughan, McKay, and Behrman (eds.): Nelson Textbook of Pediatrics. 11th Edition, W. B. Saunders, 1979.)

the gastrointestinal tract. Under normal circumstances the fetus swallows amniotic fluid, but in this instance the obstruction prevents him from doing so.

CARING FOR THE BABY WITH A
TRACHEOESOPHAGEAL FISTULA

As could be expected, the greatest preoperative problem is aspiration pneumonia. Preoperative nursing care, aside from general support, is largely aimed at preventing this difficulty. In the most common type (Fig. 8–16A), the baby's head and chest are elevated, to prevent the regurgitation of gastric juice into the lung, by elevating the floor of the isolette. The baby has to be kept in this semi-upright position at all times, including when he is being transported from a community hospital to a medical center for surgery.

Babies with each type of anomaly need frequent suctioning, but there is no purpose served by elevating the head of a baby with a type of fistula seen in B, since there is no connection between the stomach and either the trachea or the esophagus. In some instances, lowering the baby's head may be suggested to facilitate the draining of mucus and saliva that the baby is unable to swallow. The Trendelenburg position may cause respiratory distress in a newborn, and some physicians oppose using it for these tiny babies under any circumstance.

Surgery involves ligation of the fistula and anastomosis of the esophageal segments. When the segments are far apart, tissue from another area, such as the colon, must be used to bridge the gap. More than one operation may be required.

The baby returns from surgery with a chest tube and a gastrostomy tube for feeding and for relieving abdominal distention. During the first postoperative hours he needs the individual attention of one nurse. Mucus may plug the respiratory tract, so frequent suctioning is necessary. He must be turned and stimulated to cry so that his lungs will fully expand. Normally there will be a minimal amount of drainage through the chest tube, and the lungs will be expanded within a few hours.

The following standard precautions for any patient, child or adult, with a chest tube have to be observed.

1. If a bottle is used for drainage it is taped to the floor. Some newer types of setups use a heavy plastic bag that can be attached to the lower part of the isolette; the advantage here is that the bag moves automatically with the isolette when it is moved, so there is no danger of forgetting to move the bag and causing tension on the chest tube. The bag, like the bottle, must never be raised.

2. No part of the tubing should ever be disconnected nor should it be compressed or kinked. When the isolette hood is lifted and lowered, caution should be taken to see that the tubing is not caught between the hood and the metal framework.

3. If there are clots of blood in the tube, the tube should be milked away from the baby.

4. Two hemostats, their ends covered with rubber tubing, must always be taped to the top of the isolette so that if for some reason there is a break in the system (e.g., a broken bottle or a hole in the tubing), the tube can be immediately clamped to prevent a pneumothorax caused by the air rushing into the chest.

5. Fluid level in the bottle should be marked on a tape and checked frequently, depending on the amount of bleeding and drainage.

In the first days following repair of a tracheoesophageal fistula, feedings are given through a gastrostomy tube (Chapter 9). Oral feedings begin in from five to 10 days in a baby who is doing well. If total repair was not possible during the initial surgery, gastrostomy feedings will continue for many months, which means that the mother will need to learn how to feed and care for her baby with the tube in place after he goes home.

Postoperatively the biggest problem facing these babies is the healing of the esophagus. Because it has a segmental blood supply, inadequate circulation in one portion of the esophagus is not well compensated. Nor does the esophagus hold sutures well. In spite of these difficulties, surgery is generally successful when (1) the baby is full term, (2) he has no other anomalies, and (3) the esophageal segments are close together. Unfortunately one or all of these requirements may not be fulfilled, and in some studies mortality rates are as high as 45 per cent. If death comes, it is usually from sepsis or pneumonia or from general debilitation.

The Baby with Diaphragmatic Hernia

When the diaphragm fails to develop properly, part of the abdominal organs may herniate through the defect into the chest. If the displacement is extensive, the baby will be in acute respiratory distress from the time of birth and is likely to die without early surgery. In addition to cyanosis and retractions, infants with diaphragmatic hernia have small, scaphoid abdomens. There are no breath sounds on the affected side, which is more often the left side, and the heart beat is heard farther to the right (in left-sided displacement).

Both pre- and postoperatively, the baby must have his head elevated to minimize the pressure of the abdominal organs on the lungs and to allow the diaphragm to move as freely as possible. Postoperatively, the baby will have a chest tube connected to waterseal drainage and either a gastrostomy or nasogastric tube to keep the stomach from becoming distended. First feedings, which will begin in the second 24 hours after surgery if the baby is doing well, will be given through the tube.

Since it often takes several days for the lung on the affected side to expand fully, postoperative respiratory distress is not unusual. Positioning the baby so the affected side is down helps the unaffected lung to expand to its fullest potential in the immediate postoperative period when it is the only one functioning.

Even with superior care, not all of these babies survive. Mortality rates range from 25 per cent in hospitals where surgeons

and nurses are specialists in infant care to higher than 50 per cent. At least part of this high mortality is due to associated anomalies of heart, lungs, or intestines.

The Baby with an Omphalocele

Failure of the viscera to return to the abdomen after the tenth week of embryonic life (Chapter 1) results in an omphalocele — a defect immediately obvious at birth that carries a high mortality rate if the omphalocele is large. Death is likely to come either from postoperative respiratory distress, which results from pressure on the diaphragm when a large amount of bowel is replaced in the abdominal cavity at one time, or from infection of the abdominal viscera.

Before surgery, every effort is made to keep the contents of the sac sterile by covering them with sterile sponges and sterile plastic. The viscera are only partially replaced during surgery and an envelope is created over the remainder, a little more bowel being returned to the abdomen each day to keep respiratory distress to a minimum. An alternative procedure involves suturing the skin over the abdominal contents and deferring return to the abdomen until both baby and abdomen have grown larger.

The Baby with an Intestinal Obstruction

Obstruction, whether due to atresia, stenosis, or malrotation, may occur in the small or large intestine. Meconium ileus, an early symptom of cystic fibrosis, can also cause obstruction in the newborn. Careful nursing observations of vomitus and stools are most important in recognizing an obstruction and pinpointing its location. Green vomitus, i.e., vomitus containing bile, is the classic symptom. Absence of stool, abdominal distention, and, occasionally, peristaltic waves from right to left are also significant observations. The lower in the gastrointestinal tract the obstruction is located, the more likely it is that symptoms will be delayed.

As was true of babies with tracheoesophageal fistulas (and for the same reason) the mothers of babies with intestinal obstructions often have excessive amounts of amniotic fluid. Surgery is the only treatment. Since an obstruction is not likely to be recognized as early as most other anomalies of the gastrointestinal tract, the baby may have vomited several times and lost electrolytes as well as fluid, a situation that must be corrected before he goes to the operating room.

Postoperatively as well as preoperatively, vomiting and aspiration are the chief dangers for these babies. Because of this, they should be positioned on their abdomens or sides. A nasogastric tube is inserted before surgery and either a gastrostomy tube or a nasogastric tube will be in place afterward to prevent air and intestinal secretions from accumulating in the stomach until bowel peristalsis is restored. The return of peristalsis is indicated by normal stools and minimal gastric drainage.

The Baby with an Imperforate Anus

The simple expedient of taking an initial temperature on every newborn will detect the absence of a patent anus. If the anus is imperforate, urine is tested for the presence of meconium to determine whether or not there is a fistula to the urinary system. Rectovaginal or rectourinary fistulas are common. Nearly half of all infants with an imperforate anus have urinary tract infections as well.

Surgical repair is relatively simple in those instances in which the rectum ends close to the perineum (more commonly in females) and more complicated when the end of the rectum is high and there is a fistula to the bladder or urethra. In the latter instance a temporary colostomy is created, more extensive surgery being delayed until the baby is several months old.

Following perineal repair, specific nursing care is directed toward keeping the suture line free of feces. A diaper is not used so that any stool will be observed immediately and washed away. Newborns, when they lie on their abdomens, have a tendency to pull their legs up under them, creating tension in the perineal area. Because of this, following perineal surgery, the baby should be positioned on either side and his position changed frequently.

Colostomy care for infants does not differ from that given to older persons with colostomy. The mother needs a chance to become accustomed to the colostomy before she takes her baby home. The biggest problem is probably the mother's psychological reaction, i.e., the acceptance of her baby with his colostomy. Knowing that it is only temporary (for about three to six months) and discovering, through practice in the nursery, that care is not really difficult, should help to relieve her anxiety so that she can love her baby and treat him normally.

The Baby with a Meningocele, Meningomyelocele, or Encephalocele

Although these obvious defects pose no immediate threat to the baby's life, most neurosurgeons prefer to eliminate them as soon after birth as possible. Not only does early surgery reduce the risk of infection with subsequent meningitis and make baby care far less difficult, it also seems to make it easier for the mother to accept her baby. There is some evidence that rapidly progressing damage may occur in the malformed and partially exposed spinal cord of a meningomyelocele.

Before surgery the sac has to be protected. If it is relatively small, the baby can be kept in a prone position, but when the sac is large, it is difficult to place him in this position; in this case the baby may be more easily positioned on his side.

The ultimate success of surgery depends to a large extent on the kind of defect that is involved. There are no nerves in the dura mater sac of a *meningocele;* hence there is no loss of either sensory or motor function. The baby should be perfectly normal following surgery.

In a *meningomyelocele*, however, the sac does contain a portion of the spinal cord and terminal nerves. In addition, nearly three-fourths of these babies have, or will have, hydrocephalus. There will be varying degrees of paralysis due to motor nerve involvement and loss of sensation related to sensory involvement. One of the first questions the neurosurgeon is likely to ask is, "Does he move his legs?" If meconium continually oozes from the anus and urine appears to dribble, it is likely that the baby lacks sphincter control, another significant observation.

An *encephalocele* is far less common than a meningocele. The sac may contain fluid, nervous tissue, or a portion of the brain.

If the baby is born in a hospital where there is no neurosurgeon, the sac must be protected during transportation to a medical center. The area is covered with a sterile dressing and sterile plastic and is protected by a "doughnut" of foam rubber that has been wrapped in sterile gauze and secured with a binder.

Surgery for a meningomyelocele involves the excision of the sac and the replacement of nerve tissue into the spinal canal. Wound healing takes from a week to 10 days. During this time the area has to be kept scrupulously free of urine and stool, which is often more difficult to achieve than with normal newborns because of the common lack of sphincter control. To facilitate this aspect of care, the baby is kept unclothed and prone in an isolette; frequently sterile plastic is used to cover the area of the incision.

Because postoperative hydrocephalus is not unusual, daily head and chest measurements must be recorded. By plotting these measurements graphically, the nurse or doctor can detect rapid increases in head size, and a shunting procedure can be performed early, before there is opportunity for brain damage. The most common shunts are ventriculoatrial, ventriculojugular, and ventriculoperitoneal. Pudenz and Holter valves allow spinal fluid to be drained from the ventricles but prevent a backflow from the blood stream. They can become blocked by blood clots, particularly those that go to the right atrium of the heart. Blockage is sometimes overcome by a pump in the valve that can be pressed through the skin surface. Thus it is important for both nurse and parents to know what kind of apparatus has been inserted. Parents also have to learn to recognize the signs of increased intracranial pressure, which is a possibility at any time in a baby who has had a shunt. These symptoms are failure to feed well, vomiting, irritability, lethargy, and a bulging fontanelle.

Other important observations in a baby who has had surgery to correct a meningomyelocele are:

1. The amount of movement in feet and legs (passive exercise is in order when no such movement exists).

2. Presence of clubbed feet.

3. Urinary retention, which if unrecognized and untreated can eventually lead to impairment of renal function.

4. Skin breakdown when urine and feces continually dribble.

THE INFANT OF A MOTHER ADDICTED TO NARCOTICS

As drug use among young women increases, as it has during recent years, the incidence of infants being born to mothers addicted to narcotics has increased. In some urban medical centers relatively large numbers of newborns addicted to morphine, heroin, and methadone are currently being seen. The problem for the nurse is to recognize these babies.

The most prominent sign is central nervous system irritability: the baby is frantic and inconsolable, he may have tremors, and the Moro response may be incomplete. His shrill cry is not unlike that of a baby with central nervous system damage. In addition, there may be a large amount of mucus or such generalized symptoms as diarrhea and vomiting. Either excessive weight loss, due to fluid loss from vomiting or diarrhea, or failure to gain weight, because of a very high expenditure of energy, prevents these babies from growing normally in the nursery.

Since all these symptoms are common to many other kinds of newborn problems, it is important that the nurse be alert to signs of addiction in mothers, such as scarred veins and withdrawal symptoms, in order to evaluate the symptoms in babies. Addiction can be suspected and the possibility should be evaluated in mothers with venereal disease, hepatitis, cellulitis, and thrombophlebitis.

The diagnosis in the baby is confirmed by the discovery of narcotic breakdown products in the blood and urine. Specimens need to be collected shortly after birth because these narcotic metabolites disappear quickly.

Nursing approaches to common problems in infants of addicted mothers are described in Table 8–17.

TRANSPORT OF THE HIGH RISK NEWBORN

The intensive level of care that a small number of high risk mothers and newborns require is difficult to achieve at every hospital providing maternity care. For this reason, mothers and infants who are at high risk are more frequently being transferred to regional medical centers.

When the delivery of a high risk infant can be determined in advance, transport of the mother (who is usually not in acute distress) before delivery to the regional center offers many advantages over transport of a critically ill newborn. Which mother should be transported will vary with the ability of the community hospital to care for the mother and infant (see Regionalization, Chapter 12), with the status of the mother at the time transport is considered (is she in early labor or does she have hypertension, which requires intensive care and possible early delivery of an infant who will be preterm), and with the distance to the regional center.

Even with a commitment to maternal transport, there will still be a need for infant transport as well. Not all high risk births can be anticipated. Although some mothers can be identified as likely to deliver babies needing special care even before they become pregnant (e.g., the mother who has previously delivered a child with erythroblastosis), other mothers have sudden premature labor or unanticipated difficulty during labor or delivery or have a child with a major congenital anomaly without any prior indication. Infant transport will always be essential under these circumstances.

Table 8–17   The Passively Addicted Infant

Characteristics and Problems	Nursing Approach

Central nervous system irritability
  Shrill high-pitched cry
  Sleep disturbances
  Incomplete Moro response
  Increased sucking needs
	Explain behavior to parents (behavior will
	  not last)
	Help parents discover ways of soothing infant
	  (preferred position, manner of holding, etc.)
	Provide pacifier for nonnutritive sucking needs

Gastrointestinal dysfunction
  Vomiting, regurgitation, diarrhea
	Avoid overfeeding
	Assess weight loss or failure to gain, signs of
	  dehydration

Behavioral variations
  Highly sensitive to auditory stimuli
  Decreased visual orientation and following
	Provide quiet environment
	Talk to baby with quiet voice
	Provide visual stimulation

Potential disturbance in parent-infant interaction
  Inability of mother to care for infant
	Provide opportunities for parent-infant
	  interaction
	Assess parent-infant interaction
	Refer to community health nursing for long-term
	  follow-up

*Based, in part, on Kantor: MCN 3:281, 1978.

In addition, even when a high risk baby is expected, it will not always be possible for the mother to leave her own community to be cared for in a hospital many miles away for one to two weeks or longer. Not only the economic costs but the social costs in terms of separation from husband and family may be too high. Planning for hospitalization of such a mother will have to include planning for all the needs of the family, not just the mother's (and later the baby's) medical problems. In transporting high risk newborns, the same principles apply as in in-hospital care. The baby must be kept warm and ventilation, fluid, and glucose must be provided. Many transport teams are able to give a more sophisticated level of care that includes continuous monitoring of temperature, heart rate, and FiO_2 and assessment and correction of acid-base status as well as emergency intervention.

Transport Teams: Who Transports

An infant may be transported by a team from the hospital in which the baby was delivered or by a team from the regional center. Teams may consist of nurses or a nurse and/or respiratory therapist and/or physician. The regional center team must, of course, travel twice as far as a team from the community hospital, which delays the arrival of the infant at the regional center. However, if that time is used in the community hospital to stabilize the infant and to allow parents contact with their baby, it is by no means wasted. The regional center team, which participates in many transports, will frequently be more skilled than personnel from a hospital that transports only a few babies a month. At this time, regional center teams are not available in all communities. In some communities, the regional team may be called to transport the very critically ill infant (e.g., a 900 g baby with respiratory distress), whereas the community hospital may transport a baby less critically ill (e.g., a term infant with a myelomeningocele).

Whether a Baby Should be Transported

The resources that the hospital has affects the decision to transport a high risk infant. The community hospital must be able to provide not only nursing care and medical surveillance but also assisted ventilation (CPAP or respirator). The hospital also must be able to closely monitor oxygen therapy through blood gases using a micro technique (a small amount of blood) and be able to give precise amounts of intravenous fluid.

In general, the following situations indicate that an infant should receive care at a regional center: (1) weight of less than 1500 g; (2) emergency surgery required (e.g., for tracheoesophageal fistula, diaphragmatic hernia, gastroschisis); (3) congenital heart disease suspected; (4) major complications during delivery (e.g., meconium aspiration, birth asphyxia); (5) infant appears to be doing poorly for some unknown reason.

Resuscitation, Stabilization, and Preparation for Transport

The immediate resuscitation of the newborn is described in Chapter 5.

Stabilization prior to transport can be a significant factor in reducing mortality and morbidity. There is an understandable inclination to get the baby to the regional center as soon as possible. However, speed should never be at the expense of stabilization. Stabilization includes:

1. Maintenance of a thermoneutral environment to keep the infant's skin temperature at 36.3 to 36.5°C (97.5 to 97.7°F).
2. Provision of oxygen and appropriate assistance in ventilation.
3. Provision of fluid and electrolytes.
4. Correction of acidosis and hypoglycemia.
5. Specific treatment of emergency conditions (e.g., pneumothorax).
6. Specific treatment for the baby's

problem (e.g., tracheoesophageal fistula, myelomeningocele).

In addition, parents need the opportunity to see and touch their baby prior to transport. The mother may have to remain at the community hospital for one or two days (longer if she has had a cesarean birth) and will miss much early contact with her baby. Although some mothers are transported with the baby and are cared for at regional centers, some regional centers (e.g., hospitals for children) may have no facilities for maternal care.

An explanation of why the baby must be transported is also essential. Parents may not understand a great deal of what nurses tell them at this time. They may hear nothing more than "We feel your baby should be transferred to the intensive care unit at the Medical Center." Later, nurses will need to go back over what they have told the parents. It is nevertheless important to give honest, realistic information prior to the transport of their baby.

A polaroid picture of the baby can be quickly made before transport so that the mother will have tangible evidence of the reality of her baby. The father and other family members may be able to visit the baby at the regional center before the mother's discharge, but she can feel very left out. A picture may seem an inadequate substitute for a real baby, but mothers have said that it does help.

In addition to care aimed at stabilization, prophylactic vitamin K and silver nitrate should be given and charted so that the dose will not be repeated at the receiving hospital. A gavage tube is passed into the stomach and the contents are gently aspirated to prevent aspiration during transport. The baby must be properly identified. Records must be available to send to the receiving hospital. These include:

1. Xeroxed copies of the baby's and mother's records.

2. All infant x-rays (to be returned to the referring hospital).

3. 10 ml of maternal blood (clotted).

4. Infant cord blood.

5. A consent form, signed by the parents, for transport and care during transport.

Equipment and Supplies for Transport

Although some transport vehicles lack little that is available in an intensive care unit, the cost of such transport capability is prohibitive in many areas, and such a vehicle is not necessary for all transports. The equipment needed for transport can be thought of in terms of the specific needs of the baby (Table 8–18).

WARMTH

A transport incubator that provides warmth as well as visibility and has a servocontrol to adjust the temperature to the baby's skin temperature is ideal. If there is no servocontrol, the incubator temperature should be set 2 to 3°F above the infant's thermoneutral environment (see Table 8–2) and the baby's axillary temperature monitored and recorded every 15 minutes. If skin temperature is normal, incubator temperature may be set in the infant's thermoneutral range, again with 15-minute checks to ensure continuous stability.

Covering the incubator with a sheet or blanket will help prevent radiant heat loss during outside movement to and from the transport vehicle. Within the transport vehicle, increased temperature will also be required in cold weather to reduce radiant heat loss. Additional measures to provide warmth include the careful use of hot water bottles filled with water 40.5°C (105°F) (not really satisfactory but better than nothing at all), wrapping aluminum foil or plastic wrap around the baby's blanket (good insulation but visibility, which is very important, is compromised), and wrapping the baby's arms and legs in cotton batting. This last measure, frequently used in infant surgery, is a useful adjunct to other methods and will reduce heat loss without compromising visibility.

Table 8–18 Equipment Needed for Transport of High Risk Infants

Need	Equipment
Warmth	Transport incubator with servomechanism Thermometer Blankets Additional wrapping materials: plastic wrap, cotton batting, foil
Ventilation	Oxygen supply Laryngoscope with blades – #0, #1 (include spare batteries) Oral airways Endotracheal tubes (2.5–4.0 mm) Resuscitation bag and mask Stethoscope Adhesive tape Scissors Suction catheters with suction equipment Oxygen concentration monitor to monitor FIO_2 Flashlight CPAP* Mechanical ventilator* Equipment for in-transport monitoring of blood* gases and correction of acid-base imbalance
Prevention of hypoglycemia	Dextrostix Intravenous fluids and supplies (scalp vein needles, alcohol swabs, collodion, tape, cotton balls) Infusion pump Glucagon (if unable to start IV)
Assessment of vital signs	Thermometer (noted above) Stethoscope (noted above) Infant blood pressure equipment
Preparation for potential in-transport emergency	Drugs Sodium bicarbonate Calcium gluconate Epinephrine 1:10,000 Furosemide KCl Saline Heparin Syringes (tuberculin, 3 cc, 10 cc, 20 cc) Needle thoracocentesis 30 cc syringe Three-way stopcock Scalp vein needle (19–23)

*Additional equipment (not required)

Ventilation

Ventilation is provided by bag and mask or bag and endotracheal tube when needed. An extra full cylinder of oxygen should be taken along during transport because any lapse in oxygenation, even of short duration, can lead to brain damage. Plan for twice the amount of oxygen that you would appear to need (based on flow rate and amount of time in transport). The trip may be prolonged beyond the anticipated time. In a trip of more than 30 minutes, it is ideal to monitor oxygen concentration. Some infant transport systems allow the use of continuous positive airway pressure or mechanical ventilation during transport.

Prevention of Hypoglycemia

Hypoglycemia during transport is a major concern. A baby often arrives at a medical center with an initial Dextrostix of 0 with no indication of how long his blood sugar has been that low. As noted above, glucose may be given through umbilical artery catheter or through a peripheral line. Ten or 15 per cent is the common solution, given at approximately 10 ml per hour for term infants and 2 to 4 ml per hour for preterm babies. A battery-run infusion pump will ensure a constant rate. Extra sterile supplies (both fluids and peripheral intravenous equipment) should be taken on the trip.

Conditions Presenting Special Problems in Transport

Pneumothorax

A pneumothorax exists when air is trapped in the pleural cavity outside the parenchyma of the lung. Many of the respiratory problems of newborns, including RDS and meconium aspiration syndrome, predispose to pneumothorax. When positive pressure in excess of 30 cm H_2O is applied to the lungs, the risk of pneumothorax is increased.

The baby may become restless, irritable, and apneic and have bradycardia and/or cyanosis and falling blood pressure. Breath sounds may be diminished or absent on the affected side and heart sounds may shift. The abdomen may be distended.

Prior to transport, a suspected pneumothorax should be confirmed by x-ray (this is usually not possible during transport).

Emergency aspiration is accomplished by attaching a syringe with a three-way stopcock to a scalp vein needle — 19 to 23 gauge (Fig. 8–17). The needle is pointed toward the baby's feet and inserted into the second, third, or fourth intercostal space in the anterior axillary line (over the top of the rib), avoiding the nipple. Air is withdrawn from the pleural space and then expelled from the syringe via the stopcock. Withdrawal of air should continue until resistance occurs.

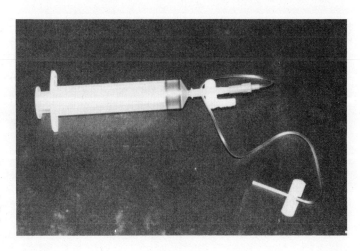

Figure 8–17. A syringe, a stopcock, and a scalp vein needle can be used to aspirate air from a pneumothorax.

Table 8–19 Additional Nursing Care for Infants with
Specific Problems During Transport

Condition	Special Points in Care
Tracheoesophageal fistula Esophageal atresia	Elevate head at a 45° angle at all times to prevent chemical pneumonia from gastric acid reflux to lungs (use an infant seat) Suction bubbly secretions in mouth and oropharynx Insert a catheter (#10 French) into blind pouch (or into stomach if tracheoesophageal fistula occurs without esophageal atresia) and connect to low intermittent suction Avoid crying (air forced into stomach may cause gastric reflux to lungs)
Pneumothorax	Transport with normal side uppermost Aspirate air Watch for sudden worsening of respiration and/or shift in position of apical heart sounds
Diaphragmatic hernia	Transport with side with better lung function uppermost (usually the right side) Elevate head so abdominal organs do not compromise limited lung function Pass orogastric tube to decompress bowel Avoid positive pressure ventilation if possible, because bowel in chest will fill with air and further compromise respiration Intubate, if essential, into main stem bronchus of unaffected side Observe carefully for pneumothorax in unaffected lung
Abdominal distention (e.g., intestinal block)	Insert nasogastric tube; aspirate gently with syringe and record amount aspirated; administer low intermittent suction if possible Observe carefully for signs of shock
Exposed internal organs (e.g. gastroschisis, ectopic bladder)	Cover exposed internal organs with warm sterile saline dressing, then Vaseline gauze; an outer wrapping of plastic drape provides further insulation (infant is at high risk of heat loss because of exposed organs)
Meningocele	Transport prone Use doughnut support around meningocele Cover with sterile saline dressing or dry sterile dressing
Hypognathia, Pierre Robin syndrome	Transport face down so that tongue will fall forward; tongue falling back will lead to respiratory obstruction
Choanal atresia or stuffy nose for some reason	Baby is obligate nose breather; to assist him to breathe through mouth, insert oral airway or cut a large hole in a nipple and tape it to mouth
Eyelids open (as in severe facial palsy, occasionally in hydrocephalus)	Administer eye drops and ophthalmic ointment

CONGENITAL ANOMALIES

A number of congenital anomalies present special problems or require specific care prior to and during transport. These con-ditions are discussed in detail in other sections of this chapter; Table 8–19 summarizes specific needs of these babies during transport.

Sensory Stimulation of the Preterm Infant

An appreciation of the effects of sensory stimulation on the development of preterm infants is growing among nurses as well as others concerned with infancy, primarily as a result of research in the past decade. If the preterm infant had remained in utero, a variety of stimuli would have been provided. Auditory stimulation comes from the mother's heartbeat, her digestive tract, and perhaps from other sources as well. As the mother moves, there is vestibular and kinesthetic stimulation, and the amniotic fluid, the walls of the uterus, the cord, and the fetal body provide tactile stimulation. Only visual stimulation is lacking.

The infant born prior to term is deprived of this intrauterine stimulation. Although the nursery environment certainly provides a variety of stimuli, including many that are painful, we need to examine the types of stimulation that we provide or fail to provide each day in relation to short-term and long-term developmental needs.

Tactile Stimulation

The skin appears to be the most highly developed of the sense organs of the preterm baby. Montagu (1971) describes skin sensitivity in embryos of less than eight weeks of age. Animal studies support the importance of tactile stimulation not only for behavioral development but even for survival.

Solkoff and his associates (1969) explored the effects of handling on 10 white preterm babies; the mean birth weight for the experimental group was 3.00 lbs and 3.02 lbs for the control group. The "handling" consisted of gently rubbing the infant's back, neck, and arms for five minutes each hour (24 hours a day) for a 10-day experimental period. Following the experimental period both experimental and control infants were handled in the same manner, with handling confined largely to burping and diaper changing. Although the sample was too small for statistical tests, the handled infants appeared more active and regained birth weight in 10.8 days as compared with 15.4 days for the control group.

Seven to eight months following discharge from the preterm nursery, each infant was given a complete physical examination and the Bayley test of Mental and Motor Development. All the handled infants were described as active and physically healthy. Of the five nonhandled infants, three were rated more than two standard deviations below the growth mean for their age and one was at the lower limit of normal. There was a suspicion of potential cerebral palsy in two. Only one infant in the control group was considered to be developing normally. One of the handled babies showed poor gross and fine motor development; four of the nonhandled infants were rated as below the mean.

It is interesting that this study, in spite of the small number of infants tested, was not only published but was accompanied by an editorial note recognizing the importance of the findings for the care of preterm infants. It is, in a sense, a landmark study in that research attention was focused on the stimulation of the preterm infant.

Powell (1974) examined tactile stimulation in a study of 36 black infants weighing between 1000 and 2000 g at birth. Powell hypothesized that (1) increased handling during hospitalization would lead to increased weight gain and higher developmental quotients for the handled infants, and (2) maternal handling of the infant during hospitalization would lead to "better" maternal behavior. Powell found that increased handling did lead to slight differences in initial weight gain but to no difference in height at two, four, or six months. The handled infants did have higher developmental quotients on all but one comparison of the Bayley infant development scale at two, four, and six months.

Proprioceptive-Vestibular-Kinesthetic Stimulation

Any receptor that is sensitive to the position and movement of the body is called a *proprioceptor*. Proprioceptors in the semicircular canals and the vestibule of the inner ear are sensitive to the orientation of the body in space and to body rotation. Proprioceptors in the muscles, tendons, and joints are sensitive to the position and movement of body members and give rise to kinesthetic sensations.

Movement as a means of quieting a fretful baby is practiced in many cultures. Movement may involve rocking the baby in a cradle or in the mother's arms in a chair, or movement may come from being strapped to the mother's body or carried on her hip as she walks. Van der Daele's (1970) studies of term infants in a rockerbox demonstrated that rocking led to a marked reduction in infant activity and distress (a fact to which generations of mothers can attest).

Preterm infants miss the rocking experience in their early days and weeks to a large extent. They lie in incubators or open beds under radiant warmers, often attached to one or more pieces of equipment such as heart rate monitors, respiratory support equipment, thermistor probes, and a variety of other devices. Two studies, Korner and associates (1975) and Kramer and Pierpoint (1976), used waterbeds to provide vestibular stimulation for preterm infants.

The logic behind the use of waterbeds is simple: the preterm infant, were he not delivered early, would be floating in amniotic fluid. Through his own movement within the fluid and through the changes in position that result from his mother's activities, his vestibular system would be stimulated during the normal course of development. Born prior to term, the premature infant loses this stimulation before the vestibular system is fully mature.

The importance of vestibular stimulation has been demonstrated in animal studies in the work of Harlow (1958) and Mason (1968). Harlow's monkeys, raised with cloth surrogate mothers and deprived of vestibular stimulation, were autistic and self-mutilating and engaged in rocking behavior. Mason's monkeys, also reared in isolation but with swinging surrogate mothers, did not show such severe behavioral changes.

Korner and her colleagues (1975) studied 21 infants with gestational ages of 34 weeks or less who were not severely ill. Infants were randomly assigned to experimental and control groups. Significant differences were found between the experimental and control babies in relation to the incidence of apnea (defined in this study as a respiratory rate of less than 20 breaths per minute), which was the primary purpose of the study.

Although Korner's group considered this a pilot study of the safety of oscillating waterbeds for use in future research and thus drew no conclusions about long-term development, the marked difference in apneic episodes could be a factor in subsequent development. Frequent apnea potentially compromises the oxygen supply of the brain and may physiologically affect development. Moreover, parents are frequently more hesitant to "attach" to babies they perceive as very sick, and thus frequent apnea could possibly affect the long-term parent-child relationship.

Kramer and Pierpont (1976) utilized both rocking waterbeds and auditory stimuli (a taped simulated heartbeat and a woman's voice) in their study of the growth patterns of preterm infants. Their sample consisted of 20 healthy preterm infants of less than 34 weeks gestation, gestational age being determined by the Dubowitz method.

They found that in their sample:

1. Stimulated infants on waterbeds gained significantly more weight than control infants.

2. Head circumference and biparietal diameters also increased significantly. The heads of the stimulated infants were both larger and more well rounded. Head size is a parameter believed to be related to brain growth and is considered by some neonatologists to be even more important than weight gain.

3. There was no difference in maturation as assessed by Dubowitz.

Because two types of stimuli were used, it is impossible to determine which, if either, was more important in determining outcome or if the combination of more than one stimulus was significant.

White and Labarba (1975) employed a combination of tactile and kinesthetic stimulation. Infants with gestational ages of less than 36 weeks received stimulation for 15 minutes every four hours. Experimental infants began to gain weight on the second day of treatment and gained at a significantly greater rate over the 10-day period. Mean increase in weight was 251 g for the experimental group and 67 g for the control group. Moreover, there was a marked shortening of the weight loss period characteristic of most newborns, whether born at term or prematurely. Significantly more formula was ingested by the experimental group. Although the nurses caring for the babies did not know which infants were in the experimental group, nurses' notes for the experimental infants included statements such as "eager eater" and "retains feedings well," whereas the charts of control infants included such notations as "takes formula poorly" and "often spits up."

Auditory Stimulation

The preterm baby spends from one to several weeks in an auditory milieu that differs markedly from both the intrauterine environment and the home setting of the term baby after the first days of life. Two studies, one by Katz (1971) and the other by Segall (1972), explored the relationship between auditory stimulation and the behavior of infants who were between 28 and 32 weeks gestational age. The criteria for determining gestational age were not described in either study. All the infants were cared for in incubators.

Katz hypothesized that the infants in her experimental group who heard their mother's voice for five minutes, six times a day beginning on the fifth day of life until they were 36 weeks gestational age, would demonstrate significantly greater maturational development, greater auditory and visual response, and less irritability than control infants. At 36 weeks gestational age the developmental levels of the infants were evaluated in terms of general maturation, audiovisual response, muscle tension, and irritability. The developmental levels of the experimental group exceeded those of the control group in motor scores, tactile adaptive behavior, and auditory and visual responses at a statistically significant level.

Segall exposed experimental infants to the sound of their mother's voice on tape for 30 minutes each day. During testing at 36 weeks, experimental infants showed a significantly greater decrease in heart rate in response to hearing a female voice. If decreases in heart rate can be considered evidence of "attending" to stimuli, auditory stimulation may facilitate arousal, attention, and the ability to habituate, i.e., to ignore stimuli after originally attending to them, a very necessary trait. All these behaviors are important in normal neurological development.

Visual Stimulation

Vision differs from the other senses in that there are no visual stimuli in utero. Although no studies have examined the effect of visual stimuli alone on the subsequent development of preterm infants, visual stimuli were included with other sources of stimulation in the research of Scarr-Salapatek and Williams (1973) described below. Something is known about the visual preferences of term and preterm infants.

1. Infants see objects best that are seven to nine inches from their face (Fantz, 1963),

2. Preterm infants will attend to a checkerboard design placed on the side of the isolette (Fantz 1963),

3. Faces promote visual attention (Lewis, 1969),

4. The ventro-ventral position (i..e, the position in which the baby is held to one's shoulder to burp) stimulates visual orientation (Korner and Grobstein 1966).

Multiple Stimuli

Scarr-Salapatek and Williams (1973) followed all the infants born alive at Philadelphia General Hospital in a year who weighed between 1300 and 1800 g (N =

30). Although the infants were randomly assigned, by chance several factors favored the development of the infants in the control (C) group. The control infants were heavier, required less oxygen, and had a lower incidence of sepsis than those in the experimental (E) group. At one week the control infants demonstrated more hand-to-mouth movements and less of a startle response. In other words, one would expect (on the basis of their condition at birth and their behavior at one week) that the prognosis for the control group would be better than that of the experimental group.

The stimulation program for the E group consisted of: (1) suspending nursery birds in a focal plane about nine inches from the baby's eyes inside the incubator; (2) thirty minutes of rocking, fondling, and talking to the baby at each feeding period (eight times in 24 hours); and (3) holding the baby in a ventro-ventral position for burping. The C group infants received minimal handling, which was generally believed most appropriate for low birth weight infants at the time of the study (1968–1969).

Following discharge, infant stimulation at home for the E group included: (1) weekly home visits by the child guidance social worker; (2) an infant seat so the baby could be out of his bed while awake, wall posters and a mobile near the baby's crib, rattles and other appropriate toys and books; and (3) demonstrations and instructions of games and various forms of stimulation by the social worker.

Assessment of the infants included the use of the Brazelton neonatal assessment scale at one and four weeks and the Cattell Infant Intelligence Scale at one year of age. The authors reported the following results.

1. At one week the C group demonstrated higher scores than the E group on most of the Brazelton criteria, as noted above.

2. At four weeks the reverse was true (the E group was superior to the C group on every scale).

3. Weight gain at four weeks was significantly higher for the E group.

4. At one year the E group had significantly higher developmental status. Developmental levels for the E group were nearly normal, unlike any previously tested low birth weight infants at Pennsylvania General Hospital. The C group remained one standard deviation (SD) below the norm of 100 for developmental status at one year.

5. The mean IQ for the E group was 95.3 (SD 11.0); the mean IQ for the C group was 85.7 (SD 15.9). Although 22 per cent of the E group scored below 20, 67 per cent of the C group did.

6. Within the E group, better developmental status was related to maternal play stimulation.

INTEGRATING SENSORY STIMULATION INTO NURSING CARE

Tactile and Kinesthetic-Vestibular Stimulation

Preterm infants are certainly touched frequently, but what is the quality of the touch they receive? Is it only to hold them while capillary blood is extracted from a heel or an intravenous needle is placed in the hand or scalp? Is time provided for gentle stroking and caressing? If tactile and kinesthetic stimulation is as important as the studies reviewed suggest, it should be incorporated into the nursing care plan and not left merely to chance when there is extra time and someone feels like playing with a cute baby.

Encouraging parents to stroke their infants gently not only provides tactile stimulation but increases opportunities for closeness between parents and infants. When parents cannot be present, stroking needs must be met by the nursing staff. Combining stroking with feeding periods is one way of assuring the stimulation of those babies who are fed, because feedings in special and intensive care nurseries are usually as frequent as every three hours and are evenly spaced throughout the 24-hour period. Special care must be taken to meet the needs of babies who are NPO.

For babies who remain in the nursery past 40 weeks gestation and for older infants who may be admitted because of illness, tactile stimulation should include objects of different textures, such as a washcloth, a smooth piece of material, or the smooth feel of a tongue blade.

Kinesthetic stimulation is provided by changing the baby's position frequently if he must remain in bed (e.g., the infant who has an endotracheal tube or nasal CPAP). Infants who can be removed from their beds should be rocked and carried about. Again, these activities should be part of the infant's nursing care plan, just as assisting the older patient to get out of bed is an essential part of the care plan for that individual. Otherwise, when the nursery is particularly busy and/or understaffed, kinesthetic needs may not be met. In some nurseries infants who can be out of bed are carried about in cloth infant carriers, similar to those many mothers use at home. The carrier should be designed so that the infant's head is always supported. A nursery swing may be used for older infants.

Auditory Stimulation

In the consideration of auditory stimulation both the negative effects of sounds that are part of the infant's environment as well as the need to provide auditory stimulation must be examined. An environmental sound of particular concern is the noise produced by the motor of the isolette. Although there are other sounds in the infant's home environment that are as loud, exposure to these sounds is almost never constant over a 24-hour period, day after day. Research is needed to assess the effect of this constant sound on infant hearing and behavior.

Given the evidence that preterm infants attend to voices and that their development and behavior is thereby affected, talking to infants and encouraging parents to talk to them should be a specific part of the nursing care plan. Sometimes parents

may feel self-conscious about talking aloud to their infants in full view of other people. Others feel it would be "silly" to talk to a tiny baby who may give no visible sign of response. Working class parents may express this view more frequently than middle class parents (Tulkin and Kagan 1972). The conviction that the sound of their voices is important, the model nurses provide by talking to each infant as they care for him, and the encouragement they give to mothers and fathers can help them to overcome these barriers. Moreover, the habit of talking to their baby, begun in the intensive care nursery, may encourage more verbal behavior after discharge, behavior many developmentalists feel is of value to long-term cognitive development.

In a few nurseries, the sound of the mother's voice on tape has been used for auditory stimulation, as in the research described. One apparent advantage of a live voice over one on tape is that auditory stimulation can then be combined with tactile and visual stimulation.

Visual Stimulation

During the time I was writing this chapter, I was caring for twins, Amy and Jamie, born at 28 weeks gestation and weighing 851 and 879 g respectively. I was continually amazed by the extended periods of time Jamie spent in the quiet alert state. At 31 weeks gestation she would lie, her eyes open but uncrying, appearing to examine her environment. I cite this example because there is a tendency to believe that premature infants sleep most of the time and rarely open their eyes, probably because the quiet alert state is briefer in most preterm infants than in term infants and may be less frequently observed. Jamie's twin sister, Amy, slept more of the time I was present.

Visual stimulation may be provided by cutouts (placed in the round doors and on the inside of the top of the isolette or on the sides of an open bed) to provide an interesting environment for the baby. At the University of Virginia, where a great deal of research has been conducted in preterm stimulation, cutouts of checkerboards and faces are used (Van Devender, Elder, and Hastings 1978). Since stimuli that are constantly present may cease to stimulate (due to habituation), a change in pictures would seem advisable for the infant who spends a long time in the nursery.

Mobiles can be useful if they are appropriate. In general, a homemade mobile is a better visual stimulus than a commercial mobile. Most commercial mobiles are attractive to adults who view them at their own eye level and from the side. If we were to lie on our backs and look up at a commercial mobile from the bottom, we would find the view from beneath very uninteresting. Mobiles hung above the bed should be no more than seven to nine inches away from the baby's eyes. A mobile that the baby will view from the side should be the same distance from his eyes, but the orientation of the design should be different. Encouraging parents to construct simple mobiles of construction paper and string not only involves them in their baby's care but also reinforces the principle that they needn't buy expensive toys for their infant; the simple toys they construct are still the best.

The human face, probably the best visual stimulus of all, may be the face of the nurse but here again, letting the mother and father know that their faces, along with their voices, are important to their baby's development involves them in his care. Nurses can assure them, "He may not look at you each time you speak to him, but he will come to know your voice and face." When a face is the visual stimulus, it should confront the baby's face. Infants appear to be very attracted to the eyes of another, and eye-to-eye contact appears important to parental attachment.

Special consideration must be given to the baby receiving phototherapy because his eyes are covered to protect him from the light. Term babies receiving phototherapy usually have their eyes uncovered at feeding time, so there are fairly frequent opportunities for visual stimulation. Preterm babies, however, may be receiving continuous feedings and may have their eyes covered throughout the day if there is no plan for visual stimulation.

THE CONCEPT OF STIMULATION

In reviewing the studies as a group, the fact of weight gain in the stimulated infant is present in all instances where weight is measured, although in one study (Powell 1974) the difference is only slight. This finding is the converse of studies of deprivation dwarfism, i.e., infants who are not stimulated fail to thrive. Since acceleration of growth may be associated with a variety of benefits to the infant including shortened hospital stay with less separation of infant from parents and siblings, decreased hospital costs, and a decreased opportunity to develop nosocomial infection, practices that facilitate such acceleration seem highly desirable.

The possibility that increased weight gain may also represent increased brain growth may be even more important, since a major long-term goal of nurses who care for preterm infants is the achievement of the infant's genetic potential in terms of intellectual development. In the study that looked at head circumference (Kramer and Pierpont 1976), the circumference significantly increased in stimulated babies. In each of the three studies in which there was postneonatal follow-up (Slokoff et al. 1969; Powell 1974; Scarr-Salapatek and Williams 1973) differences were found in the babies who received specific stimulation when compared with controls.

Further evidence of the effect of stimulation on brain growth comes from animal studies. Rosenzweig, Bennett, and Diamond (1972) reported on a series of experiments, spanning more than two decades, in which they found that the cortex in rats increased in weight quite readily in response to a stimulating environment, although the weight of the rest of the brain changed very little. Fourteen of 16 experiments demonstrated this result clearly and reliably. Specific findings included an increase in the size of nerve cell bodies and their nuclei, a change in the ratio of RNA to DNA (both factors suggesting increased metabolic activity), an increase in the number of glial cells, which perform a variety of neural functions, and changes in the activity of certain enzymes. Additional studies in this are are reviewed by Wallace (1974).

OVERSTIMULATION: A CONCERN

For many years, nurses have been concerned about the potential for overstimulation of infants. Nursing care traditionally has been planned to minimize handling. Continuous monitoring of Po_2 has shown that in infants with severe RDS, handling results in lowered Po_2. In all of the studies reported here, severely ill infants were excluded. Additional research is needed at this time to determine the short- and long-term effects of both planned stimulation and stimulation that is a by-product of being in an intensive care nursery and to determine relationships between types of stimulation and gestational age so that the specific needs of each baby can best be met.

Bibliography

Avery, M., Fletcher, B.: The Lung and its Disorders in the Newborn Infant. 3rd Edition. Philadelphia: W. B. Saunders, 1974.

Bligh, J., Johnson, K.: Glossary of terms for thermal physiology. J Appl Physiol 35:949, 1973.

Carson, B., Losey, R., Bowes, W. et al.: Combined obstetric and pediatric approach to prevent meconium aspiration syndrome. Am J Obstet Gynecol 126:712, 1976.

Cole, V., Normand, I., Reynolds, E. et al.: Pathogenesis of hemorrhagic pulmonary edema and massive pulmonary hemorrhage in the newborn. Pediatrics 51:175, 1973.

Cremer, R., Perryman, P., Richards, D.: Influence of light on hyperbilirubinemia of infants. Lancet 1:1094, 1958.

Curran, C., Kachoyeanos, M.: The effects on neonates of two methods of chest physical therapy. MCN 4(5):309, 1979.

Fantz, R.: Pattern vision in newborn infants. Science 140:296, 1963.

Field, T., Hallock, N., Ting, G. et al.: A first-year follow-up of high-risk infants: formulating a cumulative risk index. Child Dev 49:119, 1978.

Fitzhardinge, P. M., Ramsay, M.: The improving outlook for the small prematurely born infant. Dev Med Child Neurol 15:447, 1973.

Gerhardt, T., McCarthy, J., Bancalari, E.: Effect of aminophylline on respiratory center activity and metabolic rate in premature infants with idiopathic apnea. Pediatrics 63:537, 1979.

Gersony, W.: Indomethacin therapy for patent ductus arteriosus. J Pediatr 91:624, 1977.

Goldstein, G., Chaplin, E., Maitland, J.: Transient hydrocephalus in premature infants: treatment by lumbar puncture. Lancet 1:512, 1976.

Gottesfeld, I.: The family of the child with congenital heart disease. MCN 4:101, 1979.

Haddock, N.: Blood pressure monitoring in neonates. MCN 5:131, 1980.

Harlow, H.: The nature of love. Am Psychol 13:673, 1958.

Hutchison, A., Ross, K., Russell, G.: The effect of posture on ventilation and lung mechanics in preterm and light-for-date infants. Pediatrics 64(4):429, 1979.

Jackson, P.: Digoxin therapy at home: keeping the child safe. MCN 4:105, 1979.

Jones, R., Rochefort, M., Baum, J.: Increased insensible water loss in newborn infants nursed under radiant heaters. Br Med J 2:6048, 1976.

Kantor, G.: Addicted mother, addicted baby — a challenge to health care providers. MCN 3:281, 1978.

Kattwinkel, J., Nearman, H., Fanaroff, A. et al.: Apnea of prematurity: Comparative therapeutic effects of cutaneous stimulation and continuous positive airway pressure. J Pediatr 86:588, 1975.

Katz, V.: Auditory stimulus and developmental behavior of the preterm infant. Nurs Res 20:196, 1971.

Kennell, J., Jerauld, R., Wolfe, H., Chesler, D., Kreger, N., McAlpine, W., Steffa, M., Klaus, M.: Maternal behavior one year after early and extended post-partum contact. Dev Med Child Neurol 16:172, 1974.

Kitterman, J., Phibbs, R., Tooley, W.: Aortic blood pressure in normal newborn infants during the first 12 hours of life. Pediatrics 44:959, 1969.

Klaus, M., Jerauld, R., Kreger, N.: Maternal attachment: importance of the first post-partum days. N Engl J Med 286:440, 1972.

Klaus, M., Fanaroff, A.: Care of the High-Risk Neonate. 2nd Edition. Philadelphia: W. B. Saunders, 1979.

Korner, A. F., Grobstein, R.: Visual alertness as related to soothing in neonates: implications for maternal stimulation and early deprivation. Child Dev 37:867, 1966.

Korner, A., Kraemer, H., Hoffner, M., Cosper, L.: Effects of waterbed flotation on premature infants: a pilot study. Pediatrics 56:361, 1975.

Kramer, L., Pierpont, M.: Rocking waterbeds and auditory stimuli to enhance growth of preterm infants. J Pediatr 88:297, 1976.

Kuhns, L., Bednarek, F., Wyman, M. et al.: Diagnosis of pneumothorax or pneumomediastinum in the neonate by transillumination. Pediatrics 56:355, 1975.

Kuzemko, J., Paala, J.: Apnoeic attacks in the newborn treated with aminophylline. Arch Dis Child 48:404, 1973.

Lewis, M.: Infants' responses to facial stimuli during the first year of life. Dev Psychol 1:75, 1969.

Lubchenco, L., Delevoria-Papadopoulos, M., Searls, D.: Long-term follow-up studies of prematurely born infants. II. Influence of birth weight and gestational age on sequelae. J Pediatr 80:509, 1972.

Lubman, J., Borkat, G., and Hirschfeld, S.: The heart. In Care of the High-Risk Neonate, 2nd Edition, M. Klaus and A. Fanaroff (eds.). Philadelphia: W. B. Saunders, 1979.

Maisels, M.: Neonatal jaundice. In Neonatalogy, G. Avery (ed.). Philadelphia: J. B. Lippincott, 1975.

Markowitz, M.: Disorders of the cardiovascular system: general considerations. In Diseases of the Newborn, 4th Edition. A. Shaffer and M. Avery (eds.). Philadelphia: W. B. Saunders, 1977.

Martin, R., Herrell, N., Rubin, D., Fanaroff, A.: Effect of supine and prone positions on arterial oxygen tension in the preterm infant. Pediatrics 63(4):528, 1979.

Martin, R., Okken, A.: Correlation between transcutaneous and arterial oxygen tension measurements. In Care of the High-Risk Neonate, M. Klaus and A. Fanaroff (eds.): Philadelphia: W. B. Saunders, 1979, p. 178.

Mason, W.: Early social deprivation in the nonhuman primates. In Environmental Influences, Glass, D. C. New York: Rockefeller University Press, 1968.

Meier, P.: CPT — Which method if any. MCN 4(5):310, 1979.

Mizer, H.: Group B streptococci in neonatal infection. MCN 3:21, 1978.

Montagu, A.: Touching: The Human Significance of the Skin. New York: Harper & Row Perennial Library, 1972.

Moss, A.: What every primary physician should know about the postoperative cardiac patient. Pediatrics 63:320, 1979.

Nalepka, C.: Understanding thermoregulation in newborns. JOGN Nurs 5:17, 1976.

Nora, J.: Multifactorial inheritance hypothesis for the etiology of congenital heart disease. Circulation 38:604, 1968.

Northway, W. H., Jr., Rosan, R. C., Porter, D. Y.: Pulmonary disease following respiratory therapy of hyaline-membrane disease. Bronchopulmonary dysplasia. N Engl J Med 276:357, 1967.

Oh, W., Williams, P., Yao, A., Lind, J.: The effects of phototherapy on insensible water loss and peripheral blood flow. Birth Defects 12(2):114, 1976.

Papile, L., Burstein, R., Koffler, H., Koops, B.: Non-surgical treatment of acquired hydrocephalus: evaluation of serial lumbar puncture (Abstract). Ped Res 12:554, 1978.

Perlstein, P., Edwards, N., Sutherland, J.: Apnea in premature infants and incubator-air-temperature changes. N Engl J Med 282:461, 1970.

Poland, R., Ostrea, E.: Neonatal hyperbilirubinemia. In Care of the High-Risk Neonate, M. Klaus and A. Fanaroff (eds.). Philadelphia: W. B. Saunders, 1979.

Porth, C., Kaylor, L.: Temperature regulation in the newborn. Am J Nurs 78:1691, 1978.

Powell, L.: The effect of extra stimulation and maternal invovement on the development of low-birth-weight infants and on maternal behavior. Child Dev 45:106, 1974.

Ringler, N. M., Kennell, J., Jorvella, R., Navojosky, B., Klaus, M.: Mother-to-child speech at two years — effects of early postnatal contact. J Pediatr 86:141, 1975.

Rosenzweig, M., Bennett, E., Diamond, M.: Brain changes in response to experience. Sci Am 226:22, 1972.

Scarr-Salapatek, S., Williams, M. L.: The effects of early stimulation on low birth-weight infants. Child Dev 44:94, 1973.

Schechner, S.: For the 1980's: how small is too small? Clin Perinatol 7(1):135, 1980.

Segall, M.: Cardiac responsibility to auditory stimulation in premature infants. Nurs Res 21:15, 1972.

Sham, B., Messerly, A.: Apnea in the premature infant. Nurs Clin North Am 13(1):29, 1978.

Shannon, D., Gotay, F., Stein, I. et al.: Prevention of apnea and bradycardia in low birthweight infants. Pediatrics 55:589, 1975.

Smith, K.: Recognizing cardiac failure in neonates. MCN 4:98, 1979.

Solokoff, Y., Yaffe, S., Weintraub, D., Blase, B.: Effects of handling on subsequent development of premature infants. Dev Psychol 1:765, 1969.

Stairs, R., Krauss, A.: Complications of neonatal intensive care. Clin Perinatol. 7(1):107, 1980.

Stern, L.: Environmental temperature, oxygen consumption, and catecholamine excretion in newborn infants. Pediatrics 36:367, 1965.

Thompson, T., Reynolds, J.: The results of intensive care therapy for neonates. J Perinat Med 5:59, 1977.

Ting, P., Brady, J.: Tracheal suction in meconium aspiration. Am J Obstet Gynecol 122:767, 1975.

Tulkin, S., Kagan, J.: Mother-child interaction in the first year of life. Child Dev 43:31, 1972.

Uauy, R., Shapiro, D., Smith, B. et al.: Effect of theophylline on severe primary apnea of prematurity: a preliminary report. Pediatrics 55:595, 1975.

Usher, R.: The special problems of the premature infant. In Neonataology, G. Avery (ed.). Philadelphia, J. B. Lippincott, 1975.

Van der Daele, L.: Modification of infant state by treatment in a rockerbox. J Psychol 74:161, 1970.

Van Devender, T., Elder, W., Hastings, S.: The EMI-ART high-risk nursery intervention model. Charlottesville: University of Virginia Medical Center, 1978.

Wallace, P.: Complex environments: effects on brain development. Science, September 20, 1974, p. 76.

Washington, S.: Temperature control of the neonate. Nurs Clin North Am 13(1):23, 1978.

White, J., Labarba, R.: The effects of tactile and kinesthetic stimulation on neonatal development in the premature infant. Dev Psychobiol 9:569, 1976.

Whiteside, D.: Proper use of radiant warmers. Am J Nurs 78:1964, 1978.

Williams, J., Lancaster, J.: Thermoregulation of the newborn. MCN 1:355, 1976.

Wu, P., Hodgmen, J.: Insensible water loss in preterm infants: changes with postnatal development and non-ionizing radiant energy. Pediatrics 54:704, 1974.

Yek, T., Vidyasagar, D., Pildes, R.: Critical care problems of the newborn: insensible water loss in small premature infants. Crit Care Med 3(6):238, 1975.

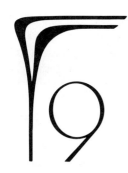

THE NUTRITIONAL NEEDS OF NEWBORNS

9

Nutrition for newborns, whether they are term or preterm, apparently normal or obviously ill, involves providing water, electrolytes, and nutrients in adequate but not excessive amounts.

Water and Fluid Balance

For several reasons fluid balance in newborns is much more precarious than in older children and adults.

1. Metabolic rates in the newborn are higher. A newborn produces 45 to 50 calories per kilogram of body weight every 24 hours. The basal metabolic level for adults in the same period is from 25 to 30 calories per kilogram. Since metabolism utilizes water, a higher rate of metabolism utilizes a proportionately higher quantity of water.

2. The larger surface area of the newborn in relation to his body mass means a higher ratio of water loss through evaporation, the rate of loss per kilogram being twice that of an adult. Evaporative loss is even higher in preterm infants.

3. The proportion of water in relation to total body mass is greater than at any other period of life — a total of 70 to 75 per cent in term infants and 85 per cent in infants of 28 weeks gestation. About 30 to 35 per cent of total body weight in the newborn is extracellular water, compared with 25 per cent in the older infant and 20 per cent in adults. Because of this, the infant has proportionately less reserve; any fluid loss or lack of intake will deplete his extracellular fluid very rapidly. In a 24-hour period an infant puts out about 50 per cent of his extracellular water; in the same period an adult excretes only about 14 per cent of his extracellular water. A large part of the difference between the newborn and the older infant disappears by the time the baby is 10 days old, for it is the loss of this large proportion of extracellular water that accounts for much of the weight loss that occurs in the first three days of life.

4. The kidneys of both preterm and term infants have about half the concentrating capacity of the normal adult kidney. They function satisfactorily under usual conditions, but they are less able to conserve fluid when the baby is stressed. In an older individual, scanty urine is a fairly reliable sign of dehydration, but because of the newborn's limited ability to conserve water by concentrating urine, his urinary output may not decrease. His normally higher blood levels of phosphate and potassium are also related to renal immaturity.

231

WATER REQUIREMENTS

The amount of water a newborn needs is related to a number of factors; among the most important are age, weight, and environmental temperature. Term infants require approximately 140 to 160 ml of water per kilogram of body weight by the third or fourth day after birth; low birth weight babies may require a somewhat greater intake because of greater fluid losses. Consider the following example:

> If the weight of the baby is 1600 g (1.6 kg), then the fluid needed would be as follows:
>
> 150 ml/kg/day
> 150 ml × 1.6 kg = 240 ml/day

If this is divided by 24 hours, the baby would require 10 ml/hour (IV) or 30 ml every three hours. If the baby is receiving all fluids intravenously, he would need 10 ml of fluid per hour. But if the baby is also taking 15 ml of formula every three hours (120 ml per 24 hours), the need for intravenous fluid is decreased to 120 ml (240−120) and only 5 ml/hour is required. When the baby is taking 30 ml of oral feeding every three hours, intravenous fluids should no longer be necessary.

Remember that this example is based on an "average" need of 150 ml/kg/24 hours and there may be slight variations. Be alert, however, to intakes that vary significantly. Intravenous fluids may be given through umbilical arteries or veins or through peripheral veins.

WATER LOSS

Urine Urine is produced beginning in the twelfth week of gestation and is a principal component of amniotic fluid. During the first 48 hours after birth urine output may be limited to 30 to 60 ml. After the third day of life, output is normally between 100 and 300 ml per 24 hours, or approximately 1 to 3 ml per kilogram per 24 hours.

In apparently healthy newborns, a check on the number of wet diapers in a 24-hour period is sufficient to indicate urinary output. When a baby is preterm or ill, more careful records may be necessary. Accurate output may be assessed in two ways. A newborn urine bag may be used, with urine withdrawn with a syringe and measured. An advantage of this method is the ease of obtaining urine for urinalysis and specific gravity, sugar, and protein checks as well as for measurement. The major disadvantage is the effect of the adhesive material of the urine bag on the skin of some newborns, especially small preterm infants. An alternative is to weigh diapers before they are placed beneath the baby, marking the weight on the diaper (each one will be different), and then weigh them again immediately after the baby voids. A sensitive scale that measures in grams is used, and a nonabsorbent diaper (e.g., a diaper wrapped in plastic wrap) is placed beneath the diaper to be weighed. The difference in weight between dry and wet diaper is recorded as the output. If the baby wets an area other than the weighed diaper, the record will be incorrect, of course. With small preterm infants this is not often a problem because of the small amounts of urine voided at one time.

INSENSIBLE WATER LOSS

Insensible water loss is fluid that is excreted through routes other than the urinary tract.

Insensible water loss is particularly high in the small preterm infant because the skin is more permeable and has a higher water content and the epidermis is thinner than in term infants or older children. Moreover, it is the small preterm infant who is more likely to be under a radiant warmer, to be receiving phototherapy, or to have a labile body temperature, all of which contribute to insensible water loss. Other important factors include diarrhea, vomiting, and losses through drainage from gastrostomy, chest, or other drainage tubes.

Table 9–1   Assessing Water Loss

Measurement	Assessment		
Weight (once or twice daily)	Weight loss should not exceed 10% in first 3 to 4 days; no weight loss after 4 days.		
Intake/Output	Diapers are weighed (wet and dry) Precise record of fluid intake is kept All fluid loss (chest tube drainage, colostomy, etc.) is measured		
Urine specific gravity	1.002 to 1.015 range		
Electrolytes		*Preterm*	*Term*
Sodium (mEq/liter)		128–148	134–144
Potassium (mEq/liter)		3.0–6.0	3.7–5.0
Chloride (mEq/liter)		95–110	96–107
Blood urea nitrogen (BUN) (mg/100 ml)		3–25	4–18
Urine osmolarity (milliosmoles/liter)	Maximum concentration 600–700 (may be higher in breast-fed infant)		
Hematocrit	Normal 45–58% (increased in dehydration)		

Weighing the baby is the most common method of determining insensible water loss. Usually weighing the baby every 12 or 24 hours will be sufficient. Other means of assessing insensible water loss are summarized in Table 9–1.

ELECTROLYTES

As might be expected because of the rapid exchange of water during infancy and the ease with which water balance is upset, electrolytes are also exchanged rapidly so that electrolyte balance is relatively unstable. Changes in sodium and potassium balance are especially likely to be affected. Any loss of fluids and secretions, caused by vomiting, diarrhea, and gastric suction, also results in the loss of sodium, chloride, and potassium. The amounts needed for replacement are determined from laboratory reports of electrolyte blood levels.

Babies with the salt-losing form of congenital adrenal hyperplasia (about 30 per cent of all infants with this condition) must receive sodium chloride (usually 4 to 8 g as an initial 24-hour dose followed by 2 to 6 g per day maintenance) as well as desoxycorticosterone acetate (DOCA) and hydrocortisone throughout their lives.

Since the condition is an autosomal recessive trait it may be suspected from family history, but there is just as likely to be no such clue. Girls with adrenal hyperplasia often have hermaphroditic external genitalia, but there is no similar indication in affected newborn boys. Symptoms that may occur in the newborn nursery or in the first month include anorexia, vomiting, and diarrhea which lead to extreme dehydration and weight loss.

PARENTERAL FLUID THERAPY

Once fluid or electrolyte balance is upset, parenteral fluid therapy is usually necessary. In a nursery caring for healthy term infants, parenteral fluid therapy would be a rare exception. But in low birth weight and intensive care nurseries the administration of intravenous fluids is very much in evidence — for the tiny infant who is unable to take sufficient food and calories orally, for the baby who is being prepared for surgery or who is a recent "postop," and for the baby with persistent vomiting or diarrhea whose fluid and electrolyte losses are substantial.

Once fluids are started, their maintenance at the proper rate becomes a nursing responsibility that involves the monitoring of both baby and intravenous equipment at the minimum of once every hour. If too small an amount of fluid is given, the baby will become increasingly dehydrated and circulating fluid volume will be decreased; if the proper fluid level is not restored, he will die in a relatively short time. On the other hand, too much fluid in too short a time will lead to pulmonary edema and water intoxication, and again, if uncorrected, death. The margin for error is narrow in a newborn.

The first requirement for assuring accurate intake is an intravenous set designed specifically for pediatric patients. A small amount of fluid can be transferred from the main fluid bottle to the burette — not more than the baby is to receive in a three-hour period. In this way, even if by some accident the fluid should begin to run at a faster rate than ordered, the baby will be protected against an overwhelming fluid intake. From 5 to 10 ml of fluid should remain in the burette at all times as a buffer so that if an emergency does arise and fluid intake cannot be checked exactly on the hour all the fluid will not be gone and the needle clogged with blood.

The amount of fluid the baby receives should be checked and charted each hour. Readings are made at the fluid level at the bottom of the meniscus. The chart should be kept at the baby's bedside so that it can be quickly checked to see the kind of fluid he is receiving, the amount he has received, and the flow rate being used.

The pediatric intravenous set is commonly calibrated so that if the baby is to recieve 3 ml per hour, for example, a rate of three drops per minute is used. The correct rate of flow can be maintained with a small pump, which is attached to the tubing between the fluid bottle and the burette and which adjusts the rate to keep it constant.

Equipment varies from one institution to another. It is essential for each nurse to be thoroughly familiar with the use and special requirements of the available equipment so that it may be used to maximum benefit. Using a monitor for any reason, however, does not eliminate the need to check the baby personally and keep complete and accurate records of fluid intake.

The fluid site is one area to be observed on the baby. The site needs to be checked for swelling at least once every hour. Occasionally, in adults, the continued position of a needle in a vein is ascertained by lowering the fluid bottle to see if blood returns in the tubing. This should not be done in newborns because of the small gauge of the needle; the back-up blood may easily clog the needle and the fluids will have to be restarted at another site. Swelling at the fluid site may indicate infiltration of fluids or merely that the tape holding the needle in place is too tight.

Umbilical artery catheterization, which allows frequent blood sampling as well as the administration of fluids, is a procedure that was developed in the early 1960s. It is usually reserved for very small preterm babies who have tiny, fragile veins and respiratory distress syndrome or other serious illness that will require fluid therapy for several days. An umbilical catheter can minimize the number of times a sick baby must be handled in the first week, which is decidedly to his advantage. After the cord and surrounding area are washed with an antiseptic solution, a catheter is inserted into one of the umbilical arteries and fixed in place with a silk thread. The tip of the catheter may be between T6 and T10 or between L3 and L4. Opinion is equally divided as to the preferable site (Stavis and Krauss 1980). The position of the catheter is confirmed by x ray.

Because there is always the possibility of infection through the cord stump (even in healthy newborns), an antibiotic ointment may be ordered for the area surrounding the stump.

Babies with umbilical catheters should be checked for leg blanching due to arterial thrombosis, which can occur shortly after the insertion of the catheter, during the time the catheter is in place, or after the removal of the catheter. The baby's leg may appear cold and white with no pulse or it may be mottled, pale, and dusky.

After an umbilical catheter has been removed there may be bleeding from the cord stump.

Even a small baby has to be restrained while receiving fluids. As with any patient with restraints, the baby's position should be changed frequently and the restraints should be checked often. The skin under the restraint should also be checked, because the skin is very delicate and can easily be injured. If the baby is to receive oral fluids while he is restrained, his head should be lifted for feeding, and after feeding he should be turned on his side or abdomen depending on the fluid site. Each time the baby is turned or moved, the site and flow must be rechecked.

If medications are added to fluids this must also be included in the record, just as any other medications would be. Some medications (e.g., calcium gluconate) may have a sclerotic effect on surrounding tissues if the needle becomes dislodged from the vein.

Other Necessary Nutrients

In addition to fluids and electrolytes, newborns, like all of us, need protein, carbohydrate, fats, vitamins, and minerals in amounts suited to their needs.

PROTEIN

Recommended protein intake for term infants is 2.2 g per kilogram of body weight per day, or 1 g per pound. Slightly less than half of this intake provides for growth; the remaining protein intake covers losses through urine and skin.

The need for increased protein in low birth weight infants is controversial. Current practice is to provide somewhat higher levels (2.5 to 4.0 g per kilogram of body weight) than for term infants. Raiha and colleagues (1976) fed human milk (which provides 1.63 g/kg of protein) and formulas that ranged from 2.25 to 4.5 g of protein per kg to 106 preterm infants in a controlled study. No significant differ-

ences were found in the growth rate of crown-rump length, head circumference, or femoral length, or in the rate of weight gain from the time of regaining birth weight until discharge at 2400 g.

Goldman and colleagues (1974) found an increased incidence of low IQ scores and strabismus when protein intake exceeded 6 g/kg/day.

The kind of protein as well as the quantity may also be significant. In human milk and in certain formulas, the whey/casein ratio is 60:40; in cow milk and other formulas the ratio is 18:82. Raiha and colleagues found metabolic acidosis to be more frequent, more severe, and more prolonged in infants who were fed formulas in which casein predominated. Many preterm infants receive intravenous protein.

There are several conditions, like PKU and other disorders of amino acid metabolism, in which the advisable level of protein intake is reduced to a lower level than that generally required. In nations where dietary sources of protein are limited, achieving minimum levels becomes the goal, with even this level being out of reach at times. This can have a deleterious effect on growth because protein malnutrition in the early months has serious consequences.

CARBOHYDRATE

Approximately 40 to 50 per cent of an infant's caloric intake should come from carbohydrates. In human milk, 37 per cent of the calories comes from carbohydrates. Since cow milk derives only 29 per cent of its calories from carbohydrates, cow milk formulas are sometimes supplemented with some form of sugar. The carbohydrate used in preparing formulas may be lactose, polycose, sucrose, corn syrup, tapioca starch, or glucose polymers (Table 9–2). Some infants are unable to tolerate lactose because their intestinal lactase (an enzyme) has not matured. For these infants, a formula without lactose is necessary.

Commercially prepared formulas vary

Table 9-2 Composition of Human Milk and Commercial Formulas

	Calories per Liter	Protein g/Liter	Type	Carbohydrate g/Liter	Source
Human milk	740	10.7	lactalbumin/casein 60:40	71.7	lactose
Similac PM 60/40	680	15.8	lactalbumin/casein 60:40	68.8	lactose
Similac 20	680	15.5	lactalbumin/casein 18:80	72.3	lactose
Similac with Iron 20					
Similac 24 LBW	810	22.0	lactalbumin/casein 18:80	84.9	lactose and corn syrup
MF Premature Formula 24	810	22.0		92.0	lactose and sucrose
Enfamil 20	680	15.0	lactalbumin/casein 18:80	70.0	lactose
Enfamil with Iron 20					
Enfamil 24	810	18.0	lactalbumin/casein 18:80	83.0	lactose
SMA 20	680	15.0	lactalbumin/casein 60:40	72.0	lactose
SMA 24	810	22.0	lactalbumin/casein 60:40	86.4	lactose
Pregestimil	680	22.0	casein hydrolysate	88.0	corn syrup and tapioca starch
Isomil 20	680	20.0	soy protein	68.0	corn syrup and sucrose
Portagen	680	23.6	casein	77.4	corn syrup and sucrose
Nutramigen	680	22.0	casein hydrolysate	87.6	sucrose and tapioca starch
ProSobee	680	25.0	soy protein	68.0	sucrose and corn syrup

Table 9–2 Composition of Human Milk and Commercial Formulas (*Continued*)

	Fat g/Liter	Fat Source	Comments
Human milk	45.6		
Similac PM 60/40	37.6	coconut and corn oil	Calcium/phosphorus ratio is close to that of human milk for preterm infants; low in sodium
Similac 20	36.1	coconut and soy oil	For infants over 1800 g
Similac with Iron 20			
Similac 24 LBW	44.9	MCT and coconut and soy oil	MCT—easily absorbed fat; low renal solute load
MF Premature Formula 24	41.0	MCT and corn and coconut oil	MCT easily absorbed
Enfamil 20	37.0	soy and coconut oil	For infants over 1800 g
Enfamil with Iron 20			
Enfamil 24	45.0	soy and coconut oil	Increased calories
SMA 20	36.0	oleo, coconut, safflower, and soy oil	Composition similar to that of human milk: low sodium, calcium/phosphorus ratio
SMA 24	43.2	oleo, coconut, safflower, and soy oil	
Pregestimil	28.0	corn and MCT oil	For infants with problems in digestion or absorption (e.g., cystic fibrosis, allergies, intestinal resection)
Isomil 20	36.0	coconut and soy oil	Used when infant does not tolerate milk protein or lactose
Portagen	32.0	MCT and corn oil	For infants with digestive or absorptive problems (e.g., pancreatic insufficiency, intestinal resection)
Nutramigen	26.0	corn oil	For infants with chronic diarrhea, allergy to milk protein, galactosemia, GI malabsorption
ProSobee	34.0	soy oil	Used when infant does not tolerate milk protein or lactose

MCT = medium-chain triglyceride

from 32 to 51 per cent in percentage of carbohydrate calories, with the majority ranging from 40 to 45 per cent. When the proportion of calories from carbohydrate is too low, i.e., below 20 per cent, babies are not able to tolerate the high percentage of protein and fat that would then constitute their formula. On the other hand, carbohydrate in excess of 50 per cent of the total caloric content can lead to loose stools because of the baby's inability to hydrolyze disaccharides, resulting in impaired growth and development.

FAT

Just as neither too much nor too little carbohydrate is well tolerated, so too the proportion of caloric intake from fats needs to fall within certain margins. From the standpoint of fats alone, a formula providing 1 per cent of the caloric intake of the essential fatty acids, linoleic and arachidonic acids, is evidently sufficient for healthy development. But such a formula would necessarily be so high in protein that the renal solute load would be excessive or the carbohydrate content would be so high that diarrhea would result. Too high a fat content is also poorly tolerated. Those formulas that derive 30 to 35 per cent of their calories from fat are generally the most acceptable. Fat provides about 50 per cent of the calories in human milk.

In preterm infants, immaturity of the intestines, liver, and pancreas may affect the digestion of fats and consequently limit growth. Medium-chain triglycerides that are already included in the infant's formula improve absorption in low birth weight infants and thereby enhance weight gain. Medium-chain triglycerides may also be given as a supplement to feedings. The use of parenteral fat is discussed below. Signs of fatty acid deficiency include scaliness of the skin, slow growth, and poor wound healing.

VITAMINS

In the United States a great many babies receive vitamin supplements during their early months in addition to the vitamins and minerals with which many formulas are supplemented. As a result, vitamin deficiencies are rare, although rickets (due to insufficient vitamin D) and scurvy (due to too little vitamin C) still occur occasionally. A mild vitamin K deficiency is not unusual in newborns but appears more frequently in preterm babies. Chemical substances that promote vitamin K activity (blood clotting) are synthesized by normal intestinal flora, which are established after birth. In many hospitals a single dose of vitamin K is given as a prophylactic measure to all babies shortly after birth.

Folic acid deficiency may occur more frequently than is generally thought because megaloblastic anemia, that is caused by inadequate folic acid and is due to a failure of the primordial erythrocytes to mature normally, may be masked by iron deficiency anemia, which is rather common in infants.

The danger with *vitamin A* is not of deficiency but of overdosage. Healthy infants who are receiving human milk, cow milk, or most commercial formulas do not need additional vitamin A. About 600 I.U. per day is considered an adequate intake; many commercial formulas contain from 1500 to more than 2700 I.U. per liter. Babies receiving skim-milk formulas or milk free formulas not supplemented with vitamin A and infants with chronic steatorrhea do need to receive supplementary vitamin A in a water-miscible preparation.

The possibility of toxicity due to excessive *vitamin D* has been suggested but is unproved. The recommended daily intake of vitamin D is 400 I.U. In the 1950s some British pediatricians recognized that the fortification of milks and cereals and the use of supplementary vitamins were raising vitamin D intakes of many British infants to a level of 3000 to 4000 I.U. per day, nearly 10 times the amount recommended. There was a suspicion that these high dosages were related to infantile idiopathic hypercalcemia, and the fortification of food with vitamin D was subsequently reduced, although no definite link between the vitamin and the condition was established. The reduction brought the maximum daily intake of vitamin D to less than 1500 I.U. without increasing the incidence of rickets, a matter of some concern at the time.

In the United States evaporated milk, most fresh whole milk, and most commercial formulas are fortified at the level of at least 400 I.U. of vitamin D per quart. Human milk, however, contains less than 100 I.U. of vitamin D per quart, and some commercial formulas contain less than 400 I.U. Infants receiving these formulas and those who are breast-fed will need supplementary vitamin D.

Vitamin E deficiency may occur in preterm infants. An infant weighing 1000 g at birth has 3 mg of vitamin E in comparison with 20 mg of vitamin E in a 3500-gram infant. Thus, for the small preterm infant, vitamin E supplementation appears to be necessary.

What is the role of vitamin E? Its major metabolic role appears to be the protection of biological membranes, including the membrane of the red blood cell, from oxidative breakdown. Vitamin E thus exerts an antioxidant effect. A vitamin E deficiency leads to oxidative damage to the red cell membrane and subsequent hemolysis and anemia. Melhorn and colleagues (1971) found that infants receiving ferrous sulfate alone (iron in an oxidant) were significantly more anemic at six, eight, and 10 weeks than infants given iron and vitamin E, vitamin E alone or no supplement at all. Small preterm infants (less than 2000 g) are given vitamin E in the form of alpha-tocopherol, which is an oral water-soluble preparation, during the first 12 weeks of life. After that time the amount of vitamin E in formula is considered adequate.

MINERALS

A number of minerals play a role in newborn nutrition, but the need for most of them is apparently met with little difficulty. An exception is iron. Various studies have shown that the incidence of iron deficiency anemia (defined as a hemoglo-

bin concentration of 10 g per cent or less) ranges from 25 to 76 per cent in infants older than six months from economically deprived areas to 1 to 2 per cent in babies from more affluent families. Preterm infants may develop iron deficiency anemia regardless of socioeconomic status.

Iron needs in term infants A term infant whose mother's iron stores were adequate during pregnancy will have sufficient iron stores until he doubles his birth weight in approximately four to six months. At that point the combination of rapid body growth and depletion of iron stores may lead to iron deficiency and subsequent hypochromic microcytic anemia (red blood cells are decreased in size and hemoglobin content) unless iron is given to the infant (Fig. 9–1). Breast-fed infants, however, appear to have larger stores of iron.

Iron-fortified formula or supplemental iron (e.g., ferrous sulfate drops) is given to formula-fed infants shortly after birth (preferably) and certainly no later than four months (timing remains controversial.) Iron-fortified cereal may also be given after four months and may become a good source of iron in the second half of the first year if two portions a day are fed consistently.

Ferrous sulfate drops are best absorbed when given between meals, although the small doses that are given for the prevention of iron deficiency anemia (1 mg/kg/day in term infants up to a maximum of 15 mg/day) are believed to result in adequate absorption. Gastrointestinal distress is rare at this dosage level. Be-

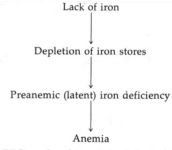

Lack of iron

Depletion of iron stores

Preanemic (latent) iron deficiency

Anemia

(RBCs replaced in substantial number by cells produced when serum iron was low; therefore RBCs are hyperchromic and microcytic.)

Figure 9–1. Development of iron deficiency anemia.

Table 9–3 Percentage of Infants Breast-Fed at Varying Ages in 1971 and 1978*

Age of Infant	1971	1978	Percentage of Change (1971–1978)	Seven-year ARG†
1 week	24.7	46.6	21.9	9.5
2 months	13.9	34.9	21.0	14.1
3 to 4 months	8.2	26.8	18.6	18.4
5 to 6 months	5.5	20.5	15.0	20.7

*Developed from data in Martinez and Nalezienski: Pediatrics 64:686, 1979.
†ARG = average annual rate of gain.

cause of the risk of accidental poisoning in siblings, no more than one month's supply of ferrous sulfate should be kept in the house.

Screening for anemia should occur between nine and 12 months; anemia is defined as a hemoglobin level of less than 11 g/100 ml or a hematocrit of less than 33 per cent. Serum ferritin levels, which reflect iron stores, fall to subnormal concentrations before other evidence of iron deficiency develops.

Iron needs in preterm infants Iron stores are depleted much more rapidly in preterm infants, who had less opportunity to store iron in utero, than in term infants. Iron stores drop rapidly after two months, and by three months of age preterm infants may have iron deficiency anemia. Therefore, either iron-fortified formula or ferrous sulfate drops are given to preterm infants beginning between two weeks and two months of age. The dosage of ferrous sulfate is 2 mg/kg/day, twice the dosage given to term infants. Lower doses have not been found to prevent iron deficiency anemia; higher doses given to preterm infants may result in hemolytic anemia because of vitamin E deficiency.

CALORIC NEEDS

Calories are supplied by protein, carbohydrate, and fat. For the healthy term infant, 110 calories per kilogram per 24 hours is recommended. Consider the following example:

If the weight of the baby is 7 lb (3200 g or 3.2 kg), then the caloric need would be as follows:

110 cal/kg × 3.2 kg = 352 cal per 24 hours
352 cal ÷ 6 feedings/day = 60 cal/feeding

If breast milk or most formulas for term infants provide 20 cal/oz, then the baby would require:

60 cal/feeding ÷20 cal/oz
= 3 oz/feeding, or
3 oz/feeding × 6 feedings/day
= 18 oz/day

Compare this need with the need for fluid (approximately 150 ml/kg). This same 7-pound infant would need:

3.2 kg × 150 ml fluid/kg
= 480 ml (16 oz) total fluid needed

Thus, approximately 18 oz a day will usually be adequate to meet fluid and caloric needs. Fluid needs are increased when environmental temperature is high. Caloric needs will vary somewhat with the individual baby; the best indicators of adequate but not excessive caloric intake are growth parameters: weight, head circumference, and length. Caloric needs are increased in preterm infants and in some infants with health problems.

BREAST OR BOTTLE

Breast-feeding is recommended for all healthy term infants and vigorous preterm infants (Standards and Recommendations 1974). Nevertheless, the decision of a mother to breast- or bottle-feed her baby

Table 9-4 Incidence of Breast-Feeding in Relation to Selected Demographic Characteristics*

| | Percentage of Breast-Fed Infants | | | | Percentage of Change (1971–1978) | | Seven-Year ARG† | |
	1971		1978					
	In Hospital	At 2 Mos.	In Hospital	At 2 Mos.	In Hospital	At 2 Mos.	In Hospital	At 2 Mos.
Education								
Grade or high school	19.4	9.8	40.2	28.5	20.8	18.7	11.0	16.5
College	42.1	27.6	63.4	52.0	21.3	24.4	6.0	9.5
Residence								
Urban	25.9	14.6	47.5	35.9	21.6	21.3	9.1	13.7
Rural	21.9	12.2	43.8	32.6	21.9	20.4	10.4	15.1
Income								
Less than $7000	22.3	10.2	34.0	23.1	11.7	12.9	6.2	12.4
$7000–14,999	26.7	16.4	47.3	34.5	20.6	18.1	8.5	11.2
$15,000 and above	NA‡	NA	50.0	39.1	NA	NA	NA	NA
Parity								
Primiparous	28.1	14.2	51.3	36.3	23.2	22.1	9.0	14.3
Multiparous	21.9	13.8	42.6	33.7	20.7	19.9	10.0	13.6

*Developed from data in Martinez and Nalezienski: Pediatrics 64:686, 1979.
†ARG = average annual rate of gain.
‡Income classification stopped at above $10,000.

is almost always a culturally based decision rather than a medical one. In societies that are just beginning to develop technologically there is no real choice but breast-feeding, either by the infant's own mother or by another lactating female. But even in traditional societies breast-feeding is on the decline as mothers become aware of Western practices. This is hardly surprising; cultural change in one aspect of life does not take place in isolation from the rest of life. But it is unfortunate that the switch from breast- to bottle-feeding has taken place in many countries before water has become safe and before adequate sanitary conditions and practices are established. Thus, gastrointestinal disease remains the major cause of infant mortality in many dveloping nations.

There was little choice in the manner of feeding infants in our own country until late in the nineteenth century when technology made bottle-feeding a reasonable alternative to breast-feeding. As recently as 1946 approximately 65 per cent of American infants were breast-fed during the newborn period. By 1965 the figure had dropped to 26 per cent and by 1970 to 25 per cent. However, since 1971 breast-feeding has become increasingly common, with 33 per cent of infants of one week of age reported to be breast-fed in 1975 and 45 per cent reported to be breast-fed at one week in 1978 (Martinez and Nalezienski 1979). Although the actual percentages are based on responses to mailed questionnaires and thus may not reflect the exact incidence in the population, the fact of an increased incidence of breast-beeding does seem evident.

Not only are more mothers initially breast-feeding but many mothers seem to be breast-feeding for longer periods of time (Table 9–3). In 1971 only 5.5 per cent of infants were breast-fed at five to six months of age. By 1978 over 20 per cent of mothers continued to breast-feed at five to six months. These data suggest that support for breast-feeding mothers must not be limited to a brief period in the hospital when one mother in three continues to breast-feed for two months and one in four continues for three to four months.

Although the incidence of breast-feeding remains higher in women with at least some college education (Table 9–4), between 1971 and 1978 the most rapid increase in breast-feeding, both initially and at two months, was in mothers with less education and mothers living in rural areas. The percentage of mothers with incomes of less than $7,000 and those with incomes of between $7,000 and $14,999 who were breast-feeding at two months postdelivery doubled between 1971 and 1978. (Note that primiparous mothers breast-feed more frequently than multiparous mothers. The reasons for this finding need to be explored.)

A variety of studies indicate that several factors influence the decision to breast- or

Table 9–5   Characteristics of Mothers Who Choose Breast- and Bottle-Feeding*

Mothers Who Choose Breast-Feeding	Mothers Who Choose Bottle-Feeding
Breast-fed as an infant	Bottle-fed as an infant
Husband supports breast-feeding	Higher incidence among single mothers
Education beyond high school	Grade or high school education
Higher socioeconomic status	Lower socioeconimic status
Successful previous breast-feeding experience	Higher incidence among smokers
Friends breast-feed their infants	Physical or emotional illness such as medical complications
Health-care personnel support breast-feeding	of pregnancy (e.g., diabetes, preeclampsia)
	More likely to work outside home or receive government financial support

*Adapted from Sauls: Pediatrics 64:523, 1979.

bottle-feed. Many of these factors are summarized in Table 9–5. Although nurses obviously cannot influence some of these variables (such as whether a mother was breast-fed herself when she was an infant or the years of education a mother has completed) special attention given during the prenatal period to mothers less likely to breast-feed (e.g., mothers who are single, who will be working outside the home soon after delivery — an ever growing number of mothers in all socio-economic groups — and mothers with medical complications during pregnancy) may encourage some of these mothers to breast-feed.

Prenatal nutritional education, such as that offered by the WIC (Women, Infants and Children's) Program does encourage breast-feeding in the prenatal period as well as offers continued education, encouragement, and incentives in the post-natal months. The WIC Program is designed for women with limited income; women from families with higher incomes should have access to the same information and encouragement.

Nutritional Comparison: Human and Cow Milk

A nutritional comparison of human and cow milk can be made on several counts. In making such a comparison it is necessary to realize that there is wide variation in human milk. This applies not only to the milk from different women but also to milk from different breasts of the same woman and milk of the same woman at different times of the day. This is true of cow milk as well, but in our urban society where most milk is obtained from the grocery store rather than from the family cow, a child will be getting milk from many cows and usually many herds of cows, so that this difference becomes insignificant.

The reasons for these differences are not known. They do not seem to be related to changes in the mother's diet. Poor nutrition affects the quantity of milk produced, but it does not appear to affect the relative proportions of carbohydrate, fat, and protein. Only vitamin content seems to be directly related to maternal intake.

PROTEIN

One of the major differences between human and cow milk is the protein content. Cow milk contains approximately three times the protein in grams per liter that human milk contains. The type of protein also differs. The principal protein in human milk is lactalbumin, whereas the primary protein of cow milk is casein. The fact that breast-fed infants have historically had a lower incidence of disease and a better growth record was at one time attributed to the differences in protein. But now it seems that at least part of this difference in infant health was caused by the bacterial contamination of bottled milk and the relatively high curd tension of the formulas. The curd tension is related to the amount of casein, and the curd in fresh, unprocessed cow milk is tough and rubbery in comparison with the soft, more easily digested curd of human milk. However, the modern processing of cow milk results in a softer curd and eliminates the major cause of its indigestibility.

CARBOHYDRATE

Carbohydrate accounts for 37 per cent of the calories in human milk and 29 per cent of the calories in unprocessed cow milk. Many formulas increase the amount of calories from carbohydrate by adding some form of simple sugar (Table 9–2).

FAT

The fat content of cow milk is higher than that of human milk and is composed of different proportions of fatty acids. As a result, the fat of human milk is more easily digested by an infant than the fat of cow milk in the early weeks of life.

VITAMINS

As for vitamins, human milk in adequate quantities satisfies the infant's requirements with the exception of vitamin D, in which cow milk is also deficient. Cow milk contains more thiamine, riboflavin, pyridoxine, vitamin B_{12}, and folic acid than does human milk. Because of the length of time between when the cow is milked and when the baby is fed, some of these vitamins are lost. The losses are, as far as we now know, of little nutritional significance where the B vitamins are concerned, but in the case of vitamin C it has been shown that the level of vitamin C (24 hours after the milk is drawn) drops from 20 mg per liter to 5 mg per liter. The vitamin C content of human milk, provided that the mother's intake of vitamin C is adequate, is in the range of 40 mg per liter, a level that satisfies the baby's requirements.

MINERALS

Human milk has long been recognized to supply adequate amounts of all minerals except iron and fluoride.

Although breast milk contains *iron* in small quantities (approximately 1 mg/liter), there is recent evidence that breast milk facilitates the absorption of iron. Saarinen, Siimes, and Dallmann (1977) found that term infants absorbed an average of 49 per cent of a trace dose of extrinsic iron administered during breastfeeding in contrast to about 10 per cent reported to be absorbed from cow milk. McMillan, Landaw, and Oski (1976) found an increased iron absorption from human milk in the adults they studied. Several possible reasons for this exist. Iron absorption appears to be increased when protein is lower (Gross 1968), when lactose is increased (Amine and Hegstead 1975), when phosphorus, which decreases iron absorption, is lower (Peters, Apt, and Ross 1971), and when vitamin C content is high. Breast milk meets all of these qualifications. Although further research is necessary, breast milk does appear to play

a more significant role in meeting iron needs during the first year of life than might be suspected from the amount of iron it contains.

Fluoride is considered the most effective dietary deterrent against tooth decay available today. Because of the low fluoride content of breast milk, supplementation with 0.25 mg/day of fluoride is frequently recommended (Thompson 1978).

Other Comparisons Between Human and Cow Milk

IMMUNOLOGICAL FACTORS IN HUMAN MILK

The immunological properties of human milk, summarized in Table 9–6, appear impressive. Undoubtedly life-saving among many peoples living in developing countries, they would appear to offer some advantage to any infant. A great deal of recent interest has focused on the immunological value of breast milk in the prevention of necrotizing enterocolitis (NEC). Although animal studies suggest the possibility that human milk may protect against NEC, there is no definite proof from human studies at this time.

Many of the antibodies transferred from the mother are probably involved in the digestive process and are more important in terms of local immunity in the gastrointestinal tract than they are in protection against generalized infection. Stools of breast-fed babies have been shown to have significant amounts of antibody to pathogenic strains of E. coli, which play such a major role in infant infection. When mothers have a high serum titer of poliomyelitis antibodies, their infants show a resistance to the attenuated live polio vaccine virus, indicating some transfer of immunity. Antibodies for mumps, vaccinia, influenza, and a Japanese B encephalitis have also been found in human milk, but the extent to which these antibodies protect the baby has not been determined. The effects of heat on the immunological components of milk are summarized in Table 9–6. This informa-

Table 9–6 Immunological Factors in Human Milk

Factor	Function (in vitro)	Effects of heating*
Lactoferrin	Inhibits growth of organisms, e.g., *E. coli* and *Candida albicans*, by chelating metabolically active iron	Two-thirds destroyed by pasteurization
Lysozyme	Acts with IgA and complement to destroy *E. coli*	Activity reduced 97 per cent by boiling for 15 minutes
Complement (C3, C4)	Enhances chemotaxis and phagocytosis by WBCs	Destroyed by pasteurization
Secretory IgA and other immunoglobulins	Contain antibodies to many common bacterial and viral pathogens including polio virus types 1, 2, and 3, *E. coli*, *Salmonella*, and *Shigella*	Destroyed by boiling; 0–30 per cent loss with pasteurization
Growth factor *Lactobacillus bifidus*	*L. bifidus* produces organic acids that lower pH of feces and impede colonization by *E. coli* and other pathogens	Stable to boiling
Antistaphylococcal factor	Inhibits staphylococci	Not known
Lactoperoxidase	Kills streptococci	Not known; presumably destroyed by boiling
Leukocytes Macrophages (80–90 per cent of leukocytes) monocytic phagocytes	Highly phagocytic Produce lysozyme, C3, C4	Destroyed by pasteurization; also destroyed by freezing
Lymphocytes (10% + of leukocytes)	Produce secretory IgA antibodies, interferon	
B_{12} and folic acid–binding proteins	May interfere with the growth of microorganisms depending on folic acid or vitamin B_{12}	
Lipids (unsaturated fatty acids)	Active against *S. aureus* and multiple viruses including herpex simplex	Stable after boiling for 30 minutes

*After Welsh and May: J Pediatr *1*:94, 1979.

tion is particularly important when milk is collected for use with preterm and sick infants.

RENAL SOLUTE LOAD

Renal solute load refers to the quantity of urea and electrolytes excreted in the urine. The renal solute load of cow milk, even when it is diluted with water and carbohydrate, is considerably greater than that of human milk. In the healthy infant this difference is of little practical concern, but it becomes significant in a number of pathological conditions, such as the inability of the kidney to concentrate properly, and in conditions in which there is a high insensible water loss, such as high fever or exposure to high environmental temperatures.

Commercially Prepared Formulas

In the United States today a great many infants, instead of receiving human or cow milk in unmodified form, are given commercially prepared formulas of various types. Some of these formulas are designed for the "average" baby under normal circumstances; others are planned to meet very specific needs, such as those of the baby with PKU or galactosemia, or are used for the baby who does not tolerate cow milk. Some formulas, although initially designed for babies with no special problems, are more adaptable than others for babies who do have special needs, such as the baby with a congenital heart defect.

The type of formula the baby will take in the hospital is prescribed by the doctor. It does, however, seem just as important that a nurse understand why a certain formula is chosen for a particular baby as it is for her to know why she is giving a particular medication. When any baby goes home on formula, especially a baby who has been ill or has special dietary needs, the mother needs to know why that particular formula has been chosen for her baby. Without that kind of understanding,

mothers may change formulas on the advice of their grandmother or sister. Or they may add sugar to a formula already supplied with carbohydrate or omit sugar when it is needed on the basis of the formula used for a neighbor's baby. Table 9–2 summarizes some major commercial formulas currently available.

The Anatomy and Physiology of Breast-Feeding

Milk is produced by the gland-secreting cells (Fig. 9–2) of the alveolus, which surround a central ductule opening. Each alveolus is partially surrounded by a contractile cell. As the infant begins to suck, nerve endings in the nipple and areolar margin of the breast are stimulated, and impulses are sent to the hypothalamus via the central nervous system and somatic afferent nerves. The hypothalamus first stimulates the anterior pituitary to secrete prolactin, which in turn induces the alveoli to produce milk. Then, within two or three minutes, the hypothalamus stimulates the posterior pituitary to secrete oxytocin. Oxytocin causes the contractile cell to contract, squeezing milk through the duct system to the milk reservoir in the areola. This second process is known as the "let-down" reflex.

Prior to let-down, i.e., when the baby first sucks, he receives the fore-milk. The let-down allows the hind-milk, with its fat particles, to be consumed by the infant. This higher caloric milk is essential to the baby's growth. The mother may experience let-down as a tingling sensation, as a pins-and-needles sensation, or as a filling of the breast or she may initially have no special feeling. Leaking or spraying from one breast while the baby nurses at the other is also a sign of let-down.

Let-down is highly sensitive to environmental stimuli. A quiet environment, a comfortable position for the mother, a warm drink — measures that promote relaxation facilitate let-down. A warm shower or warm cloths (washcloths or small towels) applied to the breast for a

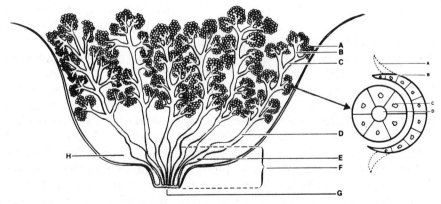

Figure 9–2. *Left,* diagram of the breast. *A,* alveolus; *B,* ductule; *C,* duct; *D,* lactiferous duct; *E,* lactiferous sinus; *F,* ampulla; *G,* nipple pore; *H,* areolar margin.
  Right, diagram of an alveolus. *A,* uncontracted myoepithelial cell; *B,* contracted myoepithelial cell, *C,* gland-secreting cell, *D,* ductule opening. Gland-secreting cells are arranged in a circle about the ductule opening. About the alveolus is a contractile cell. When sucking begins, this cell, under the influence of oxytocin from the pituitary gland, contracts and squeezes milk into the duct system. This is the "let-down" reflex. (From Applebaum: Pediatr Clin North Am 17:205.)

few minutes prior to nursing can also be helpful. Once let-down is well established, the sound of her crying baby can start the flow of milk in a nursing mother.

Fear, tension, and anxiety are the principal enemies of successful let-down. The mother may lack confidence in her ability to breast-feed. Since many mothers today were not themselves breast-fed, their mothers and mothers-in-law may undermine their confidence. Factors that interfere with the baby's sucking, such as medications given to the mother that crossed the placenta prior to delivery or that are ingested along with breast milk, or a rigid schedule rather than feedings suited to the infant's hunger, may further undermine the mother's confidence.

The nurse's supportive role is essential. Mothers not only need support during the first days in the hospital, but they need to know where to turn for help after they return home. Help after discharge may come from nurses at the hospital or in public health services, lay groups such as the La Leche League, or a physician who is interested in, knowledgeable about, and supportive of breast-feeding.

Building confidence is very supportive. Information about facilitating let-down in the manner described is also supportive.

Many mothers try to do too much too soon following discharge and need help in finding sufficient time for relaxation as well as help in accepting a less than dust free home during the weeks in which breast-feeding is being established.

When other measures have been tried and let-down still is difficult, the use of an oxytocin nasal spray may be helpful in providing initial success upon which future successes can be built.

Frequently, as the baby begins to nurse at one breast, a let-down of milk occurs in the other breast as well. This excess and sometimes copious flow of milk is disturbing to some mothers. One reported that she felt like an "unwashed milk bottle" most of the time. If the mother exposes both breasts when she feeds her baby and places a hand towel beneath the second breast so that it can catch the overflow, the major part of the problem can be solved. Soft cotton liners can be made or bought for nursing bras (old cotton handkerchiefs make fine ones) to absorb overflow between feedings. Just realizing that this reflex is an indication of adequate milk supply can help a mother to view it in a somewhat positive light. After the first weeks of breast-feeding, the let-down occurs only in the breast at which the baby is feeding.

FIRST FEEDINGS

The maxim in breast-feeding is the sooner the better. Allowing the baby to nurse while the mother is still on the delivery table, in the recovery room, or in the birthing room has several advantages. It assures rapid drainage of colostrum that is in the duct system and allows the milk, as it forms, to move down the system to the milk reservoirs (see Fig. 9–2). It is believed that colostrum may also aid in the peristalsis of meconium. Lactation is stimulated when the infant begins to suck. From the standpoint of the mother's well-being, oxytocin, in addition to causing the contraction of the contractile cells of the breast, also causes uterine smooth muscle to contract and helps to prevent postpartum hemorrhage. (It is this same mechanism that causes the mother to experience the uterine contractions commonly called "afterbirth pains" in the days immediately following delivery.)

The practice of putting the baby to breast immediately following birth is becoming more common in the United States. The use of anesthesia during delivery, however, makes this difficult, not only because the mother is asleep or groggy but also because large amounts of anesthesia make the infant suck poorly, both immediately after delivery and in the first days of life. Minimum analgesia and anesthesia is recommended for mothers who plan to breast-feed.

Before the baby begins to nurse, his mother needs to be in a relaxed, comfortable position. For the first feedings following delivery, she may prefer to lie on her side, supported by pillows behind her. This is particularly helpful if the mother has a considerable amount of discomfort from her episiotomy or if there is a contraindication to raising her head.

Later, the mother may prefer to sit with the head of the bed raised and the knee support elevated slightly. After she is able to be out of bed, she may sit in an armchair or a rocker, with a footstool for propping her feet. One advantage to a sitting position, other than personal preference, is the ease it affords in switching the baby from one breast to another if he is to be nursed on both sides. Mothers breast-feeding for the first time will need to experiment to find the position most comfortable for them.

The reason some mothers, especially multiparas, experience rather severe uterine contractions while nursing has already been mentioned. Physiologically these contractions are very beneficial to the mother and lead to more rapid involution of the uterus. But occasionally the discomfort is so severe that the mother is found nursing her baby with tears running down her face — she is truly miserable. If the mother is taught to massage her uterus so that it will be firm and well contracted prior to breast-feeding, much of the discomfort caused by contraction of the uterus will be diminished. If she continues to experience strong discomfort in spite of massage, the nurse might suggest that medication be taken in advance of the breast-feeding period. The mother should know, too, that these strong contractions will last only a few days and not as long as she is nursing her baby.

PROCEDURE IN BREAST-FEEDING

In putting the baby to breast, the following points should be remembered:

1. Stroking the infant's mouth with the nipple will cause him to root and find the nipple with his mouth. Rooting, sucking, and swallowing are examples of true instinctive behavior. Rooting refers to the instinct by which the baby tries to find the source of milk he has smelled. If his cheek touches something, he will turn his face in that direction, open his mouth to grasp the breast, and begin to suck. Holding his head rigidly in an attempt to push him toward the nipple is more likely to make him turn toward the hand.

2. The entire areolar area must be in the baby's mouth so that the milk reservoirs will be compressed as the baby sucks (see Fig. 9–2). The baby can be helped to grasp the areolar margin rather than the nipple if it is held between the thumb and forefinger. Not only is this

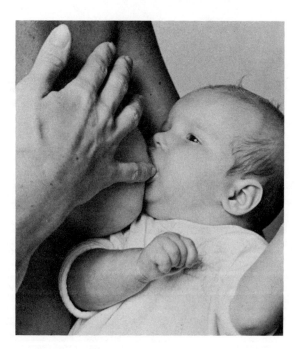

Figure 9–3. Breaking suction by placing a finger at the corner of the baby's mouth before pulling him away will help prevent sore nipples. (From Applebaum: Pediatr Clin North Am 17:211.)

necessary if the baby is to get any milk, but if the baby grasps only the nipple and chews on it, the result may be cracked and fissured nipples.

3. The breast must not press against the infant's nose. Babies can breathe only through their noses; they can't nurse if they can't breathe.

4. When nursing is completed, the baby may be asleep but still clinging tenaciously to the breast. The suction can be broken by placing the tip of a finger at the corner of the baby's mouth *before* pulling him away, thereby preventing sore nipples (Fig. 9–3).

How long should the baby be nursed at the first feeding? It has been fairly common practice to limit the first feeding to two minutes, but the most recent literature suggests nursing each breast for five minutes at each feeding on the first day, increasing the length of time on each following day. These longer periods are believed to lead to more complete drainage of colostrum and consequently better access to milk as it forms and moves down the duct system.

Milk begins to replace colostrum in the second to fourth day after birth. The baby needs to nurse for longer periods now — for as long as 15 minutes on each side at each feeding. He will probably need to nurse about every three hours since breast milk is more readily assimilated than cow milk. Breast-fed babies should be fed on demand. The baby should not be wakened and taken to his mother when he is not hungry, to be nursed briefly and then returned to the nursery only to be genuinely awake and hungry an hour later. If he is then given a supplemental feeding, the whole mechanism of milk production adequate to meet the baby's needs becomes jeopardized. Moreover, sucking from a rubber nipple requires the use of different muscles from those used in nursing at the breast (Fig. 9–4).

If breast-feeding must be interrupted temporarily for some reason, such as a mother with a fever or a tubal ligation or perhaps a mother who returns home before the baby can be discharged, it can be resumed with a minimum of problems if, first, the mother's breasts are pumped so that she can continue to produce milk and, second, the baby is fed with a rubber-tipped medicine dropper rather than a nipple so that he does not become accustomed to the kind of sucking action nipple feeding requires.

A mother who is nursing her baby should not be given sleeping medications.

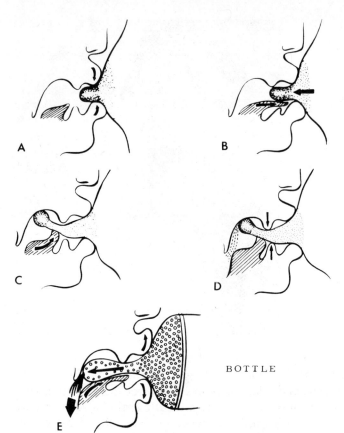

BOTTLE

Figure 9–4. The use of muscles in breast and bottle feeding is distinctly different. (From Applebaum: Pediatr Clin North Am 17:216.)

Not only will such medications make it more difficult to wake her for a middle of the night feeding, but sedatives lower the baby's basal metabolic rate and in so doing also lower the mother's milk production.

Most mothers, and especially those breast-feeding for the first time, are concerned about whether the baby is getting enough milk. It has already been mentioned that a good let-down reflex is one indication of adequate milk supply. A second indication is the infant's behavior. If he seems satisfied, sleeps well between feedings, and is gaining weight there is little doubt that he is being adequately fed. At one time it was popular to weigh breast-fed babies immediately before and after feedings. Except in rare instances this is not considered a good idea today. The amount of milk an infant takes varies from feeding to feeding by as much as several ounces. Focusing such close attention on each feeding can add to a mother's

anxiety, which may in turn reduce the milk supply.

POSSIBLE BREAST-FEEDING PROBLEMS

Difficulties in breast-feeding may be physiological or psychological. Nurses can offer specific help in both instances.

Sore nipples Sore nipples at the very beginning of a nursing period are not unusual. Before the let-down occurs, the pressure of the baby's lips on the nipple is stronger than the pressure of the milk in the nipple. Within a couple of minutes, the milk reservoirs fill with milk, the negative pressure is decreased, and the discomfort disappears. Even this initial discomfort diminishes in the second week or soon afterward.

The nipples of some mothers, especially those with very fair skin, are more tender than those of other mothers. Exposing the nipples to air or to a heat lamp for very brief periods helps to overcome this temporary tenderness. Some physicians prescribe an ointment for nipple soreness; such an ointment is harmless to the baby and does not have to be washed off before feeding. No drying substance, including soap, should be used on the nipples.

Breast engorgement In referring again to Figure 9–2, it is easy to see that when the breast is not emptied milk will accumulate in the duct system. This leads to a rise in pressure not only in the affected duct but in adjacent ducts as well because of the way in which the ducts are interconnected. There will be "caking" of the breast tissue and a decrease in milk production. If the tension is not relieved, redness, swelling, and eventual mastitis can result. Engorgement creates breathing difficulties for the baby during nursing and can lead to sore nipples for the mother (Fig. 9–5).

The major factor in the prevention and relief of engorgement is drainage of at least one breast at each feeding. Breast massage while the baby is nursing helps achieve this, although many babies seem to drain the breasts adequately without massage. Massage is used toward the end of the nursing period when the baby begins to suck intermittently with shallow movements. The mother massages her breast with her fingertips, beginning near the armpits. This helps the milk still in the alveoli to move down the ducts to the milk reservoirs so that the baby will have access to it. As one area of the breast softens, the fingers are moved to an adjacent area until the whole breast is soft. Breast massage is not used in the first minutes of nursing when the baby is making long, continuous sucking movements because it would make the milk flow faster than the baby can handle. Moist heat in the form of warm showers and warm cloths helps to dilate the lactiferous ducts and facilitate the excretion of milk.

Mothers who are nursing their babies will have many questions after they return home. Some hospitals and physicians provide excellent guide sheets to reinforce what nurses and physicians have told the mothers in the hospital. A comprehensive and very readable book, *The Womanly Art of Breastfeeding*, is available from La Leche

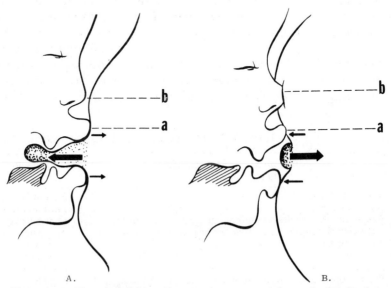

Figure 9–5.   The relationship of breast engorgement and sore nipples. *A,* when an infant sucks at a normal breast, his lips compress the areola and fit neatly against the concave nipple-areola junction (a). He also has room to breathe (b). When breasts are engorged, as in *B,* the baby can neither breathe (b) nor grasp the nipple properly (a). Attempts at sucking then damage the nipple. (From Applebaum: Pediatr Clin North Am, 17:218.)

League, Franklin Park, Illinois, 60131. La Leche also has a folder, *When You Breast-feed Your Baby,* that briefly summarizes most of the essential information and is available at a minimal cost. No matter how good a job the nursing and medical staffs have done, the mother needs some reference she can use after she returns home.

Physiologically, the chief contraindication to breast-feeding is chronic maternal disease such as tuberculosis, nephritis, or rheumatic carditis. Postpartum psychosis or chronic emotional illness would also seem to make breast-feeding undesirable. In the instance of acute infection, breast-feeding may have to be suspended temporarily, but if breast milk is expressed by hand or pump during the period, the mother can return to nursing after she is well. Not every mother who breast-feeds feels so strongly about it that she will want to do this. But some do, and they should receive any support and assistance they need so as not to jeopardize their own health. The mother who is too ill to have breast milk expressed may need reassurance that her baby will not be handicapped by formula feedings, that by breast-feeding even briefly she has contributed to his well-being, and that now her main concern is to get well herself so she can once again care for him.

Mastitis Infection of the breast (mastitis) may be due to one of several organisms including both *staphylococcus* and *strepto-coccus*. Mastitis may occur at any time during the breast-feeding period but is most frequent two to three weeks after the baby's birth. Signs of mastitis may be both local (redness, tenderness, and increased temperature of the affected breast) and systemic (nausea, aching, and sometimes fever and malaise —similar to the symptoms of flu).

Breast-feeding should continue during mastitis. Using moist heat to dilate the lactiferous ducts prior to feeding and nursing frequently on both the affected and unaffected breasts should begin at the first suspicion of mastitis. The mother should be on bed rest for the majority of the day. Frequent soaking of the entire breast in warm water (in tub or basin) is comforting and promotes circulation, which in turn aids in resolving mastitis. Antibiotics are prescribed when the symptoms are systemic; the antibiotic must be one that will not harm the infant. Ampicillin is frequently the drug of choice; antistaphylococcal drugs such as dicloxacillin are also used (Rawlins, 1980).

It has recently been recognized that sodium and chloride levels may be elevated in the human milk from a mastitic breast, a fact long known in cows. This may cause the baby to nurse poorly on the affected side (Conner 1979). Awareness of this possibility and the possibility of hypernatremic dehydration suggests that mothers who have had mastitis need frequent assessment and support over a period of

Table 9–7 Drugs and the Breast-Feeding Mother

Drugs that do not Appear Harmful to the Infant	Drugs Requiring Close Supervision of the Mother
Most antibiotics	Steroids (taken longer than one week)
Antihistamines	Lithium carbonate
Simple cough remedies (in normal prescribed quantities)	Oral diuretics (chlorothiazide, Diuril)
Antipyretics (aspirin, acetaminophen) in occasional dosages	Amphetamines
Barbiturates	Isoniazid
Analgesics	Oral hypoglycemic agents
Insulin	Antiepileptic agents (for long-term use)
Psychotropic agents *except* diazepam (Valium)	Digitalis
Cathartics (milk of magnesia, methyl cellulose)	Antiarrhythmic agents
Fecal softeners (dioctyl sodium sulfate)	Primidone (Mysoline)
Laxatives	Ampicillin
Heparin, warfarin	Cough medicines with codeine
Antidiarrheal agents	

Table 9–8   Drugs That Should Be Avoided by a Breast-Feeding Mother

Drug	Potential Effect
Ergot	Vomiting, diarrhea, convulsions, weak pulse, unstable blood pressure, suppression of lactation
Atropine	Decreases milk production
Radioactive iodine and iodides	Suppress development of thyroid
Antithyroid drugs (e.g., thiouracil, propythiouracil)	Inhibit thyroid function
Antineoplastic agents	May cause bone marrow depression
Heroin	Withdrawal symptoms in infant when feeding is delayed or discontinued
Oral contraceptives	May inhibit lactation
Reserpine	Lethargy, diarrhea, nasal stuffiness
Chloramphenicol (Chloromycetin)	Bone marrow depression in infants
Tetracycline	Discoloration of teeth; enamel hypoplasia
Metronidazole (Flagyl)	Blood dyscrasia, neurologic disorders; carcinogenic in rodents
Meprobamate (Miltown, Equanil)	2 to 4 times more concentrated in blood than plasma
Chlorthalidone (Hygroton)	Antihypertensive
Lithium	Hypotonia, hypothermia, cyanosis, ECG changes
Phenindione; ethyl biscoumacetate (Tromexan)	Anticoagulants
Diazepam (Valium)	Drowsiness
Chlorpromazine	Drowsiness, lethargy
Radiopharmaceuticals	May resume administration after varying periods of time

several weeks from public health nurses or nurses giving follow-up care.

Bilateral mastitis is rare but may be due to group B-(β-hemolytic) streptococcus infection, which is so serious that it is a contraindication to breast-feeding (Schreiner, Coates, and Shackelford 1977). Immediate evaluation is essential.

Circumstances that may contribute to mastitis are the failure to drain the milk ducts completely in both breasts and interference with circulation in the breast. Breast shields, as well as faulty nursing practices, may limit drainage of milk. A nursing bra that is too tight may interfere with circulation. In a large woman the pressure of the breast itself may be a problem; nursing bras must also offer good support.

Following the described regimen should prevent breast abscess in most instances. If abscess does occur, incision and drainage as well as antibiotics may be necessary.

Hypernatremic dehydration in breast-fed infants   Hypernatremia can occur because of increased sodium intake or decreased fluid intake with a greater loss of water than of sodium. Permanent neurological damage and even death may result. Clarke and his associates (1979) reported an instance of severe dehydration in an infant breast-fed only three times a day from 48 hours until two weeks of age. (I have seen two similar infants in our nursery in the past two years.) Mothers report their infants would rather sleep than eat. As infants become dehydrated, they become progressively more lethargic and feed even less well. Hospitalization of the infant is usually required to restore fluid and electrolyte balance. Education of mothers about breast-feeding (three feedings a day is not normal during the first weeks of life) and improved supervision of breast-feeding mothers are indicated. In the known instances of hypernatremic dehydration, the mothers were middle-class, had high school or college education, and would be considered of above average intelligence, suggesting that these mothers have as much need for education as mothers from lower income families.

The excretion of drugs in breast milk Drugs taken by a breast-feeding mother may be passed to the baby through the milk. The amount of drug passed to the infant will vary according to the plasma/milk ratio and the ability of the breast to detoxify the particular drug. The molecular weight of the drug, binding to plasma and milk proteins, the degree of ionization, and the amount of fat in the mother's body are some additional factors. The effect of the drug on an individual infant will also be influenced by the age of the baby and his genetic constitution. As during pregnancy, nursing mothers should take as few medications as possible. But medications are not necessarily a contraindication to breast-feeding. Tables 9–7 and 9–8 group drugs in three categories: those that do not appear to be harmful, those that require close supervision of the mother, and those that should definitely be avoided. The categories are not rigid and there are differences of opinion about the appropriate category for certain drugs. In some instances knowledge about a drug is based on a small number of case studies rather than controlled experiments. Like many areas that concern human infants, controlled studies present problems. In each instance, the risk of

affecting the infant is balanced with the needs of the mother.

Helping the Mother Who Wants to Breast-Feed Her Baby

To assume that breast-feeding is instinctive and that the mother who wants to nurse her baby will automatically know how to do so is pure fallacy. Very little human behavior can be considered truly instinctive; most of what we do is dictated by the culture of the society in which we live. In tribal societies and traditional villages where a girl grows up observing her mother, her aunts, and her sisters feeding infants at the breast, she will have learned almost unconsciously a great deal about nursing before she has an infant of her own. But many young mothers in our own society have never seen another infant breast-fed. They may live many miles from any female relative, and it is very possible that none of their friends have breast-fed their babies. A nurse cannot walk in, hand these mothers their babies, and expect them to know how to begin breast-feeding with any degree of success.

Usually (and ideally) the decision to breast-feed is made at least several weeks before the baby is born. In the time that remains before delivery the mother can learn something of breast anatomy and physiology and the most effective way to breast-feed. The breasts should be bathed only in plain water both before and after delivery. Soap can cause sore, cracked nipples and may also destroy normal skin flora, which are a defense against pathogenic bacteria.

Atkinson (1979) found that six weeks of prenatal nipple conditioning significantly reduced nipple pain ($p < .01$). The regimen used by the women studied included: (1) gently rolling each nipple for two minutes twice daily, using the thumb and first finger while applying gentle traction to the nipple; (2) gently rubbing each nipple with a terry cloth towel for about 15 seconds once a day; and (3) exposing the nipples to gentle friction and airing by allowing the nipples to rub against outer clothing for two hours daily. The effect of skin color on the amount of nipple pain was also investigated, with fair-skinned women reporting more nipple soreness. Atkinson's results vary from those of Brown and Hurlock (1975), who found no advantage to prenatal conditioning. However, women in their study conditioned their nipples for only three weeks. Whitley (1978) retrospectively reviewed the experience of 34 nursing mothers who prepared their nipples for varying lengths of time and found no advantage. Further nursing research should clarify the value of nipple conditioning and other variables related to nipple pain.

When nipples are inverted, a Woolwich breast shield, worn inside the mother's bra during the last four to five months of pregnancy, will exert gentle pressure and draw the nipples out (Auerbach 1979). Breast massage and hand expression are two additional aspects of prenatal preparation for breast-feeding.

BREAST MASSAGE

Before touching her breasts for any reason, the mother should wash her hands with hot soapy water and rinse them thoroughly. Using the fingertips and starting in the upper portion of her breasts, the mother should begin to massage milk from the outer breast to the nipples with small circular motions.

HAND EXPRESSION

Cupping the breast in her hand with the thumb above and the forefinger below the nipple, the mother gently squeezes her thumb and forefinger together as she presses inward toward the chest wall and then slightly pulls forward. The fingers are rotated so that all the milk ducts are reached. Expression should be alternated between breasts every few minutes.

Helping the Mother Who Wants to Bottle-Feed Her Baby

Just as we cannot hand a mother her baby and expect her to nurse it without some instruction and assistance, neither can we assume that the mother who plans to bottle-feed her baby can do so without guidance, as to both feeding techniques and the method of preparing the formula. The mother should be aware that while the baby is being fed he needs (1) to be warm and dry, (2) to be held in a semi-sitting position, (3) to drink from a nipple that is always filled with milk, and (4) to be given frequent opportunities to burp.

Most mothers seem to be familiar with "over-the-shoulder" burping. There is nothing wrong with this; it is very satisfying to have a warm, well-fed sleepy baby lying with his head on your shoulder. An alternate method is to hold the infant in a sitting position, his chest supported with one hand while his back is gently rubbed or patted with the other hand. After feeding, the baby should be laid on his side or stomach, so that if there should be some regurgitation, the milk will not be aspirated.

Many hospitals now buy formula already prepared and in bottles, a procedure that is apparently more economical than running a hospital formula room and that seems to have the added advantages of greater sterility and safety. Once the bottles and nipples are used they are thrown away. Bottles are kept at room temperature and are not warmed. Occasionally this may disturb a mother because our traditions tell us that baby's milk should be warm, although studies some years ago demonstrated that babies who were fed only formula taken directly from the refrigerator could thrive. A formula that is too hot poses many more dangers than one that is cool or cold.

When do bottle feedings begin? The trend is toward earlier feeding, within the first four to six hours. Plain water, rather than glucose water, is now considered best for the first two to three feedings because the aspiration of glucose water has been found to be as damaging to lung tissue as the aspiration of milk. First feedings usually measure 5 to 15 ml (depending on how awake the baby is), with increases of about 15 ml each day so that by the end of the first week the baby is taking approximately 2½ oz (75 ml). The size of the baby has a direct bearing on the amount of formula he needs and often on the amount he seems to want. The ideas that "if a little is good, a lot is wonderful" and "bigger babies are better babies" seem to be a part of our cultural heritage, but there are distinct disadvantages to overfeeding a newborn. An immediate danger is that the infant's stomach may become distended, causing him to vomit and aspirate. As a long-range consideration, the possibility has been advanced that overfeeding in infancy conditions the baby physiologically to eat more food than he actually needs and is one factor responsible for the high incidence of obesity in the population of the United States. Whether obesity results because the baby overeats in his first weeks or because the mother who takes pride in the large quantities consumed by her newborn continues to overfeed the child throughout infancy is a moot question at this time. However, the presence of obesity in our society is in itself reason enough to give mothers some guidance about feeding and a philosophy of feeding.

After the first week, about 2 to 2½ oz of formula per pound of body weight is the rough rule for feeding in the first month. The length of time between feedings and the amount of formula taken at each feeding vary; the mother needs to know this so that she will not be overly concerned. Consistent failure to feed well at nearly every feeding, on the other hand, is often the first indication of illness — infection or congenital heart disease, for example — and needs to be reported to a physician.

A baby who begins gaining weight on the fourth day of life, who has regained his birth weight somewhere between seven and 12 days, and who gains, on the average, six to eight ounces a week after that is likely to be well nourished. The fact that he also sleeps well between feedings and is generally content also confirms that probability. Fluctuations in weight gain are normal, periods of rapid growth being followed by slower gains and vice versa. Baby scales at home can sometimes do more harm than good when they focus undue attention on daily and even weekly changes.

FORMULA PREPARATION

There are several alternatives in formula preparation today. The entire formula may be purchased in a disposable nurser, a system that is easy, aseptic — and somewhat expensive, so that most likely it is the upper-middle-class mother who is able to take advantage of this convenience and who is also able to prepare the formula correctly and with a minimum of difficulty.

Expense can be minimized by using two to three bottles that are washed thoroughly after each feeding with cold and then warm water and then are boiled and kept sterile in the same pan. (The high temperature of the water in an automatic dishwasher is excellent for sterilization.) Bottles are prepared individually as the baby requires them, a single can of formula or evaporated milk being opened at a time and kept refrigerated. Powdered formulas have the advantage of not requiring refrigeration, making them ideal where cold storage space is limited or inadequate. They are also very useful for the occasional supplementary feeding of a breast-fed baby, since the unused portion will not spoil. Boiled water is used if the formula requires the addition of water. Such a method eliminates the need for a large sterilizer and extensive refrigerator room for a number of prepared bottles and saves a good deal of time each morning.

Perhaps the hardest thing for the mother in financial distress to do is throw away that portion of the formula that the baby leaves in the bottle, particularly if a great deal remains. The temptation is to refrigerate it and then rewarm it and offer it again at the next feeding. Meanwhile, bacteria have had several hours in which to multiply. The mother not only needs to understand why this can be harmful to her baby, but she needs concrete suggestions as to how the leftover milk can be used, such as in the making of puddings. In addition, filling the bottle with only slightly more formula than the baby usually drinks prevents most leftover milk.

FEEDING SCHEDULES

Whether the baby is breast- or bottle-fed, a constant concern of mothers leaving the hospital is how often the baby should be fed. "Feeding by the clock and not by guess or when the baby cries" was the advice in a 1922 nutrition text, *Dietetics for Nurses*. After that we went through a period in which food was offered at every cry, but now we have come to the conclusion that the answer lies somewhere between the two extremes. Parents need to know that not every cry represents hunger. They also need to understand that because babies have relatively immature central nervous and digestive systems, they are somewhat erratic in their eating habits in the first couple of months.

Feeding on demand, as it is currently understood, does not mean a complete absence of any schedule. It is more nearly a substitution of a schedule suited to the needs of an individual baby rather than an arbitrary schedule based on the assumption that certain hours of the day are the best ones in which to feed every infant. The parents of Baby C, an 8½-pound boy born two weeks before his expected date, kept a record of how often their baby ate during his first weeks home from the hospital. They found he was nursing every three hours except for one two-hour interval which occurred at approximately the same time each day and one four-hour interval, resulting in a total of seven feedings. By the beginning of his fourth week he had lengthened the time between feedings so that he was nursing six times in 24 hours. Still the intervals were not equal; there was a three-hour span in the afternoon followed by a five- to six-hour stretch after supper.

Parental response to crying has been discussed in Chapter 6. Crying that is accompanied by rooting behavior, as if the baby were searching for the nipple, and is not relieved, even when the baby is held, probably means that he is hungry. If he is truly hungry, allowing him to cry for 20 or 30 minutes until he is exhausted will generally mean that he will go to sleep before he has had as much milk as he really needs and will then awaken in a fairly short time to begin the cycle again.

It seems worth considering whether "demand" feeding might not be a possibility in hospital units in which rooming-in is not available. It is particularly important for breast-fed babies, as we have already discussed, but it has something to offer to every baby.

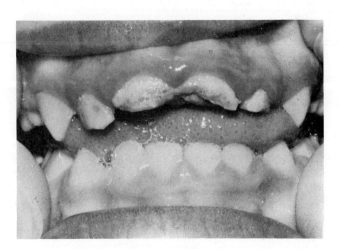

Figure 9–6. The difference in the upper and lower incisors is characteristic of bottle caries. (From Trippie, R., Jennings, R.: Nursing bottle syndrome. Keep Abreast J 3(2):114, 1978.)

NURSING BOTTLE SYNDROME

Nursing bottle syndrome, also called *bottle caries* or *bottle mouth,* is a type of tooth decay that occurs in approximately 1 per cent of children who take a bottle of milk, juice, or carbohydrate-containing liquid to bed with them at naptime or bedtime (Fass 1962; Kroll and Stone 1967; Michal 1969; Trippie and Jennings 1977). As a result, a particular pattern of tooth decay results, with the maxillary incisors affected most severely. Other affected teeth are the maxillary first primary molars, the maxillary primary cuspids, and the mandibular first primary molars (Figs. 9–6, 9–7).

The infant who takes a bottle to bed usually lies down with the nipple held against his palate. His tongue protects the lower (mandibular) incisors. As he becomes sleepy and swallows less frequently the carbohydrate-containing liquid pools around the teeth and acid formation begins. Caries are usually first seen when the baby is 10 to 12 months old.

Breast-feeding may be one form of prevention, although there are some conflicting reports about the relationship of breast-feeding and dental caries. When infants are bottle-fed, they should not be allowed to take a bottle to bed with them that holds any liquid other than clear water. Checking an infant's mouth at each health checkup and querying parents about feeding practices is also important because caries develop long before children normally have their first dental visit (at about three years of age).

Position of Infants Following Feeding

Regardless of the method of oral feeding (breast, bottle, or gavage), the issue of the best position for the infant following feeding is an appropriate concern. Traditional nursery practice, based on a series of x-ray studies, has favored a prone or right lateral position as the one in which stomach emptying is facilitated (Smith and LeWald 1915; DeBuys and Henriques 1918; Hood 1964). Yu (1975) found less retention of a test meal of 10% dextrose in infants in a prone or right lateral position. Blumenthal, Ebel, and Pildes (1979) were unable to confirm these results, however, and found no differences in stomach emptying in relation to position in 14 infants tested at 20-minute intervals. Blumenthal's studies also indicate something about the pattern of stomach emptying, with nearly half of the volume emptied within the first 20 minutes (Fig. 9–8).

Although further research will be necessary to confirm Blumenthal's results, there is no apparent disadvantage in placing infants in either the prone or right lateral position. Moreover, the prone position has been shown to enhance respiratory function in preterm infants (Martin et al. 1979); decrease diaper rash (Kietel, Cohn, and Harnish 1960); reduce aspiration (Hewitt 1976); and promote sleep (Brackbill, Douthitt, and West 1973).

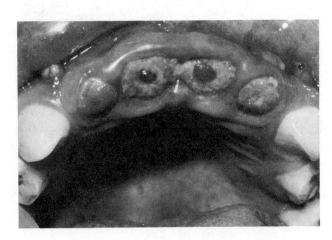

Figure 9–7. This child's teeth are so badly destroyed that they will have to be removed surgically. (From Trippie, R., Jennings, R.: Nursing bottle syndrome. Keep Abreast J 3(2):114, 1978.)

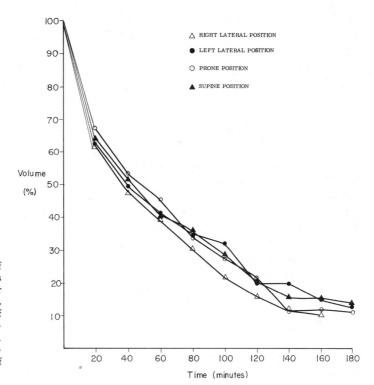

Figure 9–8. The percentage of volume of stomach contents emptied per unit of time in four positions. (From Blumenthal, I., Ebel, A., Pildes, R.: Effect of posture on the pattern of stomach emptying in the newborn. Pediatrics 63:532, 1979. Copyright American Academy of Pediatrics 1979.)

INFANTS WITH SPECIAL FEEDING PROBLEMS

As the discussion of formulas indicated, there are a number of instances — some of them fairly common, others relatively rare — in which special kinds of feedings are necessary. Low birth weight infants, babies with congenital heart disease, babies with cleft lips or palates, and infants with inborn errors of metabolism such as PKU and galactosemia need special attention. Later in the neonatal period evidence of allergy to cow milk or conditions with associated vomiting and diarrhea may also require special kinds of feedings.

The Preterm Infant

Preterm infants have several potential problems with feeding. Even more than term newborns, preterm infants can differ greatly from one another, and so their feeding must be planned on a very individualized basis.

Since neither the skeletal muscles nor the smooth muscles of the gastrointestinal tract are as well developed in the preterm baby as in the term baby, the preterm baby sucks less vigorously and has a greater tendency toward abdominal distention. In addition, sucking, swallowing, and gag reflexes are less well developed and may be entirely absent in a very young infant (in terms of gestational age).

The smaller the baby, the smaller his stomach capacity, hence the necessity for smaller, more frequent feedings. If the baby is overfed the likelihood of regurgitation and the associated danger of aspiration are very real.

There also appears to be a difference in the physiology of digestion in preterm infants in that they are less able to handle fats than preterm infants. Protein and carbohydrate digestion is similar to that of term infants, but if preterm infants are fed cow milk with none of the fat removed, a great deal of fat is then excreted in the stool.

What is the best type of feeding for preterm and low birth weight babies, particularly those below 1500 g? There is no totally satisfactory answer to this question. In a very real sense, any feeding other than via the placenta is "unnatural" for babies of less than 36 to 37 weeks gestation. Historically, breast milk was used in early preterm nurseries. Breast milk for preterm infants became unpopular in the United States during much of this century because it was felt that the amount of protein was inadequate for growth. Many physicians in England continued to utilize breast milk, however, and now there has been renewed interest in the United States in breast milk for preterm infants. Advantages and problems of using breast milk as a feeding for preterm infants are summarized in Table 9–9.

PSYCHOLOGICAL CONSIDERATIONS

A major advantage of human milk is the opportunity given the mother to participate in the care of her own baby in a very special way. Mothers who deliver preterm or ill infants frequently suffer a blow to their self-esteem. If they had planned to breast-feed and feel that it is now impossible, they can be doubly disappointed. Providing milk for the baby can promote feelings of self-worth and attachment.

An enhancement of self-esteem, however, is related to a successful experience in providing breast milk. Nurses (in the postpartum unit, the special care nursery, in ambulatory settings, or visiting at home) can be a major factor in that success. The means of providing support is detailed in this chapter.

IMMUNOLOGICAL CONSIDERATIONS AND PREVENTION OF CONTAMINATION

The immunological advantages of breast milk have been described previously. As indicated in Table 9–6, heating the milk to a level sufficient to destroy microorganisms also destroys many immune factors. Yet raw breast milk expressed into a container may contain microorganisms from the donor's nipples and hands and from the container. The method of collection was found to be significant (p <.001) by Liebhaber and colleagues (1978); milk collected by manual expression was found to have a bacterial colony count of 2500 colonies/ml. Milk collected with a rubber bulb breast pump had a bacterial colony count of 135,000 colonies/ml. Ninety-four per cent of the hand-expressed samples as compared to 53 per cent of the pump-expressed samples could have been used without pasteurization (a bacterial count of less than 10,000 colonies/ml). *Staphylococcus aureus* and *Pseudomonas* were cultured from the pump-expressed samples.

Table 9–9   Breast Milk for Low Birth Weight Infants

Advantages	Problems
Participation of the mother in infant care through provision of milk	For some mothers, difficulty in expressing milk, leading to frustration and disappointment
Immunological properties (Table 9–6)	Freezing/pasteurizing destroys many immune components Viral infection in mother may be passed to infant Possibility of contamination of collected milk *Potential* graft vs host reaction in donor milk; little evidence of occurrence
High biological level of protein	Sodium, calcium, and protein levels may be inadequate for baby weighing less than 2000 g
Better fat absorption	Composition varies Immune components higher in colostrum Fat content and calories higher in hind-milk Caloric density declines over period of time
Low renal solute load	

Washes of the "clean" rubber bulbs, which were either immersed in boiling water for 10 minutes or washed in a home dishwasher with a water temperature of 60° C (140° F) or greater, revealed bacterial counts of more than 1,000,000 colonies/ml.

Similar studies must be undertaken with other methods of collection (e.g., electric breast pump, Kaneson breast pump, Lloyd-B pump). From a bacterial standpoint, manual expression seems to have some advantage, yet some mothers find manual expression more difficult than pump expression. If milk can be collected with minimum contamination, immune factor–destroying processes will not usually be necessary.

The passage of a virus from mother to baby through her milk can be avoided if viral disease is recognized in the mother. During illness, the mother can express her milk to maintain milk production, discard the milk, and resume providing milk for the baby after the infection is past.

NUTRITIONAL CONSIDERATIONS

Lower amounts of *protein* in human milk are partially offset by the high biological value of human milk protein (Raiha et al. 1976). The ratio of lactalbumin to casein, important to digestibility, is 60:40 in human milk and certain formulas. Currently, very small preterm infants receiving human milk usually receive protein from other sources as well.

The fat of human milk is well absorbed. In human milk, fat provides approximately 50 per cent of the calories (the recommended amount for preterm infants). Fat in human milk is predominantly in the hind-milk, i.e., the milk expressed after let-down has occurred. Breast milk in a bottle should be shaken or mixed so that the fat does not remain on the sides of the container.

In infants born before 32 weeks gestation or those weighing 1500 g at birth, hyponatremia is common during the first six weeks of life and sodium needs are 3 to 4 mEq/kg of body weight each day (compared to 1 to 1½ mEq/kg/day in term infants). Since human milk supplies only 7 mEq of sodium per liter, the amount of human milk ingested is inadequate to meet *sodium* needs.

Human milk does not meet the preterm infant's need for calcium; a better calcium/phosphorus ratio results in higher serum calcium levels in term infants (Wald 1979). Nevertheless, small preterm infants usually require calcium supplementation.

SUPPORTING AND INSTRUCTING THE MOTHER WHO WANTS TO PROVIDE BREAST MILK FOR HER PRETERM OR SICK INFANT

A key factor in successful breast-feeding, and especially in successful letdown, is relaxation. When the mother is separated from the baby or when the baby is ill, relaxation is not always achieved easily. A number of techniques to enhance relaxation have already been described; it is with a discussion of these techniques that nursing instruction of the mother begins. Warm cloths placed next to the breasts increase circulation and enhance milk production.

Whether hand massage or a pump is used, the mother should wash her hands thoroughly with soap and warm water and rinse them before she touches her breasts. The breasts can then be wiped with sterile gauze and sterile water. (Our nursery provides mothers with sterile water in 4-oz bottles — formula bottles.)

Breast massage precedes hand expression.

Breast pumps A variety of hand-operated and electric breast pumps are available commercially. Each part of the Kaneson breast pump can be boiled, a decided advantage. The Kaneson pump is not difficult for mothers to operate; milk can be easily poured from the cylinder into a sterile plastic container for storage.

The Lloyd-B pump, by Lopuco, creates a vacuum when the pump handle is squeezed. The collection apparatus can be boiled but not the pump handle. Milk that may be pulled into the pump body must be flushed out or the pump body can be damaged.

The amount of suction on the Egnel electric breast pump can be controlled by the mother, beginning with a very gentle pulsating suction and gradually increasing.

A number of other types of pumps are available. Neither hand expression nor any single device meets the needs of every

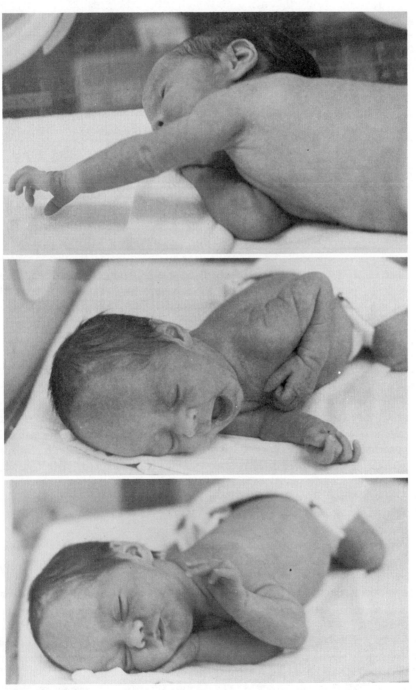

Figure 9–9. The development of feeding behavior in a premature baby. Top to bottom: prefeeding tension, rooting, and hand-mouth activity. (From O'Grady: Am J Nurs, 71:736.)

mother. Nurses must be aware of a variety of ways to assist expression of milk so that they can help each mother individually.

Storage and culture of milk Breast milk should be stored in *plastic* containers because macrophages adhere to the sides of glass containers and thus are unavailable to the baby. The container is labeled with the date and time of collection as well as the baby's name. Fresh milk should be used within 48 hours (many nurseries use fresh milk within 24 hours).

Milk that will not be used within 24 hours may be frozen for as long as four months. If milk is frozen at home, it should be transported to the nursery in a closed insulated container. When frozen milk is thawed, it should be used within 24 hours; the time of thawing should be noted on the bottle. Breast milk should be warmed immediately before feeding by placing the bottle in warm water.

The initial breast milk expressed is cul-

tured and withheld from the baby until the culture results are available. Milk is then cultured weekly.

ENCOURAGING THE MOTHER

At first, mothers of preterm infants may be able to express only very small amounts of milk. It is easy for them to become discouraged. Assurance that this is not unusual and that even small quantities are of value to the baby is important.

When a mother does not breast-feed immediately following childbirth but subsequently wishes to do so, *relactation* is a possibility for her. Relactation differs from *induced lactation*, which is defined as breast-feeding that is not preceded by pregnancy, e.g., the adoptive mother who wishes to breast-feed.

Relactation may be desired for several reasons. The baby may have been born prematurely and the mother did not know about expressing her milk or did not wish to do so at that time. Illness of the mother may have precluded breast-feeding. The baby may not be tolerating formula well. The mother may have stopped breast-feeding but now wishes to resume.

For whatever reason, the mother who wishes to induce lactation needs to be highly motivated because she will need to breast-feed approximately every two hours continuously for several weeks. Not every mother will have the patience for such a demanding schedule. To suggest that relactation will be simple and then allow the mother to fail damages her self-esteem.

The support of family members allow her adequate rest and time to be with her baby as well as support outside the family (from a nurse, the La Leche League, a neighbor) seems essential. A relactating mother will have both good and bad days and will need continuing, readily available support. The characteristics of her baby are also a factor; a very irritable baby may make a mother so tense that relactation is compromised.

Mothers who are relactating are asked to keep a daily record of the number and length of feedings, the number of ounces of supplement given and the number of wet diapers. If the baby is maintaining weight and there are eight wet diapers a day, relactation is considered to be occurring. Weight gain will occur as the milk supply increases. In general, it is estimated to take one week of relactation for each month the baby has not nursed plus one week. Thus, if the baby is two months old before relactation is started, it will take three weeks to establish lactation. Encouraging signs for the relactating mother include good sucking on the part of the baby and enlargement of the breasts with the appearance of colostrum.

METHODS OF FEEDING LOW BIRTH WEIGHT INFANTS

Careful observation of each infant can help determine the best method of feeding (Fig. 9–9). There are several alternatives for feeding the preterm infant. Direct breast-feeding or bottle-feeding is possible only for a few relatively large and vigorous preterm babies of more than 34 to 35 weeks gestational age whose sucking and swallowing reflexes are well developed.

When the baby has neither sucking nor swallowing reflexes or when sucking and swallowing seem to exhaust him, gavage feeding, continuous feeding through a gastric or nasojejunal tube, or intravenous feeding will be necessary.

The technique of gavage feeding is as follows:

1. For very small infants of 2 to 3 lbs a #8 gavage tube is used; in larger babies a #10 tube may be satisfactory.

2. The length of the tube is measured from the bridge of the nose to the ear to the xiphoid process. The catheter may be premarked, but since there are all sizes of even tiny infants, the tube should still be measured at each feeding.

3. A small quantity of sterile water run through the tube *before* it is inserted assures its patency. (This is not usually necessary if a disposable tube is used.)

4. Nasal catheters may be lubricated with sterile water; oral catheters do not need to be lubricated.

5. After the catheter is passed, the baby should be observed for a moment for signs of dyspnea, an indication that the tube may be in the trachea rather than the esophagus.

6. If the catheter is not already attached to a syringe, the syringe is attached and the formula poured into it and allowed to flow by gravity.

7. If the tube is not to be left in place it is pinched and removed when every drop of formula has passed through the tube.

8. A baby should be "burped" following gavage feeding just as he is after a bottle- or breast-feeding. If he must remain in the incubator he can be held in a sitting position and have his back gently stroked toward the neck.

If the baby begins to suck on his gavage tube during feedings, he may be ready to graduate to small nipple feedings (Fig. 9–10). Bottle-feedings should begin grad-

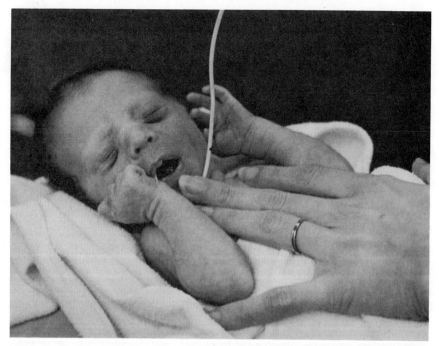

Figure 9–10. Hand-mouth gestures and a capacity to "mouth" the feeding tube are indications that this 3½-pound premature baby will soon take feedings from a nipple instead of a tube. (From O'Grady: Am J Nurs, *71:737*.)

ually, initially at only one feeding during the 24-hour period, and gradually increased when the baby shows that he is not overly tired from sucking. First breast-feedings should also be brief and should be increased gradually.

Nasojejunal feeding Although used less frequently than gavage feeding, nasojejunal feeding is an alternate feeding route for some infants (Table 9–10). Infants who have marked apnea and/or bradycardia when a gavage tube is passed, infants who have persistent tachypnea, and infants who require assisted ventilation or who aspirate formula persistently are examples of possible candidates for nasojejunal feeding. Advantages of nasojejunal feedings for certain infants are decreased aspiration and decreased vagal stimulation. The one-time passage of the nasojejunal tube may be less fatiguing.

The nasojejunal tube is frequently a radiopaque Silastic catheter. After the length of the tube is determined the catheter is passed through the baby's nose and then through the esophagus, stomach,

and duodenum until it reaches the jejunum. The infant is placed on his right side during the procedure to facilitate passage and proper placement. Abdominal x-ray confirms placement of the catheter.

Continuous feedings of a precise amount of formula each hour can be provided by using an infusion pump such as the Harvard pump. The amount of milk the baby receives should be recorded each hour just as intravenous fluids are recorded.

The syringe and tubing leading to the stopcock connected to the nasojejunal tube are usually changed every eight hours to protect the infant from bacterial contamination of milk formula at room temperature. However, Schreiner and colleagues (1979) found that the rate of bacterial colonization was not affected by the duration of time the feeding was in the tube.

Bacterial infection has been shown to be a major hazard in continuous feedings; Schreiner and colleagues found that 33 per cent of the continuous drip feedings they cultured yielded bacteria. In many

Table 9–10   Assessment and Intervention for the Infant Receiving
Gastric and Nasojejunal Feedings

Observation	Assessment	Possible Causes	Nursing Intervention
Abdominal distention	Inspection Measurement of abdominal circumference	Improper location of tube Excessive amounts of formula	Check tube every 8 hours for patency Report abdominal distention
Blood in stool	Test for occult blood (Hematest, guaiac test)	Necrotizing enterocolitis	Report presence of blood in stool Feeding may be discontinued
Emesis	Presence of bile Test for occult blood	Reflex from duodenum to stomach Improper location of tube Necrotizing enterocolitis	Report presence of bile or blood Feeding may be discontinued
Aspiration	Formula in infant's mouth and/or nose	Displacement of tube	Stop feeding Suction to remove milk
Residual	Aspirated residual	Displacement of tube Necrotizing enterocolitis	Report residuals > 0.8 to 1.0 ml

instances the organisms were similar to those cultured from the hands of nurses, strongly suggesting the need for meticulous hand washing by nurses preparing continuous feedings. Although Schreiner does not suggest the use of gloves, an experiment comparing the effectiveness of hand washing alone with hand washing plus gloves would be of value to future practice. The fluid administered for continuous feedings should be cultured at regular intervals.

Infants receiving continuous feeding, like all infants who are NPO, require oral stimulation. They should have pacifiers if they are able to suck. Oral medicines will usually not be given; if they are, an oral gastric tube may be passed for medicine administration.

The Infant with a Cleft Palate

Since a hard palate is essential to sucking, the baby with a cleft palate may have to be fed by some means other than breast or bottle. Some babies with cleft palates can be successfully bottle-fed; others seem to feed more easily with a Breck feeder. (An elongated nipple, used to feed baby lambs, is available from at least one manufacturer of infant formula and at most feed stores.) Nipple holes need to be small enough to keep the baby from being flooded with milk which would then flow into his respiratory tract, depositing curds in the nasal passages and making the danger of infection of both the nasopharynx and the ears a very real possibility. Holding the baby upright to feed him also helps to prevent this regurgitation.

If the cleft is large the baby may push the nipple up into the open area with his tongue. This can be avoided by keeping most of the nipple outside of his mouth and positioning it at an angle to the cleft.

Once the baby has begun to feed well his mother should begin to feed him under nursing supervision. I am continually amazed at how well and how quickly many mothers are able to feed their babies with a Breck feeder. The baby is ready for discharge (barring other complications) when the mother feels comfortable about caring for and feeding him.

When the cleft involves only the soft palate, some mothers who have been highly motivated to breast-feeding have been able to do so (Weatherly-White 1978; Grady 1978). An infant with a cleft lip should not be breast-fed following surgery until the suture line is healed, but the mother may express milk to be fed to the baby during the period of healing (approximately six weeks), after which the baby may nurse at the breast. Not every mother of an infant with a cleft lip and/or palate will choose to breast-feed, but the opportunity should be offered to those who strongly desire to do so.

The Infant Who is to be Fed Through a Gastrostomy Tube

The most common reason for gastrostomy feedings in newborns is the repair of a tracheoesophageal fistula. The tube is inserted during surgery and sutured in place. Initial feedings of glucose and water (5 to 10 ml) begin on the second to third day after surgery. If they are well tolerated they are followed by small amounts of milk, which are gradually increased as the baby shows his ability to handle it. Vomiting and abdominal distention are signs that feedings need to be decreased for a period.

The gastrostomy tube is connected through the hole in the top of the isolette to an asepto-syringe without the bulb. It is never clamped until the baby is taking oral feedings and then only during the feedings themselves. This allows any gas and the contents of the baby's stomach to reflux up the tube and into the syringe when the baby cries or strains. Because of this reflux there is no advantage to rinsing the tube with water after each feeding. If the baby is able to tolerate the extra amount of fluid that would be used to rinse the tube, his milk intake should be increased, giving him needed calories and nutrients as well as liquid.

Hyperalimentation as a Means of Infant Feeding

When infants cannot tolerate oral feedings or when oral feedings cannot be given in a quantity that meets the baby's nutritional needs, intravenous alimentation provides an additional source of nutrition. Protein and fat as well as glucose may be provided intravenously.

Hyperalimentation solutions may be given in a peripheral vein or through a central catheter. Peripheral alimentation is more commonly used in the small preterm infant, whereas central lines are placed in the larger infant requiring long-term parenteral nutrition, such as an infant with bowel surgery because of a large omphalocele, gastroschisis, or other congenital abnormality of the gastrointestinal tract.

When a central catheter is used, the catheter is inserted into the right external jugular vein and guided into the superior vena cava, this location being chosen because the high blood flow of the superior vena cava helps avoid inflammation and thrombosis in the vein. The proximal end of the catheter (i.e., the end that is not in the vena cava) is passed from the neck subcutaneously to a stab wound in the parietal area of the scalp (Fig. 9–11). This procedure serves three purposes:

1. By displacing the point of the catheter entrance from the skin exit site, additional protection against infection is provided.

2. Contamination by the baby's oral and nasal secretions becomes less likely.

3. The catheter is out of reach of the baby's ever-searching hands. After the catheter has been inserted an x-ray is taken to ensure proper placement.

The intravenous system includes a millipore filter, which serves to remove particles or microorganisms from the system that may have contaminated the solution before they can reach the baby, and a peristaltic constant-fusion pump to ensure that the solution is delivered at a constant rate throughout the 24 hours. Both filter and pump are changed at least as often as every three days.

Because there are a number of serious complications possible with hyperalimentation, constant nursing attention is an absolute necessity. Septicemia is a major danger because the glucose-protein solu-

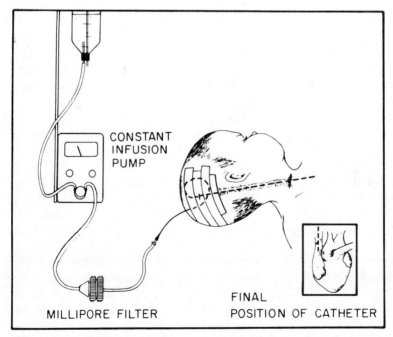

Figure 9–11. Technique of catheter insertion and delivery of fluids for total intravenous alimentation.

tion is a nearly perfect medium for the growth of bacteria, particularly *Monilia*. The prevention of infection depends on careful technique not only at the time the catheter is inserted but throughout the period it is in place. Frequent changing of the intravenous set-up has already been mentioned. The catheter should never be used for the administration of medications or for the withdrawal of blood; both procedures increase the possibility of contamination. A careful record of temperature and frequent blood cultures are important in detecting infection as early as possible. If the catheter is needed for more than 30 days it is usually reinserted on the opposite side.

Fever may occur in the baby in the absence of positive blood culture or other signs of infection. It has been suggested that fever of this nature may be an antigenic reaction to peptides in the solution. Such fever begins early, usually within four hours after therapy has been started, and may subside within a week.

The utilization of the amino acid solution by the baby's body is dependent upon the addition of a quantity of glucose sufficient to stimulate insulin production. The insulin, in turn, stimulates both the transport of amino acids into the cell and the synthesis of protein. If relatively large amounts of glucose are not given, the amino acids will be utilized for energy by the body rather than for the synthesis of protein.

However, the high quantity of glucose necessary (as much as twice that normally given to infants) can cause a rapid and severe dehydration. Urine specimens are tested for glucose at least every six hours during the first days of treatment. If two or more consecutive samples reveal a 3+ or 4+ glucose by the Clinitest method, either the rate of infusion or the glucose content of the solution is decreased. Some physicians add insulin to the solution under these circumstances. Others begin therapy with a 10% solution of glucose during the first 24 hours, followed by a 15% solution during the next 24 hours and a 20% solution thereafter to prevent this initial glycosuria.

Hypertonic sugar solutions in combination with amino acids may, after several days of administration, lead to a hypoglycemic response within the body, whether insulin has been added or not. If insulin is added it is generally not needed after the first few days. It is important to be watchful for signs of hypoglycemia at this time.

As in all newborns, weight gain is a significant observation. If the baby was not malnourished before the feedings began and has no infection, weight gain may be comparable to that of a normal infant, although it will also be influenced by the infant's original problem. If the baby was nutritionally depleted at the time therapy started, his weight is likely to remain constant for several days even though he shows other signs of improvement

A number of other side effects are possible including demineralization of bone and cerebral edema. However, in spite of the hazards, which admittedly are great, with very good care hyperalimentation does indeed mean a difference between life and death for some newborns.

INTRALIPID

Intravenous fat, in the form of Intralipid, provides a concentrated source of calories (9 cal/g) and essential fatty acids in the form of linoleic acid. Intralipid solution contains soybean oil emulsified with egg yolk and phospholipids; it is isotonic with serum.

Intralipid may be given in the same peripheral vein as hyperalimentation solution by joining the two lines with a Y-connector before they enter the vein. A common line is not used prior to that point because of the delicate nature of the lipid solution. Intralipid solution is never given through a filter.

Intralipid is given slowly; the maximum rate is 3 ml/kg/hour, but lower rates are often used.

Some infants may have an allergic reaction to Intralipid solutions. Infants should be observed for an enlarged liver; severely abnormal liver function is a contraindication to Intralipid therapy.

The Infant with Necrotizing Enterocolitis

Necrotizing enterocolitis (NEC) is a potentially life-threatening condition that occurs in approximately 3 to 8 per cent of preterm infants. Two factors are believed essential in the etiology: ischemia of the gut and feeding. Although the precise pathophysiology is unclear, the following sequence is postulated. After an episode in which circulation to the gut is impaired (e.g., perinatal asphyxia), intestinal cells that have been damaged by hypoxia stop secreting mucus. After feeding, the damaged cells are invaded by gas-forming bacteria and a characteristic picture of pneumatosis cystoides intestinalis (air in the wall of the intestine) may be seen on x-ray. Unrecognized, NEC may result in bowel perforation and death.

Early signs of NEC are most likely to be recognized through careful nursing observation. Infants at risk can frequently be identified at birth: any baby who has experienced perinatal asphyxia requiring vigorous resuscitation in the delivery room and any baby who has apnea, bradycardia, and cyanosis, sepsis, exchange transfusion, umbilical vessel catheterization, or who is young in gestational age. Obviously a great many babies in a special care nursery will be at risk.

Significant nursing observations are summarized in Table 9–11. The evaluation of abdominal distention should not rely on the eye alone; points are marked on the abdomen and the distance between those points is measured every four to six hours. An increase of more than 1 cm from the previous measurement requires further evaluation. A shiny abdominal wall is a further sign of distention.

Both frequent spitting and the presence of residual formula in the baby's stomach at the time of the next feeding are indications of failure to totally absorb a feeding and may indicate NEC. These signs may also suggest that the feedings being offered are too large. Residual formula is checked by aspirating formula from the gavage tube; the aspiration is measured and then replaced rather than discarded because it contains electrolytes normally present in the stomach.

Every stool is checked for occult blood; the use of a test strip (Hemastix) is a rapid and inexpensive way to do this in the nursery.

When NEC is suspected, abdominal x-ray may confirm the diagnosis of air in the intestinal wall. In the presence of symptoms (even without the x-ray picture), oral feedings are frequently discontinued for seven to 10 days; in addition, antibiotics are given to the baby. When feedings are resumed they are usually both small and dilute and are advanced very carefully.

There is some evidence that breast milk may decrease the incidence of NEC. Delaying the initial feeding in babies at risk and providing parenteral nutrition is the practice in some nurseries (Brown and Sweet 1978). Parenteral nutrition, of course, also poses certain risks.

Table 9–11 Observing Infants for NEC

Signs	Nursing Action
History of asphyxia or hypoxia	Identify infant at risk
Abdominal distention	Measure abdomen every 4 to 6 hours
Failure to absorb feedings	Observe and record spitting
	Measure residual at each feeding
Absence of bowel sounds	Listen with stethoscope
Blood in stools	Test stool for occult blood

The Infant with a Congenital Heart Defect

Not every baby with a congenital heart defect will have feeding problems. There are, however, two possible sources of difficulty. The baby may tire so easily that he takes an insufficient amount of formula or he may choke and become dyspneic and the mother will discontinue feeding him. Yet because of an increased cardiac workload and an increased expenditure of energy he actually needs more calories than usual. When this happens it is necessary to use a formula that increases the concentration of calories within the limits of a small fluid intake. In addition, the formula should have a fairly low concentration of sodium and a low renal solute load.

The Infant with Phenylketonuria

The inheritance and dietary treatment of phenylketonuria, an autosomal recessive trait, are described in Chapter 2.

The Infant with Galactosemia

Like PKU, galactosemia is also inherited as an autosomal recessive trait. An infant with galactosemia lacks a specific enzyme — galactose-1-phosphate uridyl transferase. Because of this he is unable to metabolize lactose and galactose so that galactose-1-phosphate accumulates in the red cells (hence galactosemia) and reducing sugars (for which specific tests are available) are found in the urine. Glucose, however, is not present in the urine.

The symptoms of galactosemia are not always easy to detect. Common findings are failure to gain weight and jaundice that persists beyond the first week (unlike physiologic jaundice). There may also be subcutaneous bleeding, vomiting, diarrhea, and subsequent dehydration. If the disease is not detected the baby usually deteriorates progressively with physical and mental retardation, signs of malnutrition, cirrhosis of the liver, and cataracts.

The treatment is simple in theory. Since lactose occurs naturally only in milk, the newborn infant who shows signs of galactosemia is fed a formula, such as Nutramigen, that does not contain milk. Soy bean formulas have also been found to be satisfactory if the baby does not have diarrhea. Problems in feeding arise as the baby grows older and needs a more varied diet since milk and milk components such as lactose, casein, and whey are incorporated into so many commercial foods. Lactose, for example, is added to many canned and frozen fruits and vegetables during processing.

The removal of lactose from the diet changes the course of galactosemia markedly, even when the condition has gone unrecognized for several months. Appetite improves, vomiting, diarrhea, and jaundice subside, and liver function improves. In some instances, cataracts disappear.

The Infant with Cystic Fibrosis

In the newborn nursery the recognition that a baby has an obstruction due to meconium ileus (Chapter 6) leads to the diagnosis of cystic fibrosis. Only about 10 per cent of cystic fibrosis babies are diagnosed this early, the remaining 90 per cent being recognized in later infancy or early childhood. Obstruction in the bronchi may not appear for weeks or even years after birth. The characteristic bulky foul stools may or may not be evident in the newborn period.

Several dietary changes are necessary for babies with cystic fibrosis. Total caloric intake has to be increased because of the abnormally high loss of calories in stools. Fecal losses are reduced, but not entirely eliminated, by giving the baby pancreatic enzymes before each feeding. A formula is chosen that is high in protein and carbohydrate but has a low to moderate fat content, the fat being one that is readily absorbed.

Water-miscible preparations of the fat-soluble vitamins (A, D, E, and K) are given to the baby. The dosage of vitamin

D is adjusted on the basis of blood levels of calcium, phosphorus, and alkaline phosphatase and evidence on wrist x-ray, whereas the dosage of vitamin E is correlated with levels of blood alpha-tocopherol. The adequacy of vitamin K intake is determined by checking prothrombin time at intervals of one to two months.

NUTRITIONAL DEPRIVATION IN THE NEWBORN PERIOD

What happens when nutrition is not adequate in the newborn period? Obvious effects may be inadequate growth in length and failure to gain weight. It is strongly suspected that nutritional deficiency may affect the central nervous system as well. The effects of nutritional deficiencies on the central nervous systems of very young animals have been demonstrated in a succession of studies over nearly 50 years. Rats with inadequate caloric intake during the period of most rapid postnatal brain growth exhibited marked retardation (Scrimshaw 1968). Severe undernutrition has been shown to influence the chemical composition of the brains of infant pigs so that their brains resemble those of considerably younger pigs (Fomon 1974).

Even more important than a lack of calories is a lack of protein. A number of animal studies have examined protein deficiency in the presence of adequate caloric intake. In a London study, weanling rats, piglets, and puppies born of well-nourished mothers were fed diets adequate in calories but severely deficient in protein. The animals showed signs of degenerative changes in their nerve cells. Electroencephalograms were abnormal; one researcher noted certain resemblances in the EEGs of these pigs and those of children with kwashiorkor, a condition involving severe protein deficiency (Nelson 1959).

The animal studies showed that the time at which nutritional restriction occurs is significant. Food restriction prior

to weaning was associated with permanent changes in the size and chemical composition of the brain in rats. Food restriction for an equal period but imposed at the time of weaning also led to brain alterations, but these later alterations disappeared during a subsequent period of adequate nutrition (Winick and Noble 1966).

Lack of specific vitamins and minerals also led to deformities in animals studied.

In human infants prodigious development of the brain occurs after birth. Head circumference increases from approximately 34 cm at birth to 46 cm at the first birthday and then at a rate of roughly 0.5 cm each succeeding year until the adult size of 52 cm is reached. Similarly, the weight of the brain, about 400 g at birth, more than doubles in the first year to 1000 g and continues to grow for many years. Brain mass increases until about 25 years of age.

In addition to these changes in size, a major change in brain structure occurs in the first years of life. At birth, the infant brain contains most of the ten billion neurons that it will have during the individual's lifetime. But the neurons are packed very densely in the small infant skull. They enlarge and the connecting links between them increase in number and complexity very rapidly until the age of four and more slowly until the age of 12. Because of this, it is believed that when nutritional deficiencies, particularly protein deficiencies, are severe enough to limit height and weight gains in the first years of life, brain development and the related motor, language, and adaptive behavior are also likely to be affected. The earlier the period of deprivation, the more serious the consequences. In studies of children with kwashiorkor, rates of progress in behavioral development were related to the age at which the children were admitted to the hospital. Relatively little progress was made by children who had kwashiorkor at the age of three to six months; there was better development in children who were 15 to 29 months at the time they were admitted. Children who were 37 to 41 months at the time of admission demonstrated the best rate of behavior development (Fomon 1974).

Maternal Deprivation and Undernutrition

Whitten, Pettit, and Fischhoff (1969) have proposed that undernutrition may not always be recognized for what it is. Studies in the 1940s suggested that emotional deprivation in an infant or young child could be directly responsible for the child's failure to grow and thrive. Whitten and colleagues point out that none of these psychological studies determined the babies' caloric intakes. This study involved 13 maternally deprived infants, 11 of whom gained weight at an accelerated rate when they were fed adequately in a hospital environment that deliberately simulated their home situations, i.e., they were confined in windowless rooms and were neither talked to nor smiled at nor held for feeding. The two babies who did not gain remained anorectic. Both of them had a history of repeated attempts by the mother to force-feed them. It was reported that one father, reacting to his baby's poor intake, had tried to "ram a hamburger down the infant's throat."

In a second group of seven infants, all seven gained weight rapidly in their own homes when they were fed an adequate diet in the presence of a public health nurse acting as observer. Whitten and colleagues believe that there was no improvement in home environment that could account for the increase in weight. For example, one infant, who was visited 42 times by the nurse (three times a day for 14 days) was found alone in a crib in a back room on every occasion. Forty-one times the baby was returned to the back room before the nurse left. Yet during the 14-day period the baby gained 26 ounces.

A second infant gained 22 ounces during an eight-day feeding program in spite of the fact that during that period his family was evicted for nonpayment of rent and he had been physically abused by his father.

When the mothers were questioned prior to the period of the observed feedings most of them had claimed that their babies ate adequately. During supervised home feeding, however, some mothers began to realize that their babies actually had been underfed.

The Environmental Contamination of Milk

As mentioned earlier, in Western society we have the knowledge and means to deal with the biological contamination of milk through pasteurization, sterilization, and refrigeration, although these means are still not used by everyone in our society. Environmental contamination, on the other hand, is a potential threat to all infants regardless of socioeconomic factors. Two sources of environmental contamination of milk given to newborns are DDT and radioactive material.

DDT

In 1969 the DDT residue level in human milk was reported to be 0.1 to 0.2 parts per million, two to four times the level permitted by the Food and Drug Administration in cow milk that is to be shipped in interstate commerce. One reason the level is higher in human milk is that DDT becomes more concentrated at each step in the food chain. Animals, poultry, and fish all store DDT in their tissues and pass it on to humans as meat and milk. Women also secrete a higher percentage of DDT in their milk than do cows. Just what effect these high levels of DDT have or will have is not directly known. Animal studies have implicated DDT as a cancer-causing substance, which at least raises the question of a similar possibility in humans. In some animal populations DDT has apparently affected reproduction and has led to a decline in some species (Wurster 1970).

Is the problem of DDT contamination of such magnitude that mothers should no longer nurse their infants? Wurster feels that this is not the answer. Other foods also contain DDT, and since DDT is also known to pass the placental barrier even before birth, the baby has already stored DDT in his tissues. Two suggestions for nursing mothers are avoiding household sprays containing DDT or other chlorinated hydrocarbons and minimizing the intake of eggs, fatty meats, and fish.

DDT is now banned in the United States as well as in many other countries. Nevertheless, it was reported in 1976 that levels of DDT in the breast milk of indigent blacks in rural Mississippi and Arkansas far exceeded WHO standards for cow milk (Woodard, Ferguson, and Wilson 1976). Other pesticides are also excreted in breast milk.

ORGANOCHLORINE COMPOUNDS

Organochlorine compounds include a variety of chemicals that have been used for more than 40 years in such diverse substances as paint, printer's ink, and electrical transformers. They include polychlorinated biphenyls (PCBs) and polybrominated biphenyls (PBBs). Because these compounds concentrate selectively in breast milk, the exposure of nursing infants is greater than that of adults. Because the compounds are very stable, they remain in the environment for long periods of time.

Maternal ingestion of PCBs is most possible in fish from contaminated waters; pregnant and lactating women should avoid such fish. Commercial fish in the United States are checked for this and other contamination. The other possible route of contamination is through accidental ingestion; this occurred in Japan when mothers ingested contaminated rice oil. In Michigan in 1973 cattle feed contaminated with PBBs entered the food chain, exposing a large part of the population to PBBs (Dunckel 1975).

Just what the risk to infants of ingestion of PCBs and PBBs may be is unclear. The Japanese children who ingested PCBs from breast milk appeared apathetic and hypotonic (Giacoia and Catz 1979).

RADIATION

Another source of potential environmental contamination of infant milk is radiation. As in the past, the major source of radiation today is from natural sources, such as cosmic rays and atmospheric and terrestrial radiation. Man-made sources, including diagnostic x-ray (the most important), therapeutic x-ray, and luminous dials account for about seven times as much radiation as fallout. Even if there should be no further testing of atomic weapons in the atmosphere, the increasing peacetime uses of atomic energy as power sources and the expanding use of radioisotopes in medicine and industry will increase radiation in the environment. The hazard from fallout, probably the most feared source, is small in comparison with the potential radioactive contamination from sources that we tend to accept as necessary.

Radioactivity relates to infant feeding on several counts. Unlike DDT residuals, the radioactive content of human milk is considerably lower than that of cow milk. The length of time during which milk is stored affects some radioisotopes. For example, since only 0.6 per cent of the original amount of iodine-131 remains in cow milk after the milk has been stored for two months, it cannot be considered a real hazard in evaporated and powdered milk formulas. Barium-140 and strontium-89 also have short half-lives and are biologically important only for a few months after a bomb has been exploded. Strontium-90, on the other hand, has a half-life of 20 years (half-life being the time required for half the atoms of a radioactive substance to disintegrate). Increases in the concentration of strontium-90 occurred in the United States in 1963 and 1964 following the atomic testing of 1961.

Bibliography

Amine, E., Hegstead D.: Effect of dietary carbohydrates and fats on inorganic iron absorption. J Agric Food Chem 23:204, 1975.

Anderson, P.: Drugs and breast feeding: a review. Drug Intell Clin Pharm 11:208, 1977.

Applebaum, R.: Breastfeeding and drugs in human milk. Keep Abreast J 2(4):292, 1977.

Atkinson, L.: Prenatal nipple conditioning for breastfeeding. Nurs Res 28:267, 1979.

Auerback, K.: The role of the nurse in support of breastfeeding. J Adv Nurs 4:263, 1979.

Berke, R., Hoops, E., Saenger, E.: Radiation dose to breastfeeding child after mother has ^{99m}TcMAA lung scan. J Nucl Med 14:51, 1973.

Bliss, V.: Nursing care for infants with neonatal necrotizing enterocolitis. MCN 1(1):37, 1976.

Blumenthal, I., Ebel, A., Pildes, R.: Effect of posture on the pattern of stomach emptying in the newborn. Pediatrics 63:532, 1979.

Brackbill, Y., Douthitt, T., West, H.: Psychophysiologic effects in the neonate of prone versus supine placement. J Pediatr 82:82, 1973.

Breast-Feeding and the Mother. New York: Ciba Foundation Symposium, 45 (new series), 1976.

Brown, M., Hurlock, J.: Preparation of the breast for breastfeeding. Nurs Res 24:448, 1975.

Brown, E., Sweet, A.: Preventing necrotizing enterocolitis in neonates. JAMA 240:2452–2454, 1978.

Catz, C., Giacoia, G.: Drugs and breast milk. Pediatr Clin North Am 19:151, 1972.

Clarke, T., Markarian, M., Griswold, W., Mendoza, S.: Hypernatremic dehydration resulting from inadequate breast feeding. Pediatrics 63:931, 1979.

Cole, A., Hailey, D.: Diazepam and active metabolite in breast milk and their transfer to the neonate. Arch Dis Child 50:741, 1975.

Conner, A.: Elevated levels of sodium and chloride in milk from mastitic breast. Pediatrics 63:910, 1979.

Counseling the mother on breast-feeding. Report of the Eleventh Ross Roundtable on Critical Approaches to Common Pediatric Problems. Columbus, Ohio: Ross Laboratories, 1980.

Cunningham, A.: Morbidity in breast-fed and artificially fed infants. J Pediatr 90:726–729, 1977.

Dallman, P.: Iron, vitamin E and folate in the preterm infant. J Pediatr 85:742–752, 1974.

DeBuys, L., Henriques: Effect of body posture on the position and emptying time of the stomach. Am J Dis Child 15:190, 1918.

Doucette, J.: Is breast-feeding still safe for babies? MCN 3(6):345, 1978.

Dunckel, A.: An updating of the polybrominated biphenyl disaster in Michigan. J Am Vet Med Assoc 167:838, 1975.

Fass, E.: Is bottle-feeding a factor in dental caries? J Dent Child 24:245, 1962.

Ferguson, B., Wilson, D., Schaffner, W.: Determination of nicotine concentrations in human milk. Am J Dis Child 130:837, 1976.

Fomon, S.: Infant Nutrition. 2nd Edition. Philadelphia: W. B. Saunders, 1974.

Giacoia, G., Catz, C.: Drugs and pollutants in breast milk. Clin Perinatol 6(1): 181, 1979.

Goldman, A.: Immunologic aspects of human milk. In Symposium on Human Lactation, L. Waletzky (ed.). Rockville, Md.: U.S. Department of Health, Education and Welfare, 1976.

Goldman, A., Smith, C.: Host resistance factors in human milk. J Pediatr 82:1082, 1974.

Goldman, H., Goldman, J., Kaufman, I., Liebman, D.: Late effects of early dietary protein intake on low-birth-weight infants. J Pediatr 85:764–769, 1974.

Grady, E.: Breastfeeding the baby with a cleft of the soft palate. Keep Abreast J 3(2):126, 1978.

Grams, K.: Breast-feeding: a means of imparting immunity? MCN, 3(6):340, 1978.

Grassley, J., Davis, K.: Common concerns of mothers who breast-feed. MCN 3(6):347, 1978.

Gross, S.: The relationship between milk protein and iron content on hematologic values in infancy. J Pediatr 73:521, 1968.

Hall, J.: Influencing breastfeeding success. JOGN Nurs 7(6):28, 1978.

Henderson, K., Newton, L.: Helping nursing mothers maintain lactation while separated from their infants. MCN 3(6):352, 1978.

Hewitt, V.: Effect of posture on the presence of fat in tracheal aspirate in neonates. Aust Paediatr J 12:267, 1976.

Hood, J.: Effects of posture on the amount and distribution of gas in the intestinal tract of infants and young children. Lancet 2:107, 1964.

Kietel, H., Cohn, R., Harnish, D.: Diaper rash, self-inflicted excoriations and crying in full-term newborn infants kept in the prone or supine position. J Pediatr 57:571, 1960.

Knoles, J.: Breast milk: a source of more than nutrition for the neonate. Clin Toxicol 7:69, 1974.

Kroll, R.G., Stone J.: Nocturnal bottle feeding as a contributory cause of rampant dental caries in the infant and young child. J Dent Child 34:454, 1967.

Lactation: A Comprehensive Treatise. Bruce Larson (ed.). New York: Academic Press, 1978.

Liebhaber, M., Lewiston, N., Asquith, M., Olds-Arroyo, L., Sunshine, P.: Alterations of lymphocytes and of antibody content of human milk after processing. J Pediatr 91:897, 1977.

Liebhaber, M., Lewiston, N., Asquith, M., Sunshine, P.: Comparison of bacterial contamination with two methods of human milk collection. J Pediatr 92:236, 1978.

Lundstrom, U., Siimes, M., Dallman, P.: At what age does iron supplementation become necessary in low-birth-weight infants? J Pediatr 91:878, 1977.

Martin, R., Herrell, N., Rubin, D., Fanaroff, A.: Effect of supine and prone positions on arterial oxygen tension in the preterm infant. Pediatrics 63:528, 1979.

Martinez, G., Nalezienski, J.: The recent trend in breast-feeding. Pediatrics 64:686, 1979.

Mata, L., Kromal, R., Urrutea, J., Garcia, B.: Effect of infection on food intake and the nutritional state: perspectives as viewed from the village. Am J Clin Nutr 30:1215, 1977.

Mata, L.: Breast-feeding: main promoter of infant health. Am J Clin Nutr 31:2058, 1978.

McMillan, J., Landaw, S., Oski, F.: Iron sufficiency in breast-fed infants and the availability of iron from human milk. Pediatrics 58:686–691, 1976.

Melhorn, D., Gross, S., Lake, G., Leu, J.: The hydrogen peroxide fragility test and serum tocopherol level in anemias of various etiologies. Blood 37:438, 1971.

Michal, B.: "Bottle mouth" caries. J La Dent Assoc 27:10, 1969.

Miller, H., Weetab, R.: The excretion of radioactive iodine in human milk. Lancet 2:1013, 1955.

Nelson, G.K., Dean, R.F.A.: The electroencephalogram in African children: effects of kwashiorkor and a note on the newborn. Bull WHO 21:779, 1959.

O'Brien, T.: Excretion of drugs in human milk. Am J Hosp Pharm 31:844, 1974.

Patrick, M., Tilstone, W., Reavy, P.: Diazepam and breast feeding. Lancet 1:543, 1972.

Peters, T., Apt, L., Ross, J.: Effects of phosphates upon iron absorption studied in normal human subjects and in an experimental model using dialysis. Gastroenterology 61:315, 1971.

Price, E., Gyotoku, S.: Using the nasojejunal feeding technique in a neonatal intensive care unit. MCN 3(6):361, 1978.

Raiha, N., Heenonen, K., Rassin, D., Gaull, G.: Milk protein quantity and quality in low-birth-weight infants. I. Metabolic responses and effect on growth. Pediatrics 57:659, 1976.

Rawlins, C.: Mastitis, and acute and chronic illness. In Counseling the Mother on Breast-feeding, R.A. Lawrence (ed.). Report of the Eleventh Ross Roundtable on Critical Approaches to Common Pediatric Problems. Columbus, Ohio: Ross Laboratories, 1980.

Saarinen, U., Siimes, M., Dallman, P.: Iron absorption in infants: High bioavailability of breast milk iron as indicated by the extrinsic tag method of iron absorption and by the concentration of serum ferritin. J Pediatr 91:36, 1977.

Sauls, H.: Potential effect of demographic and other variables in studies comparing morbidity of breast-fed and bottle-fed infants. Pediatrics 64:523, 1979.

Saxena, B., Shrimanker, K., Grudzinskas, J.: Levels of contraceptive steroids in breast milk and plasma of lactating women. Contraception 16:605, 1977.

Schou, M., Amdisen, A.: Lithium and pregnancy. III. Lithium ingestion by children breast fed by women on lithium treatment. Br Med J 2:138, 1973.

Schreiner, R., Coates, T., Shackelford, P.: Possible breast milk transmission of group-B streptococcal infection (letter). J Pediatr 91:159, 1977.

Scrimshaw, N.S.: Infant malnutrition and adult learning. Saturday Rev March 16:64, 1968.

Slattery, J.: Nutrition for the normal healthy infant. MCN 2(2):105, 1977.

Smith, C., LeWald, L.: The influence of posture on digestion in infancy. Am J Dis Child 9:261, 1915.

Standards and Recommendations for Hospital Care of Newborn Infants. 6th Edition. Evanston, Illinois: American Academy of Pediatrics, 1974.

Stavis, R., Krauss, A.: Complications of neonatal intensive care. Clin Perinatol 7(1):107, 1980.

Stokan, R.E.: The right formula for the right infant: making sense of infant nutrition. MCN 2(2):101, 1977.

Thompson, D.: Breast milk and dental caries: the question of fluoride. Keep Abreast J 3:108, 1978.

Trippie, R., Jennings, R.: Nursing bottle syndrome. Tex Med 73:47, 1977.

Tunnessen, W., Hertz, C.: Toxic effects of lithium in newborn infants: a commentary. J Pediatr 91:804, 1972.

Wald, M.: Problems in metabolic adaptation: glucose, calcium and magnesium. In Care of the High-Risk Neonate, M. Klaus and A. Fanaroff (eds.). Philadelphia: W. B. Saunders, 1979.

Weatherly-White, R.: Breastfeeding the baby with a cleft lip. Keep Abreast J 3(2):125, 1978.

Weaver, J.: Excretion of radioiodine in human milk. JAMA 173:872, 1960.

Welsh, J., May, J.: Anti-infective properties of breast milk. Pediatr 94:1, 1979.

Whitley, N.: Preparation for breastfeeding: a one year followup of 34 nursing mothers. JOGN Nurs 7(3):44, 1978.

Whitten, C., Pettit, M.G., Fischhoff, J.: Evidence that growth failure from maternal deprivation is secondary to undereating. JAMA 209:1675, 1969.

Winick, M., Noble, A.: Cellular response during malnutrition at various ages. J Nutr 89:300, 1966.

Womanly Art of Breast Feeding. Franklin Park, Illinois, La Leche League.

Woodard, B., Ferguson, B., Wilson, D.: DDT levels in milk of rural indigent blacks. Am J Dis Child 130:400, 1976.

Wurster, C.F.: DDT in mother's milk. Saturday Rev May 2, 1970, p. 58.

Wyatt, D.: Phenylketonuria: the problems vary during different developmental stages. MCN 3(5):296, 1978.

Wyburn, J.R.: Human breast milk excretion of radionuclides following administration of radiopharmaceuticals. J Nucl Med 14:117, 1973.

Yu, V.: Effect of body position on gastric emptying in the neonate. Arch Dis Child 50:500, 1975.

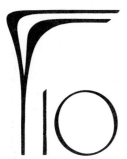# INFANTS AND FAMILIES: ATTACHMENT, FAILURE OF ATTACHMENT, AND LOSS

A newborn human is unable to survive without the care of others. Thus, to consider the newborn without considering his caregivers severely limits our understanding. In this chapter we will explore the interaction between newborns and parents and how illness of either infant or parent affects that interaction. Signs that attachment may not be developing will also be considered.

ATTACHMENT

Attachment is a bond of affection between two individuals that endures over time. Attachment is also a *process*; attachment does not happen at a specific point in time but develops gradually. The process of attachment between parent and infant is particularly unique in that it not only begins before the infant is born but, following the stages of Klaus and Kennell (1976), begins even before conception. These stages are listed in Table 10–1.

Notice that, of the nine stages, five occur before the birth of the baby. From the perspective of nursing care, this suggests, first, that assessment of attachment begins during the prenatal period and, second, that nursing intervention may foster the beginnings of attachment during the prenatal period.

A Context for Attachment

In the model of the attachment process described in Table 10–1, attachment to a newborn begins with the planning of the pregnancy. However, a vast array of past experiences in the lives of both mother and father may influence the attachment process.

The parenting received from one's own parents is important in the development of a relationship with other people including an infant. When an individual's relationships have been characterized by warmth and trust, it is more likely that future relationships will have similar characteristics. Benedek (1938, 1959) believes that one's own experience of being a child surges up when one's baby is born and influences parenting behavior.

In addition to childhood experiences, the ongoing relationship of a woman with her husband and/or other members of her family will affect attachment. Basic relationships undergo evaluation and change during the pregnancy in preparation for a new family member. Although intrafamily relationships are regarded as "fixed" in the widely used model developed by Klaus and Kennell (Fig. 10–1), family therapists or counselors might argue that certain family relationships may be altered by appropriate intervention.

Table 10–1 Steps in Attachment*

Planning the pregnancy
Confirming the pregnancy
Accepting the pregnancy
Feeling fetal movement
Accepting the fetus as an individual
Giving birth
Hearing and seeing the baby
Touching and holding the baby
Caring for the baby

*After Klaus and Kennell: Maternal-Infant Bonding: The Impact of Early Separation or Loss on Family Development. C. V. Mosby, 1976.

One characteristic of many families with dysfunction in parent-infant interaction is family isolation. The nuclear family or single mother has few family members and friends upon whom they can rely for help and/or emotional support. Kennell, Voos, and Klaus (1976) suggest the following questions as a routine part of prenatal assessments.

1. How long have you lived in this immediate area?

2. Where does most of your family live?

3. How often do you see your mother or other close relatives?

(Note who accompanies the mother to prenatal visits, if anyone, and whether she is receiving supportive help from any community agencies.)

Factors that cannot be altered include the mother's genetic endowment and her experience with previous pregnancies. At birth, which is the perspective of the Klaus model, the events of a particular pregnancy are fixed, but intervention during the prenatal phase may alter some of the events or, perhaps just as important, the mother's perception of those events. The hypothesis certainly seems testable.

The Development of Prenatal Attachment

Planning a pregnancy can be a very positive step toward attachment. Porter and

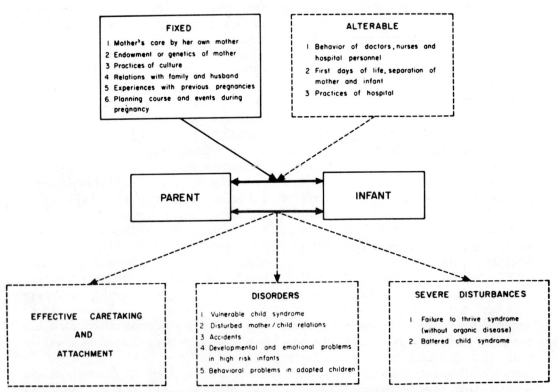

Figure 10–1. Disorders of mothering: a hypothesis of their etiology. Solid lines indicate determinants that are ingrained; dashed lines indicate factors that may be altered. (From Klaus and Kennell: Maternal-Infant Bonding: The Impact of Early Separation or Loss on Family Development. C. V. Mosby, 1979, p. 13.)

Demeuth (1979) found an association between planning pregnancy and adjustment to pregnancy in 25 white couples and stated that the deliberate decision to bear a child should make acceptance of the pregnancy predictably high. However, a pregnancy that is unplanned will not necessarily result in the failure of attachment. Conversely, neither will a planned pregnancy always result in a healthy attachment; a pregnancy may be planned to fulfill the conscious or unconscious needs of one or both parents, which may not be in the best interests of the infant (Moore 1978).

Confirmation of pregnancy makes suspicions a reality. Accepting the pregnancy fully, however, is rarely instantaneous. The idea of "being pregnant" must first be accepted. After fetal movements are felt, the fetus becomes more of an individual to the mother. In Macfarlane's (1977) study of 97 mothers, 41 per cent of the mothers indicated that they first felt love for their infants during the prenatal period.

Assessment of Prenatal Attachment

During the prenatal period both context and prenatal factors related to attachment should be assessed in a systematic way. The word *systematic* is important. Although events in medical and obstetrical history are systematically evaluated in prenatal assessment (e.g., number of pregnancies, family history of diabetes), assessment of social factors is often based on chance information and intuition.

The timing of this assessment is also important. Since many parents initially feel ambivalent about the pregnancy, particularly during the first trimester, an assessment of attitudes and behaviors must consider the stage of the pregnancy. Moreover, a certain degree of anxiety and self-questioning is normal during pregnancy and seems essential in preparing for parenthood.

Positive signs that indicate the progression of attachment include the following:

1. Gradual recognition of the fetus as a unique individual.

2. Interest in learning to care for the mother and the baby.

3. A search for baby names.

4. Attendance of classes that prepare the mother and the father for labor, delivery, and baby care.

5. Purchase of baby clothes and other supplies.

6. Decisions about infant feeding.

Individual and cultural environment and beliefs will modify behavior. The father's role in prenatal classes varies from one culture to another. Baby showers, popular in some families, are thought to be bad luck by others. Thus, assessment of behavior cannot be superficial but must be related to an understanding of the reasons for that behavior.

Other behaviors during pregnancy suggest *possible* difficulty with attachment. It cannot be overemphasized that no *single behavior* viewed in isolation can be considered a conclusive sign of difficulty with attachment. A combination of several characteristics suggests the need for further assessment and possible intervention.

When there is *undue concern with the baby's sex,* the infant may be expected to fulfill strong needs of the mother, or the mother may feel that she must please the father by giving him a child of the sex he prefers. The expectations of the parents that the child must fulfill may result in abuse and/or neglect when the infant fails to do so, as inevitably he must (if not in terms of gender then in some other way). This phenomenon, called *role reversal,* is not unusual in reports of parents who abuse or neglect their children (Morris and Gould, 1963).

Indications that the mother may be denying her pregnancy include refusal to gain weight, failure to dress appropriately, and lack of "nesting behavior" such as planning for baby clothes or equipment. Conversations with the mother may also indicate denial of pregnancy.

A mother who is depressed may have difficulty caring for an infant. Signs of depression during pregnancy include sleep disturbances other than those that may be related to the physical discomforts of pregnancy, dropping out of many former activities, and lack of affect or attempted suicide. Relating the time of onset of depressive symptoms to the time of pregnancy may indicate that pregnancy, rather than some other factor, is the cause of the depression.

If either *abortion* or *relinquishment* has been considered, it is important to know why there was a change of mind. Was the abortion not performed because the decision was delayed until a therapeutic abortion was no longer possible?

Although most mothers express anxiety about pregnancy, labor, delivery, and their ability to be good mothers, *inordinate fear* should be of concern to the nurse assessing prenatal attachment.

Fears may be a result of a lack of understanding of pregnancy, in which case education may help to dispel them. Signs of deeper fears may include overdependence on health care professionals and frequent visits to the emergency room or calls to the clinic or office with complaints for which no organic basis can be found. Such frequent visits may indicate the level of stress felt by the mother. In Elmer's (1977) study comparing mothers of 17 infants who had accidents with mothers of 17 infants who were abused (from a sample of 101 infants), five abusive mothers but only one accident mother saw the pregnancy with the index baby as stressful. Objective data from their medical records showed no difference in complications, indicating that the stress was in the mother's perception.

Prenatal Enhancement of Attachment

How do nurses help parents to develop prenatal attachment? The answer to this question is as individual as the couples nurses care for. For many couples, the nurse who finds the time to listen and assure them of her support is a major help. It is ideal when the same nurse can follow a mother through all phases of the childbearing cycle as a primary supportive person; nurse-midwives, some childbirth educators, and others are able to do this. Hopefully, in the future more nurses will develop roles in which this kind of care is possible. Close communication between nurses who care for the mother in each stage of the childbearing cycle is particularly essential when there is no single supportive professional.

Classes that allow active participation of parents in preparation for childbearing can be of value as a forum in which to share concerns with other parents as well as the childbirth educator. These classes can enhance the birth experience by preparing parents realistically for the appearance and attributes of their baby.

Labor, Delivery, and Birth

Attachment is further enhanced when labor and delivery are positive experiences in which the parents feel they received support from the professionals caring for them and they actively participated in the birth to the extent that they desired. Conversely, when labor is difficult or when the parents feel that staff is antagonistic rather than supportive, much of the mother's energy (and perhaps the father's as well) is turned from the baby toward the mother. Twenty-four per cent of the mothers interviewed in the Macfarlane study (1977) reported that they first felt love for their infants at birth.

Certain behaviors during labor and delivery may also indicate a potential for problems in parent-infant interaction. Gray and colleagues (1976) suggest that the labor-delivery record include information about how the mother *looks* (sad, happy, apathetic, disappointed, angry, exhausted, frightened, ambivalent); what the mother *says* (talks to baby, talks to baby's father, uses baby's name; and what the mother *does* (looks at baby, cuddles, touches, examines, kisses, hugs).

Behaviors that *may* indicate rejection include passive, ambivalent, or noncompliant behavior, focusing attention on self rather than the baby, refusal or reluctance to hold the baby, hostility toward the father, and verbal expressions of hostility or disparaging remarks about the baby indicating disappointment over sex or physical characteristics.

Verbal expressions need to be interpreted in relation to tone of voice, facial expression, and other behaviors. A mother can say, "You're a funny looking baby," in a way that indicates love as well as disappointment.

When the mother is herself ill following the baby's birth or when the baby must be rushed to a special care nursery, attachment is delayed and may be permanently impaired. It is difficult for a sick mother to focus much attention on her infant. The father's attention is also divided. It is also difficult to become attached to a baby you cannot touch and hold or even see and hear.

The First Hour After Birth: A Sensitive Period

Studies of both animal and human behavior suggest that the period immediately following birth is important to the development of attachment (Klopfer 1971; Barnett et al. 1970; Kennell et al. 1974). In human mother-infant pairs, differences in mother-infant interaction have been observed as late as two years after birth (Ringler et al. 1975). Early contact has been shown to be associated with longer and more successful breast-feeding in Brazil, Guatemala, and Sweden and with improved weight gain in Brazil and Guatemala (McCall 1979).

Moreover, close observation during the minutes following birth of the unique characteristics of mothers and infants who have not received medication that makes them drowsy suggests that both infants, who frequently are in a prolonged state of quiet alert, and mothers, who are also highly alert, are "primed" for interaction. Studies by Greenberg and Morris (1974) indicate that early contact also enhances the attachment of fathers.

On the basis of a body of research, hospitals throughout the country have been reviewing and changing the way in which they care for parents and infants so that parents and newborns may have as much opportunity as possible to be together during the first hour following birth. With increasing frequency, mothers and fathers are seeing, touching, and holding their newborns. If the mother plans to breast-feed, feeding begins almost immediately, a practice that also contributes to the contraction of the uterus caused by the release of oxytocin.

Examples of ways in which early maternal-infant and paternal-infant contact may be facilitated include the following:

1. Minimal use of analgesia/anesthesia so that mothers and babies will be awake and alert in the immediate postpartum period.

2. Skin-to-skin contact between mother and baby (see Thermoregulation, Chapter 5).

3. Participation of father during antenatal, intrapartal, and postpartal periods.

4. The use of birthing rooms so that parents and infants can remain in the same room during labor, delivery, and postpartum periods.

5. Delay in the administration of silver nitrate to facilitate eye contact (Chapter 5).

In some areas of the country alternative birthing sites, such as the Maternity Center Association in New York, provide family-centered care. Some couples, unable to find the family-centered atmosphere they seek within institutional walls, opt for home delivery.

WHEN IMMEDIATE CONTACT IS NOT POSSIBLE

So much emphasis has been placed on the potential long-range significance of early contact, not only in the professional literature but to some extent in books and articles read by at least a segment of the general public, that it is important to address the question, What if, for any number of reasons, immediate contact between parent and infant is not possible? Either the infant or the mother may be too ill and may require immediate care. The mother may be drowsy from medication or even asleep if general anesthesia has been used for cesarean delivery.

Although in animals these circumstances might lead to absolute failure of attachment, humans appear to be far more flexible. (If this were not true, how could one expect adoptive parents to ever develop attachment?) When the mother and/or infant is ill during the immediate postpartum period, nursing intervention, described in detail below, can certainly enhance attachment and in some instances may be necessary to achieve that attachment.

The First Days of Life

Under normal circumstances parents will have completed all the steps of attachment described in Table 10–1 by one hour after birth. Some caretaking behavior, such as breast-feeding, may also have occurred. During the next few days attachment grows as the parents see, hear, touch, hold, and care for their baby and he responds to their activities.

In Macfarlane's study, 27 per cent of the 97 mothers said they first felt love for their babies during the first week of life, whereas 8 per cent indicated that they did not have feelings of love for their baby until after the first week. Moreover, more mothers reported an increase of affection during the first two weeks of life than at birth. Robson and Moss (1970) also found that many mothers felt that their babies were strange and unfamiliar during the first weeks of life and that their affection grew as they came to know their babies.

Time spent together during these first days gives parents and infants an opportunity to become acquainted. The practice of rooming-in, in which the infant spends much of the day in his mother's room with the father present for as much time as possible, facilitates that acquaintance.

Not every mother chooses to have rooming-in when it is available. Sometimes nursing staff (and nursing policies) offer rooming-in as an "all or none" option, i.e., once the mother chooses to have her baby with her she assumes total responsibility for his care. Because she feels unable to cope with total care, she rejects the rooming-in opportunity. Policies that force mothers to make such a choice are just as much a barrier to attachment as traditional policies that keep babies in nurseries except for feeding periods.

Nurses can support parents by helping them become acquainted with the individual characteristics of their babies and by supporting their caregiving. The opportunity to bathe the baby with the nurse's support and encouragement will be far more valuable than a baby bath demonstration in which a nurse bathes a baby before a group of parents. The opportunity for parents to share their concerns about infant care and to know where to turn for support, not only while in the hospital but, even more importantly, after they return home can free their energy for caregiving and thereby enhance attachment.

Variables in Attachment During the Postpartum Period

Attachment is influenced by three individuals (or groups of individuals). The characteristics of the baby can enhance or, occasionally, be a barrier to attachment. The characteristics of the parents also influence attachment. Support, particularly from nurses (because nurses have the opportunity to spend time with parents during the first days) and also from family members and other professionals can facilitate the interaction of parents and baby.

CHARACTERISTICS OF THE BABY

The "babyish" appearance of infants is believed to be a powerful stimulus to attachment (Eibl-Eibesfeldt 1970). For example, adults showed a preference for pictures of young animals and humans over pictures of adults of the same species. Most of us have seen individuals respond to puppies or kittens in a way that is different from their response to adult dogs and cats. When the characteristic of baby-ishness is not so evident, as in the preterm infant or the infant with anomalies, attachment may take longer.

In addition to the appearance of the baby, the behavior of the baby serves as an attachment stimulus. The baby who is alert and cuddly, with whom it is possible to establish eye contact, becomes a real person to his parents more rapidly than the unresponsive infant.

Specific strategies in relation to the facilitation of parent-infant interaction and the unique characteristics of individual babies have been discussed in Chapter 6.

CHARACTERISTICS OF THE MOTHER

The mother's perception of her baby and her feelings about her ability to care for her baby, as well as her previous level of attachment, are important.

Broussard (1978, 1979) has been using her Neonatal Perception Inventory (NPI) for 16 years to measure a mother's perception of her baby as compared with her perception of the average baby on six aspects of infant behavior: crying, spitting, feeding, elimination, sleeping, and predictability (Fig. 10–2). The instructions for completing the NPI follow.

1. The mother is told: "We are interested in learning more about the experiences of mothers and their babies during the first few weeks after delivery. The more we can learn about mothers and their babies, the better we will be able to help other mothers with their babies. We would appreciate it if you would help other mothers by filling out these two forms now (first or second postpartum day) and again when your baby is one month old."
2. The mother is given the "average baby" form. The examiner remains with the mother while she is filling out the form.
3. When the mother has completed the "average baby" form, the examiner takes it from her and gives her the "your baby" form.
4. Each behavioral item is scored on a 5-point scale ranging from "a great deal" (5 points) to "none" (1 point). (This scor-

ing is used on both occasions of completing the forms.)
5. NPI scores are obtained by adding the numerical scores for each item and subtracting the total score of the "your baby" inventory from the total score of the "average baby" inventory. The difference between the two scores represents the NPI score. A positive score indicates a favorable perception of the infant; he has been rated as better than the average baby and is at low risk for subsequent developmental problems. A negative score indicates a less favorable perception; this infant is at risk for subsequent developmental problems (paraphrased from Broussard 1978, 1979).

Most mothers perceive their babies as better than the average baby; in our high risk nurseries we have found that even mothers of infants who have spent a number of weeks in intensive care perceive their infants as better than average on the NPI.

The mother's feelings about herself and her ability and the ability of the father to care for the infant may indicate future difficulties in parent-infant relationships. Cues to these feelings include: (1) frequency of mother's and father's interaction with baby; (2) progression in skills such as diapering and feeding; (3) mother's or father's views of the baby as too demanding, too interruptive, too messy; (4) tendency to ignore baby; (5) maternal or paternal difficulty in handling baby's crying; and (6) ways in which the parents refer to the baby.

The ability to console their baby, already discussed in Chapter 6, seems particularly important. When parents feel helpless and unable to comfort their baby a potential for long-term problems exists.

Using the baby's name and appropriate sex in referring to the baby indicates progress toward attachment; continuing to refer to the baby as "it" over a period of days should be of concern. Other signs of attachment difficulty may include: (1) failure to establish and maintain eye contact; (2) continued disappointment over the sex of the infant; and (3) lack of support for mother from father, other kin, or someone other than family; mother's perception of

AVERAGE BABY

Although this is your first baby, you probably have some ideas of what most little babies are like. Please check the blank you think best describes the AVERAGE baby.

How much crying do you think the average baby does?

| _____ | _____ | _____ | _____ | _____ |
| a great deal | a good bit | moderate amount | very little | none |

How much trouble do you think the average baby has in feeding?

| _____ | _____ | _____ | _____ | _____ |
| a great deal | a good bit | moderate amount | very little | none |

How much spitting up or vomiting do you think the average baby does?

| _____ | _____ | _____ | _____ | _____ |
| a great deal | a good bit | moderate amount | very little | none |

How much difficulty do you think the average baby has in sleeping?

| _____ | _____ | _____ | _____ | _____ |
| a great deal | a good bit | moderate amount | very little | none |

How much difficulty does the average baby have with bowel movements?

| _____ | _____ | _____ | _____ | _____ |
| a great deal | a good bit | moderate amount | very little | none |

How much trouble do you think the average baby has in settling down to a predictable pattern of eating and sleeping?

| _____ | _____ | _____ | _____ | _____ |
| a great deal | a good bit | moderate amount | very little | none |

YOUR BABY

While it is not possible to know for certain what your baby will be like, you probably have some ideas of what your baby will be like. Please check the blank that you think best describes what your baby will be like.

How much crying do you think your baby will do?

| _____ | _____ | _____ | _____ | _____ |
| a great deal | a good bit | moderate amount | very little | none |

How much trouble do you think your baby will have feeding?

| _____ | _____ | _____ | _____ | _____ |
| a great deal | a good bit | moderate amount | very little | none |

How much spitting up or vomiting do you think your baby will do?

| _____ | _____ | _____ | _____ | _____ |
| a great deal | a good bit | moderate amount | very little | none |

How much difficulty do you think your baby will have sleeping?

| _____ | _____ | _____ | _____ | _____ |
| a great deal | a good bit | moderate amount | very little | none |

How much difficulty do you expect your baby to have with bowel movements?

| _____ | _____ | _____ | _____ | _____ |
| a great deal | a good bit | moderate amount | very little | none |

How much trouble do you think that your baby will have settling down to a predictable pattern of eating and sleeping?

A

| _____ | _____ | _____ | _____ | _____ |
| a great deal | a good bit | moderate amount | very little | none |

Figure 10–2A

Figure 10–2.   Neonatal perception inventories. *A*, form given on the first or second postpartum day. *B*, form given when the baby is one month old. (From Broussard: Diss Abstr 26:484, 1964–1965. Copyright 1964— Retained Elsie R. Broussard, M.D.)

AVERAGE BABY

Although this is your first baby, you probably have some ideas of what most little babies are like. Please check the blank you think best describes the AVERAGE baby.

How much crying do you think the average baby does?

_____   _____   _____   _____   _____
a great deal   a good bit   moderate amount   very little   none

How much trouble do you think the average baby has in feeding?

_____   _____   _____   _____   _____
a great deal   a good bit   moderate amount   very little   none

How much spitting up or vomiting do you think the average baby does?

_____   _____   _____   _____   _____
a great deal   a good bit   moderate amount   very little   none

How much difficulty do you think the average baby has in sleeping?

_____   _____   _____   _____   _____
a great deal   a good bit   moderate amount   very little   none

How much difficulty does the average baby have with bowel movements?

_____   _____   _____   _____   _____
a great deal   a good bit   moderate amount   very little   none

How much trouble do you think the average baby has in settling down to a predictable pattern of eating and sleeping?

_____   _____   _____   _____   _____
a great deal   a good bit   moderate amount   very little   none

YOUR BABY

You have had a chance to live with your baby for about a month now. Please check the blank you think best describes your baby.

How much crying has your baby done?

_____   _____   _____   _____   _____
a great deal   a good bit   moderate amount   very little   none

How much trouble has your baby had feeding?

_____   _____   _____   _____   _____
a great deal   a good bit   moderate amount   very little   none

How much spitting up or vomiting has your baby done?

_____   _____   _____   _____   _____
a great deal   a good bit   moderate amount   very little   none

How much difficulty has your baby had in sleeping?

_____   _____   _____   _____   _____
a great deal   a good bit   moderate amount   very little   none

How much difficulty has your baby had with bowel movements?

_____   _____   _____   _____   _____
a great deal   a good bit   moderate amount   very little   none

How much trouble has your baby had in settling down to a predictable pattern of eating and sleeping?

B   _____   _____   _____   _____   _____
    a great deal   a good bit   moderate amount   very little   none

Figure 10–2B

support systems as "unhelpful" or "not much help."

Following discharge, multiple phone calls or visits for very minor problems indicate a lack of confidence in mothering skills, which is considered a high risk indicator as are multiple prenatal calls.

Supporting Attachment

Support of attachment while the mother is in the hospital has been discussed both in this chapter and in Chapter 6. But hospital stays are brief, lasting from a few hours to a few days. Occasionally, signs of difficulty in attachment have been sufficient indication for prolonging hospitalization, just as a biological problem such as sepsis is, but this is usually an exception. Mothers and/or fathers may leave the hospital without a firm bond of attachment for their baby. For most of these mothers/fathers, just being in familiar surroundings, caring for their baby without interference, allows attachment to grow. Sometimes this is not enough.

Every nursery should have some *systematic* follow-up of mothers, especially mothers at risk of attachment. The health department or visiting nurses may be utilized or follow-up may be initiated by the hospital nursing staff. Occasionally other professionals, such as social workers, will need to be involved.

SIBLINGS AND THE NEW BABY

The words *sibling* and *rivalry* commonly go together in our society. It is hard for an older child, particularly a child who is not very much older, to hold on to the "specialness" he feels when a new baby, with needs of his own, becomes a part of the family. Jealousy can begin even before the birth of the baby. "If I were only good enough, Mommy wouldn't have to go to the hospital to have a new baby," the child often feels but rarely articulates. Sometimes these feelings can be addressed by playing a game in which roles are reversed. "You be the mommy and I'll

be the baby" may provide the child with an opportunity to express his feelings about the coming birth.

Nurses can suggest to parents a number of other ways to prepare a child for a new member of the family. Obviously, the age of the child (or children) is important. Children under the age of six, and particularly children three and under, seem most vulnerable to the birth of a new baby because their own world is centered around their parents.

Children should be told about the new baby early in the pregnancy, by four months at the latest. This gives them time to become accustomed to the idea. A mother in my postpartum unit asked, "How can I 'sneak' this new baby into the house?" She had never told her son, then 16 months old, about the baby. During prenatal visits, nurses need to ask parents about "telling."

All too frequently, when the idea of a new baby is introduced, it is suggested that the baby will be a "playmate" or "someone you can help take care of." Realistically, a new baby is not much of a playmate. And there are certainly limits to the extent to which the older child (toddler or preschool child) will be able to participate in the baby's care.

Somewhat more realistic is the comparison of the new baby with the baby experience of the older child. Pictures are very helpful. "This is what you looked like when you were in the hospital (or when you first came home)." Tell the child how he was fed and held and cared for as a baby, emphasizing that he is still cared for, but in his special, more "grown-up" way. Books are available to help young children better understand pregnancy and birth (e.g., Gruenberg 1970; Sheffield 1974).

During the hospitalization, the separation from the mother is most traumatic for young children. The strongest reason for sibling visiting is not to let the child see his new brother or sister but to allow him to be with his mother. For years the problems associated with separation of young children from parents when the child is hospitalized have been recognized; we need to recognize that hospitalization of a parent can be devastating as well.

Because young children have no accurate sense of time, telling them that their mother will be away in the hospital for four days means little. Christensen (1980) suggests wrapping four dinners for the freezer (or four small packages) in advance. The child opens one package each day; when all are gone it is time for Mom to come home.

If possible, children should stay in the familiar environment of their home while their mother is in the hospital. The hospital telephone number can be posted in big numbers on the refrigerator door. Prior to hospitalization, the mother should talk on the phone to the children. Voices sound different on the phone; the mother's voice may not be recognized if the child has never heard it on the telephone before.

Sibling visiting in hospitals is becoming increasingly common. In some units siblings may visit at the mother's bedside; in others, visiting may occur only in a waiting room. One concern has been the potential effect of young children on the incidence of bacterial colonization in the newborn. Umphenour (1980) reports on a study in which nasal and umbilical cord swab specimens obtained in each newborn (N = 214) at birth and at discharge prior to the institution of sibling visiting were compared with specimens after the sibling visiting policy was changed. In addition, infant records were examined for evidence of infection at two to three weeks of age. In this institution (Dwight David Eisenhower Army Medical Center, Fort Gordon, Georgia), siblings visit at the mother's bedside with the baby present for two hours every evening and are allowed unrestricted contact with the mother and new baby after hand washing with an iodine scrub preparation. No significant difference was found in bacterial colonization, infection, or illness. Only three instances of illness were discovered in the audit of 89 charts on follow-up exam: two cases of monilial diaper rash and one case of conjunctivitis that cultured *Staphylococcus epidermidis*.

Parents need to know that not everything will go smoothly with siblings in the first weeks at home with a new baby. Parents often feel torn between the needs of older children and those of the baby. Siblings often regress in behavior, especially if a behavior is recently learned (e.g., toilet training). The older brother or sister may wonder why everyone is mad at him for "messing in my pants" when no one is mad at the baby for doing the same thing.

Even young children can hold out a finger for the baby to grasp or can hold up a shiny foil pie pan for the baby to look at; thus they may feel they are helping with infant care (consider the importance of touch in parent attachment to infants).

Siblings need reassurance that parents are in control and that their angry feelings will destroy neither parents nor baby. Parents can say, "I see you don't like babies very much today," and thereby give children an opportunity to verbalize or play out their feelings.

Siblings need to feel "special," just as the baby is special. Pointing out that they have their special foods (babies don't get hamburgers) and activities (babies don't have wagons or whatever is the child's favorite toy) shows that each age has its rewards. Some time away from home for parents and older siblings while someone baby-sits with the new baby is important. (Time for the mother and father alone is important, too.)

CRISIS AT BIRTH

A crisis may be defined as a situation that cannot be easily handled by an individual's or a family's usual problem-solving mechanisms. A reaction to a crisis may be, "I've never faced anything like this before. I just don't know what to do." It is possible for the birth of a healthy infant to a healthy mother to be thought of as a crisis under certain circumstances, but the focus of this discussion is the sick newborn and/or mother.

Crisis intervention theory, developed from the work of Lindemann (1944), Erikson (1950), and Caplan (1964), involves prevention as well as treatment. If nurses are to help parents in an optimum way, they must consider both aspects.

Preventive Crisis Intervention

Preventive crisis intervention consists of providing support for the family prior to the development of the crisis. Caplan (1951) suggests that the kinds of interactions that occur between the individual and key figures in the environment are more important to the outcome of the crisis than the emotional make-up of the individual. This principle implies that the ongoing relationship with staff as well as family and friends is significant. That staff may be in a clinic, the physician's office, the labor or delivery room, or a newborn or special care nursery, or it may be the public health nurse visiting the home. If the parents perceive the staff to be interested and caring before a crisis occurs, the support of that staff is enhanced.

When high risk mothers (e.g., mothers with severe hypertension or diabetes) are hospitalized prior to delivery, meeting nurses and physicians who care for high risk infants and visiting the nursery can be supportive (Slade, Reidl, and Mangurten 1977).

A second aspect of prevention involves the full participation of parents in each phase of the childbearing process. Parent involvement in childbearing classes and in labor and delivery may seem remote from parent involvement in an intensive care nursery, but it is a prelude. Hospital and nursing care policies must be developed to foster involvement rather than serve as a barrier.

Occasionally, a father may be asked to leave the delivery room when a complication is suspected. We have to consider whether such a practice offers psychological protection to the delivery room personnel rather than the father. If there is a serious problem to be faced, it would seem that the support that the mother and father would offer each other would be of real value. There are probably individual

exceptions to this concept, but they should be exceptions and not the rule.

Secondary preventive intervention is more appropriate to the special or intensive care nursery. Once an infant becomes ill following birth or is in need of special care because of gestational age or size, the involvement of parents in their baby's care is the next step in helping parents achieve a healthy resolution of the crisis. A number of specific policies are important.

Secondary Preventive Intervention

INITIAL COMMUNICATION

How should the parents be told that their infant has a problem? What should they be told? These questions have concerned health care professionals for many years, but changes in other aspects of maternity care have caused them to rethink the way they answer these questions.

A couple of decades ago, when many mothers were asleep during delivery and for some time afterward and when fathers were kept in distant waiting rooms, "telling" parents, especially mothers, was often postponed. Today in a growing number of hospitals, the mother is watching the delivery with her husband beside her. Such postponement obviously is not possible under these circumstances.

A second traditional practice that is fortunately on the decline (but hardly eradicated) is the explaining of the baby's condition to the father or some other member of the family but withholding part or all of the truth from the mother. The assumption here is that the father is better able to cope with reality and to make decisions than the mother who has recently delivered. Aside from the fact that this assumption is, at best, questionable and places a tremendous burden on the new father, the delay not only does not fool the mother but adds to her anxiety. Her energy is drained in wondering what is wrong . . . why she hasn't seen her baby . . . why the nurses and perhaps her husband are avoiding her . . . why no one answers her questions. Moreover, if nurses are less than honest with either parent in the hours after a problem is first recognized, the parents may easily doubt what nurses tell them later, wondering if they are still "putting them off."

What is said to the parents initially will depend, of course, on the baby's condition. In every instance it is important to be honest. However, even when the baby is quite ill, honesty can often be combined with a note of optimism such as "Many babies as sick as your baby do get well." Some optimism is helpful in encouraging parents to develop an attachment to their baby.

At this time parents need to know about some of the tests and procedures that may be carried out; hospital staff must get their written permission for these procedures. Talking with both parents together, as soon as the baby's problem is recognized, is nearly always the most helpful course. In this way, the same information is given to both parents. The physician or midwife who delivered the baby should be present; he or she may be the only member of the team who knows the parents and is known to them prior to delivery. A nurse who will be caring for the mother in the first days after delivery should also be present, not only for support but so that she, also, will know what the parents have been told. Nursing notes should include the basic information given to the family so that everyone who subsequently cares for the family will be better able to support them.

After the parents have been told about their baby's condition, nurses need to be available to them. They can stay nearby, holding a mother's hand if it seems to be the right thing to do (particularly if the father is not there). Most nurses feel at a loss for words, but words are not really necessary. "Hit and run," in which the parents are "hit" with distressing information about their baby by the doctor or nurses who then "run" away, leaving them to deal with the information in solitude, should be unthinkable.

The initial shock of their baby's condition will block out much of what is told to the parents at this time. Some written information about the nursery in which their baby will receive care should be given to them; they will turn to it in the hours and days that follow and it will help remind them of what has been said in these first minutes. Most important, this early time of communication should give parents the feeling that nurses are concerned about them and their baby and that they will be available to answer their questions or just listen whenever they wish. Nurses want the parents to know that they will be honest and open in trying to answer their questions.

If the baby is to be transferred to another hospital (e.g., from a community hospital to a medical center with an intensive care nursery), the reasons should be explained to the parents in a way they can understand. Parents should *see and touch* their baby before the transfer. This is particularly true of the mother who, because of her own hospitalization, may not be able to see her baby for several days (critically important days in terms of maternal attachment).

This initial period of communication is not a time to bring up every complication that may occur. For example, the preterm baby may develop hyperbilirubinemia in two to three days, but this can be dealt with later. To mention too much initially may raise a barrier to attachment.

PARENTAL REACTION: THE GRIEF PROCESS

Although every parent will have individual emotions when a child is born who in some way appears less than perfect to them, there seems to be some pattern of reactions. These emotions, which are those of the grief process associated with death and dying, occur even when the defect is one which to nurses may appear relatively minor and repairable (e.g., a cleft lip), as well as when the problem is major, life-threatening, or terminal. Not only is the grief process common, it seems essential that the parents grieve for the lost baby of their imagination before they can accept their baby as he really is.

The stages of grief do not necessarily occur in the order described here. The extent of each stage will also vary with the individual.

Shock and disbelief are frequent first reactions. "Why me? . . . Why us?" they ask. *Denial* is one way of coping with the shock. "I don't believe it . . . I can't believe it . . . I won't believe it." In the process of denial, external reality is rejected and replaced by wish-fulfilling fantasy. Sometimes denial leads to behavior by parents that nurses view as inappropriate. Their baby is critically ill, yet the parents seem unconcerned; they may even be laughing. Only gradually does the full impact of their baby's problem become real to them.

A second group of feelings — normal to this situation — are those of *shame, embarrassment, loss of self-esteem,* and *personal inadequacy.* "What caused this?" they ask, which may often be translated, "What is wrong with us that we couldn't have a normal child?"

Guilt about the origin of an anomaly or the prematurity is another frequent response to abnormality. Is the baby's problem the result of something they did or perhaps something they didn't do? Our long-standing beliefs about sin and punishment, a part of our heritage for many centuries, leave the nagging fear that this is a punishment for some deed or thought. Perhaps the pregnancy was originally undesired — many are, even when the baby is later accepted. Maybe an abortion was contemplated or even attempted; the feelings of guilt here can be almost overwhelming. Unresolved guilt feelings may lead to depression.

Parents are *anxious* for many reasons. What will become of this child? How will we care for him — physically, emotionally, financially? Can we love him as we love our other children? Will this child hurt our other children? A particularly big question is, Will future children have a similar defect?

Anger, also common, is probably the hardest of all the grief-related emotions

for nurses to deal with, because so often they are the target of that anger, and it seems so unjustified. Nurses may wonder, What did *we* do to deserve this? It isn't *our* fault that the baby is ill or malformed. Of course it isn't. But anger is a part of the grief process. Anger may also be directed at the marital partner or even at the baby.

Why are the parents angry? They are angry that this should have happened to them. Even though they know it is irrational, they are often angry at the baby. They may be angry at each other. And they feel guilty because they are angry. The anger will come out in many ways: the bath water is too hot, the bed is too hard, or the food is terrible.

Bargaining, the making of promises and deals, is not uncommon in the grief process. The promises may be to God or to others. Promises are not necessarily verbalized, even internally; the parents may try very hard to be perfect, spending long hours in the nursery, doing everything possible for the baby, hoping, often subconsciously, that if they behave in such a manner their baby will be spared.

Acceptance is the final step in the grief process. Nurses need to realize that it will be many months, even a year or more, before that acceptance comes. Nurses who care for infants and families in the hospital may not see the parents at this point. Acceptance should be assessed, however, by the nurse providing care to the infant after discharge from the nursery. There are clues, even in the first days, that may indicate eventual outcomes. Caplan's research, summarized in Table 10–2 suggests several.

CONTINUING SUPPORT

Parents must feel welcome in the nursery at all times, 24 hours a day, whether that nursery is in a community hospital or a regional center. If they are unable to be physically present, they need to know that their phone calls are welcome at any time of the day or night. The telephone is an important means of communication for

Table 10–2 Some Parental Responses to Preterm Births*

Responses Suggesting Healthy Outcome	Responses Suggesting Unhealthy Outcome
Parents obtain as much information as possible about infant's condition Ask frequent questions Request specific information	Parents do not seek information about infant
Parents are aware of negative feelings and able to express them; are able to accept help from family and friends	Parents deny negative feelings; are unable to accept help from family and friends
Parents are appropriately anxious about infant's condition	Parents deny that infant's life is in jeopardy; converse about less threatening subjects

*After Caplan: Psychiatry 23:365, 1960.

parents. It gives nurses a chance to tell them how much weight their baby has gained, how he is eating, and little personal bits of information such as "He opened his eyes while I was bathing him" that not only mean a lot to most parents but contribute to their feelings of attachment. An ideal situation is to provide a telephone number that can be called long distance at no charge to the family. Many parents cannot afford long-distance calls each day; some have no access to telephones at all.

Parents can be expected to ask many, many questions about their baby and his care; the answers may not have been understood or may have been forgotten in the stress surrounding the crisis. These questions should be answered with patience and care each time.

Good communication among nurses, physicians, and other workers in the nursery is also essential to good communication with the parents. Nothing can be more confusing or distressing to parents than to hear different stories from different people. The information communicated to parents should be documented and easily accessible to everyone caring for the baby.

Equally important as knowing what parents have been told is knowing what they understand about what they have been told. Nurses should listen for clues about their understanding or lack of it. For example, when the father of a baby with serious brain damage talks about his son as a future Little Leaguer, communication has certainly been ineffective for some reason. It may be that this father is not psychologically ready to accept what he has heard. Or the information may have been unclear. An important question to ask about the family each day is, "Where are they in their understanding of their baby's condition?"

In addition to picking up on clues in conversation, nurses can ask the parents what they have been told. For example, if a mother points to an intravenous line and says, "How much longer will my baby need to have that needle in his head," a nurse might first ask her what information she has already been given. Many parents will ask a question of several nurses and physicians just to see if they will get the same answer. It is a way of looking for assurance, but it can certainly be very hard on staff if their communication is not good.

Enhancing Attachment Between Parents and their High Risk Baby

Studies indicate that approximately one-third of all infants who are battered or who "fail to thrive" in the absence of physiological disease either were preterm babies or were ill following birth. The common denominator has been separation from their parents during the early days when attachments are formed. Facilitating the attachment of high risk babies and their parents is obviously important.

Attachment is equally important if the baby is expected to die. Parents will grieve, regardless of whether or not they have formed an attachment. It is far healthier for them to grieve for a specific, tangible baby than for a vague entity they never knew. Normal grief can be resolved. Undefined grief may linger — as anger or sadness or in some other form — for a very long time.

It is not surprising that parents are reluctant to form attachments to their sick or malformed baby. Their problem is then compounded by the guilt they feel about not feeling love for their baby.

As with healthy term babies, attachment formation with high risk babies involves seeing, touching, and caregiving. Many parents who will eagerly caress a term baby may shrink from a preterm infant or a child with a defect. This is one more reason why nurses need to be with them the first time they visit and need always to be close by.

Nurses may have to encourage their touch. "Would you like to hold your baby's hand?" they can say. Sometimes if a nurse holds the baby's hand or strokes his head or leg while talking he or she can encourage parents to be less fearful. Fathers often need a great deal of encouragement to handle tiny babies, although in some families the father may be less reluctant than the mother.

When a baby is very sick, it is more difficult to involve the parents in caregiving than with the term baby. At first parents may not be able to feed, bathe, or diaper their baby, but nurses can assure them that their gentle stroking and talking to him plays a real role in his care. Nurses can also use ingenuity to involve the parents in as many ways as possible. For example, if the baby is to have a gavage feeding, a nurse might insert the tube and be sure of its position; the mother might then pour the premeasured formula into the syringe. As the baby's condition improves, the parents can assume a more active role in his care.

The centralization of high risk newborns in medical centers, although obviously offering significant advantages from the standpoint of physiological care, presents some real barriers to attachment. Parents may live 50 or 100 miles from the hospital in which their baby receives care; they may live in a different state. Many times they lack transportation to travel back and forth except on weekends. Often there are other children at home who also need care. How do nurses foster attachment on a long-distance basis? No one has the answer to this question, but attempts are being made to deal with the problem.

There should be a system to help parents with housing arrangements when they are able to visit. Few parents can afford motel bills in addition to intensive care nursery bills of $300 a day or more. Hospital social workers and chaplains are important resources in finding appropriate housing.

Telephone communication, already discussed, is of great importance. Letters and photos from the hospital can be helpful if the mother and father are unable to come for several weeks at a time.

Contact through public health nurses in the parents' home area, if for some reason it is difficult to reach the parents themselves, is another avenue of communication. Certainly the public health nurse should be contacted before the baby is discharged so that she can come to know the family and be available to them for teaching and counsel.

The concept of "back-transfer," i.e., sending the baby to a hospital nearer to his home for intermediate-level care before discharge, is growing in popularity. Not only is the baby nearer his family, which facilitates visiting and their learning to care for him, but local care is often less expensive.

Siblings of High Risk Infants

In caring for parents and their dying infant it is very easy to overlook the brothers and sisters of that infant, whom nurses may never have seen. It is very easy for parents to be so caught up in their own feelings about the baby (which are a normal part of grieving) that they are unaware of the needs of the other children, who perhaps have been sent to stay with a grandmother or friends or other relatives. Even when parents are aware of the needs of their other children, they may find it difficult to answer their questions or may feel inadequate to give them support.

Preschool-age children, with their limited understanding of cause and effect and a focus that is primarily self-centered, may feel that in some way they are responsible for the baby's death. For example, a child may have said or thought "I don't want a baby brother" and may now feel that he is thereby responsible for the baby's death.

Nursing assessment includes checking with the parents about what siblings have said or what they may have observed in sibling behavior. A nurse could say, "Brothers and sisters often have worries about their baby brother (sister). Has _____ asked about the baby?"

Intensive care nurseries frequently provide opportunities for children to briefly visit their sick sibling.

THE BABY WHO IS DYING

Although perinatal mortality is decreasing, newborns will continue to die—some in a relatively short time after birth, others after weeks and months in an intensive care nursery. Support for parents is an essential part of the nursing care of babies who are dying. To provide that support, nurses must also recognize their own needs for support.

The Grief Process: Nurses

Just as family members experience both anticipatory grief and real grief after an infant dies, nurses also experience grief and demonstrate that grief in their behavior, particularly when they have cared for the baby over a period of days or weeks and have become closely attached to the infant. Table 10–3 compares the grief process in families and nurses. There is little doubt that nurses must bear the brunt of parental anxiety when an infant is ill.

Nurses, therefore, must learn to help their peers as well as families deal with grief. Such help is the responsibility of nursing administration, but it is also the responsibility of nurses. Support needs to be immediately available on a 24-hour basis. Nurses who care for dying babies

Table 10–3   Manifestations of the Grief Process in Nurses and Families

Emotion	Nurses	Families
Shock and disbelief	Particularly acute when baby who appeared to be doing well worsens—Why this baby?	Why me? Why us? Why our baby?
Shame, loss of self-esteem	Inability to prevent death seen as threat to self-esteem	Why could we not produce a healthy child?
Guilt	Guilt about care given or not given	Guilt about preterm birth or anomaly Guilt about not wanting to attach to baby
Anxiety	Fear of helplessness Coping with anxiety by remaining detached, enforcing "rules"	Fear of attaching to baby, growing to love baby Fear of loss of baby
Denial	Denial of severity of illness to self and parents	Denial of severity of infant's illness
Anger	Anger at baby Anger at parents Anger at other team members Blaming parents and team members	Anger at baby Anger at staff Anger at other family members
Bargaining	Promises to God and others	Promises to God and others
Acceptance	Need opportunities to express feelings and ask questions Require acceptance of colleagues' expressions in nonjudgmental fashion	Need opportunities to express feelings and ask questions

may come to the point of tears of anger and frustration at the end of a shift; they need to talk about those feelings at that moment. Otherwise they may become exhausted from trying to cope with their own grief and the grief of the parents as well as the continued physical and emotional needs of the other infants in the intensive care nursery.

In addition to immediate support, regularly scheduled conferences in which nurses can share both the problems and the joys of their practice are important. Careful leadership is important in these conferences, lest they disintegrate into "gripe sessions," which can be more destructive than constructive. A discussion of group dynamics is beyond the scope of this book, but help is available within most hospital settings or from other agencies in most communities in the form of individuals who can assist nurses in developing these skills or who can share their leadership with a nursing unit.

With support, experiences with dying infants and their families can lead to emotional equanimity, which enables nurses to give compassionate care without devastating their colleagues or being devastated themselves. Without support, grief experiences may lead to an emotional detachment that prevents nurses from being responsive to the special needs of these infants and families. The nurse who says "I don't let myself get involved so I won't get hurt" not only compromises care to families but denies himself or herself the satisfaction that can come from supporting families well at a difficult period of their life.

Support for Families

Duff and Campbell (1976) suggest that two philosophies underlie the way in which nurses care for dying babies and their families: (1) a "disease-oriented" philosophy, which sees death only in a highly negative context of failure, and (2) a "person-oriented" philosophy, which recognizes that under some circumstances

death is not only inevitable but not necessarily the worst of fates.

The way nurses have traditionally treated the dying newborn and his family is not much different from the way the American culture in general, and nursing and medical subcultures in particular that preside over the dying, has dealt with death at any age. With a few exceptions (e.g., the baby with anencephaly or the baby of less than 25 weeks gestation), hospital personnel make heroic efforts to save the baby, but if they fail they then feel they did all they could, and they frequently withdraw from the baby and family, emotionally if not physically.

Some newborns die in spite of everything that is done. For others, life may be prolonged but not necessarily saved by a variety of means. The intensity and duration of care given to a particular baby must take into account not only medical factors but family feelings as well. Nurses can find great satisfaction working in a nursery where the understanding and feelings of parents are discussed on daily rounds along with laboratory values and respiratory status.

All who care for sick infants should read, with sorrow, Robert and Peggy Stinson's account of the life and death of their six-month-old son Andrew in an intensive care unit (1979). Andrew weighed 800 g at birth and was, throughout his life, sustained by technology. His parents appear to have received little support and were admittedly bitter.

By way of contrast, consider the following account (Duff and Campbell 1976).

> A premature infant was believed to have a hopeless prognosis. The parents and doctor, with agreement of the medical and nursing staff, decided to stop all heroics. The parents informed their healthy three-year-old daughter that her brother probably could not live and, on her request, she was brought to see the baby. Later, after contemplating autopsy and plans for disposition of the baby's body (both discussed at the parents' request), they were asked which they preferred — to leave, to be beside their baby's incubator, or to have the baby, with all his tubes and apparatus re-

moved, brought to them in a private room. Immediately, they chose the last. In the company of the doctor, they held their infant for 55 minutes while he died. During this time, they wept, talked to their son or about him, found humor in some incongruities, or were silent. The mother cradled the baby to her bosom most of the time while the father stroked his wife and baby. He told us that the scene of mother and dying child was one of sublime beauty despite its occurrence in the midst of tragedy. He later said he believed that the time interval spent in intimacy with their baby was about two hours, not 55 minutes. She told us, "We had to say hello to him before we could say goodbye." They came to think of this experience as a fitting funeral from which they gained greater strength for living. They helped each other. They also helped their daughter over the ensuing weeks as she overcame her abnormal fears of dying and openly dealt with her guilt for feeling that her bad wishes had killed her brother.

Reference Books for Parents

When parents have difficulty talking about death with their children, they may find one of the books listed below helpful (see also Mills 1979, and Sheer, 1977). Carefully chosen, books may help parents and children describe their feelings more easily and appreciate that feelings of sadness and grief are a normal reaction to the death of someone who is loved. A nursery library might have some books available for parents and children to share. Even though parents may not be able to talk with their other children in the period immediately surrounding the infant's death, knowing that resources are available may help in the months that follow. With one exception, none of these books describes the death of an infant, but each may help parents begin a discussion of death with their other children.

Preschool-Age Children

Someone Small, by Barbara Borack. New York: Harper & Row, 1969.

The Dead Bird, by Margaret Wise Brown. Reading, Mass.: Addison-Wesley, 1958.

My Grandpa Died Today, by Joan Fassler. New York: Human Sciences Press, 1971.

Why Did He Die, by Audrey Harris. Minneapolis: Lerner Publications, 1965.

When Violet Died, by Mildred Kantrowitz. New York: Parents' Magazine Press, 1973.

School-Age Children (ages 6–9)

Nana Upstairs, Nana Downstairs, by Thomas De Paola. New York: G. P. Putnam's Sons, 1973.

Confessions of an Only Child, by Norman Klein. New York: Pantheon, 1974. (This books describes the feelings of a nine-year-old when the new baby dies.)

Death is Natural, by Lawrence Pringle. New York: Scholastic Book Service, 1977.

Preadolescent Children (ages 10–12)

Life and Death, by H. Zim and Sonia Bleeker. New York: William Morrow, 1970.

Parents

About Dying: An Open Book for Parents and Children, by Sara Stein. New York: Walker & Company, 1974.

Helping Your Child to Understand Death, by Anna Wolf. New York: Child Study Association of America, 1973.

Bibliography

Barnett, C., Leiderman, P., Grobstein, R. et al.: Neonatal separation: the maternal side of interactional deprivation. Pediatrics 45:197, 1970.

Benedek, T.: Adaptation to reality in early infancy. Psychoanal Q 7:200–215, 1938.

Benedek, T.: Parenthood as a developmental phase: a contribution to the libido theory. J Am Psychoanal Assoc 7:389–417, 1959.

Breslin, R.: Family crisis care. Clin Perinatol 3(2):447, 1976.

Broussard, E.: A study to determine the effectiveness of television as a means of providing anticipatory counseling to primiparae during the postpartum period. Diss Abstr 26:484, 1964–1965.

Broussard, E.: Psychosocial disorders in children: early assessment of infants at risk. Cont Ed February, 44–57, 1978.

Broussard, E.: Assessment of the adaptive potential of the mother-infant system: the neonatal perception inventories. Semin Perinatol 3:91–100, 1979.

Cagan, J., Meier, P.: A discharge planning tool for use with families of high-risk infants. JOGN Nurs 8:146, 1979.

Caplan, G.: A public health approach to child psychiatry. Ment Health 35:235, 1951.

Caplan, G.: Patterns of response to the crisis of premature birth. Psychiatry 23:365, 1960.

Caplan, G.: Principle of Preventive Psychiatry. New York: Basic Books, 1964.

Christensen, V.: Sibling adjustment to the newborn. Paper presented at a conference, Childbirth: A Family Experience. Charlotte ASPO, Charlotte, North Carolina, February 23, 1980.

Clark, A.: Recognizing discord between mother and child and changing it to harmony. MCN 1:100–105, 1976.

Clark, A., Affonso, D.: Infant behavior and maternal attachment: two sides to the coin. MCN 1:95–99, 1976.

Duff, R., Campbell, A.: On deciding the care of severely handicapped or dying persons: with particular reference to infants. Pediatrics 57:487, 1976.

Eibl-Eibesfeldt: Ethology, the Biology of Behavior. New York: Holt, Rinehart & Winston, 1970.

Elmer, E.: Fragile Families, Troubled Children. Pittsburgh: University of Pittsburgh Press, 1977.

Erikson, E.: Childhood and Society. New York: Norton, 1950.

Gray, J., Cutler, C., Dean, J., Kempe, C.: Perinatal assessment of mother-baby interaction. In Child Abuse and Neglect, R. Helfer and C. Kempe (eds.). Cambridge, Mass.: Ballinger, 1976.

Greenberg, M., Morris, N.: Engrossment: the newborn's impact upon the father. Orthopsychiatry 44:520, 1974.

Gruenberg, S.: The Wonderful Story of How You Were Born. New York: Doubleday, 1970.

Hardgrove, C., Warrick, L.: How shall we tell the children? Am J Nurs 74:448, 1974.

Kennell, J., Jerauld, R., Wolfe, H., Chesler, D., Kreger, N., McAlpine, W., Steffa, M., Klaus, M.: Maternal behavior one year after early and extended post-partum contact. Dev Med Child Neurol 16:172–179, 1974.

Kennell, J., Sluter, H., Klaus, M.: The mourning response of parents to the death of a newborn. N Engl J Med 283:344, 1970.

Kennell, J., Voos, D., Klaus, M.: Parent-infant bonding. In Child Abuse and Neglect, R. Helfer and C. Kempe (eds.). Cambridge, Mass.: Ballinger, 1976.

Klaus, M., Kennell, J.: Maternal-Infant Bonding: The Impact of Early Separation or Loss on Family Development. St. Louis: C. V. Mosby, 1976.

Klaus, M., Kennell, J.: Parent to infant attachment. In Mother/Child; Father/Child Relationships, J. Stevens and M. Mathews (eds.). Washington, D. C.: National Association for the Education of Young Children, 1978.

Klaus, M., Kennell, J., Plumb, N. et al.: Human maternal behavior at the first contact with her young. Pediatrics 46:187, 1970.

Klopfer, P.: Mother love: what turns it on. Am Sci 49:404, 1971.

Lindeman, E.: Symptomatology and management of acute grief. Am J Psychiatry 101:141, 1944.

Macfarlane, A.: The Psychology of Childbirth. Cambridge, Mass.: Harvard University Press, 1977.

McCall, R.: Infants. Cambridge, Mass.: Harvard University Press, 1979.

Miller, C.: Working with parents of high-risk infants. Am J Nurs 78:1228, 1978.

Mills, G.: Books to help children understand death. Am J Nurs 79:291, 1979.

Moore, M.: Realities in Childbearing. Philadelphia: W. B. Saunders, 1978.

Morris, M., Gould, R.: Role reversal: a concept in dealing with the neglected/battered child syndrome. In The Neglected-Battered Child Syndrome. New York: Child Welfare League of America, 1963.

Mullaly, L., Kervin, M.: Changing the status quo. MCN 3:75, 1978.

Opirhory, G.: Counseling the parents of a critically ill newborn. JOGN Nurs 8:179, 1979.

Porter, L., Demeuth, B.: The impact of marital adjustment on pregnancy acceptance. Maternal-Child Nurs J 8(2):103, 1979.

Ringler, N.M., Kennell, J.H., Jarvella, R., Navojosky, B.J., Klaus, M.: Mother-to-child speech at 2 years — effects of early postnatal contact. J Pediatr 86:141–144, 1975.

Robson, K.S., Moss, H.A.: Patterns and determinants of maternal attachment. J Pediatr 77:976–985, 1970.

Sheer, B.: Help for parents in a difficult job — broaching the subject of death. MCN 2(5):320, 1977.

Sheffield, M.: Where do Babies Come From? A Book for Children and Their Parents. New York: Knopf, 1974.

Slade, C., Reidl, C., Mangurten, H.: Working with parents of high-risk newborns. JOGN Nurs 6:21, 1977.

Stinson, R., Stinson, P.: On the death of a baby. Atl Monthly July, 244:64, 1979.

Umphenour, J.: Bacterial colonization in neonates with sibling visitation. JOGN Nurs 9(2):73, 1980.

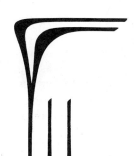

CULTURE, FAMILY, AND THE NEWBORN

Culture, the sum of a society's beliefs, customs, knowledge, and capabilities, is a significant factor in the health and well-being of every infant. Culture affects him even before his conception, as it determines the childhood experiences of his parents — their exposure to illness, the organization of their families, the amount and kind of education they have, the kind of food the mother eats as she grows up, whether she will come to pregnancy strong and healthy or ill and malnourished. Culture determines parents' beliefs about pregnancy, whether they will seek medical care or the counsel of relatives or a midwife, or whether the mother will consider herself sick or well during pregnancy. To a degree, culture will determine the age at which she first becomes pregnant, the number of children she will have, whether or not she will breast-feed her infant, how often she will hold him, and so forth.

Of course, within any society, all parents will not act identically, regardless of similar cultural backgrounds. Individual differences, determined by both heredity and environment, are always important factors in behavior. Yet culture does exert its influence; the middle-class American mother would not be likely to pin a charm on her baby's dress to protect him from the "evil eye," nor would she use a cradle board, rather than a carriage, to transport him.

The United States is a nation of many subsocieties, each with its own distinct cultural heritage. When the beliefs of these groups come in conflict with those of nurses and doctors, misunderstandings can and do arise, creating barriers, which in the long run can hurt the infant. For example, many Spanish-American parents believe in *el mal ojo*, the evil eye, which leads them to care for their babies in certain ways. Because nurses do not share their belief, they may ridicule this behavior. But consider how odd the Spanish-speaking mother would consider the previously popular American notion that babies must be "fed by the clock." She must surely think that any woman who watches the clock as her baby cries vigorously and sucks his fist is cruel and unloving. Or consider the practice of most American hospitals of separating mother and infant immediately after birth. To most of the world's women this must seem peculiar.

It is important, then, for nurses to know something of those traditional ideas of infant care that differ from their own. But it is also important that they realize the extent to which their beliefs — some of which stem from middle-class culture and some of which are taught to nursing students and passed on to patients as "scientific" principle — may themselves be products of a particular heritage.

What is the source of our own ideas about infant and child care? Wolfenstein (1953) studied the effects of changing attitudes toward child care in our society and the concomitant changes in child care practices. Using the United States government publication *Infant Care,* which was first issued in 1914 and has since undergone a number of revisions, she traced changes in the advice given about weaning, masturbation, thumb sucking, and toilet training.

Considering how rapidly our society has changed technologically in the 40-year period covered by Wolfenstein's study, it is not surprising that ideas have changed in the same period. Wolfenstein points out, however, that many of the changes in child care practices are not related so much to new knowledge as to the widespread belief in our society that new ideas are always better than old ones — the latest suggestion becomes *the* way to care for the new infant.

Breast-feeding, for example, was recommended from 1914 through 1945, with warnings about the dangers of early weaning beginning in 1921. In 1914 stress was placed on gradual weaning — it might begin as early as five months and might not be completed until the baby is a year old. By 1921 early weaning was in growing disrepute. Ideally, weaning was to be postponed until the baby was nine months old, but once begun it "need not take more than two weeks." Both in 1921 and 1929 there was emphasis on being very strict with the baby; "the child will finally yield" was the statement made in 1921, and "soon the baby will give in" was the phrasing used in 1929. Similar attitudes were expressed in 1938.

Not every pediatrician in this era was so severe in his advice. Bartlett (1932) suggests that there is no set time for weaning and that gradual weaning is more pleasant for the mother and safer for the baby unless serious illness in the mother makes rapid weaning necessary.

By the 1940s *Infant Care* was back to stressing the idea of gradual weaning; at the same time the age at which bottle-feeding was to be given up for good became a matter of "little difference." But by 1951, when gradual weaning was still advocated, there was apprehension lest weaning to the cup be delayed too long.

Wolfenstein found similar vacillation in the other areas she examined. The change in ideas is not so important as the fact that at any given time the dominant ideas expressed in the culture are accepted and professed by so many as *the* correct way to care for an infant, other methods being considered "old-fashioned" and "unscientific," if not completely damaging.

Perhaps the realization that nurses are influenced by their own cultural biases can make them more tolerant and understanding of some of the biases encountered in those families whose newborn infants they attend.

What is the reaction to beliefs that we see as based on "superstition" and folklore rather than on "fact"? Sometimes these beliefs are ignored, at other times ridiculed. Very often an attempt has been made to exorcize such ideas as one might exorcize the devil himself. Saunders and Hewes (1953) point out that "such an approach is likely to be less harmful to the persistence of folk medical beliefs than it is to the quality of the relationship between the physician and his patient, and is more effective in drawing patients deeper into a dependence on folk medicine than in drawing them into the folds of enlightened followers of science."

Even the most rural tenant farmer or the poorest resident of the urban ghetto is aware of the attitudes of many doctors and nurses toward his cultural beliefs, and he knows that he had best keep those beliefs to himself. His faith in them is no less firm; they are discussed freely within family and community, but almost never are they shared with the health team — if there is any contact with the health team at all.

THEORIES ABOUT FAMILIES: A BASIS OF NURSING PRACTICE

The concepts to which nurses subscribe, both as persons and as professionals, are major factors in their relationship with expectant and new parents.

There are three major approaches to conceptualizing what happens in families during childbearing: structure-function or functionalism, symbolic interaction, and utilitarianism (exemplified by the exchange theory). In this chapter major maternity textbooks will be examined in relation to the theories of the family, and some implications for nursing practice and research will be suggested.

Functionalism

Functionalism or structure-function was the predominant theory of family sociology in the 1940s, 1950s, and early 1960s. Parsons, Pitts, and Spiegel are major functionalist theorists; Parsons derived some of his ideas from Freud's concepts.

For functionalists, the family is a nuclear family, with the father playing an instrumental leadership role and the mother playing a subordinate expressive role; this division of labor is seen as not only true but necessary. Roles are fixed; they represent the way families *ought* to function. Variations are seen as both deviance and a threat to the social order.

Functionalists espouse male superiority. "A generalized male superiority is a basic theme of the structure of the nuclear family in all known societies" (Pitts 1964). Women are accorded little prestige. "In relation to prestige, the first observation is that housekeeping is universally an activity of low status. . . . It is repetitious, monotonous . . . [i]t remains essentially a low-skill activity which requires for successful discharge a high sense of responsibility rather than complex training. The same is true of parenthood, especially care of the prepubertal child" (Pitts 1964).

Functionalism is no longer a viable theory for most family theorists. In a recent textbook of family theory (Burr et al. 1979) there is no chapter on functionalism. The functionalist perspective almost never appears in a contemporary family journal. However, if one examines maternity nursing texts, one can see that functionalism is alive and well. Reeder and colleagues cite

Christensen's volume as an "invaluable resource for helping to delineate content in clinical nursing courses and providing conceptual frameworks for the development of assessment tools and the testing of nursing intervention techniques" (1976). Part of the Christensen volume, particularly the chapter by Pitts, was written from a structure-function perspective. Clark (1979) states, "the family is a social system with a structure that is related to the functions to be performed by family members. Statuses and roles are component parts of the structure, with roles channeling the behavior of individuals into specific statuses so that the functions of the system are performed."

Jensen, Benson, and Bobak (1977) utilize this conceptual perspective when they state that the nuclear family is the family structure considered "normal" in contemporary Western society. "The parents in this family are expected to play complementary roles of husband-wife and father-mother." They also note that "those individuals who accept and follow the family's blueprint are esteemed; those who rebel are labeled *deviant* and, depending on the power they possess, are either ignored or have sanctions directed against them."

Ziegel and Cranley's (1978) assumption of traditional family roles for all mothers is also a functionalist view. According to them, for the new mother, "the baby will take up quite a bit of time. . . . Her husband and other children will also make demands on her time. If her mental health is to be maintained, she will need some time to herself to read a book or sew, work with her plants, or get out of the house for socialization. . . . Fathers are often willing to perform household chores in order to have some time for individual attention from their wives" (Ziegel and Cranley 1978).

What is wrong with this functionalist approach? More important, does using a functionalist conceptual framework limit nursing practice? For the functionalist each role demands specific role behavior. The mother has her role and appropriate behavior as does the father. These roles are predetermined. Pitts (1964) notes Parsons' "cogent case for the importance of this type of division of labor for the socialization of the child in any society." Clark (1979) states that "the many practical attitudes necessary to take care of infants and guide learning are facilitated by characteristic qualities of a woman's personality." As for fathers, "fatherliness consists of instinctive responses of empathy for the children as the man fulfills his ultimate goal as protector and provides for his family."

Nursing approaches toward the new family, based on these concepts, would emphasize adaptation to the prescribed roles. But what if the mother is the major provider for the family, either by choice or out of necessity? For functionalists, this pattern represents deviance:

> Mothers working outside the home . . . and shifting values in our society all contribute to confusion in parental role acquisition (Clark 1979).
> "Certain social roles become stereotyped to such a degree that modification of the role by a player is construed as betrayal, and the *deviant* [italics mine] individual can be viewed with much disfavor. The roles of mother and father fall into this category. Changes in lifestyles can cause conflict in role expectations, for example, if the mother contributes to the family income and the father shares in the caretaking activities in the home. The mother can be labeled inadequate because she does not act in a "true motherly fashion" (Jensen 1977).

A nurse practicing from a functionalist perspective will assume that particular tasks, such as bathing and feeding, are a mother's responsibility. Baby bath classes will be held for mothers in the mornings, rather than at a time that may be more convenient for fathers as well. The question has been raised in nursing literature and practice whether grandmothers who are the primary caregivers should be a focus of teaching (e.g., when the mother is a younger teenager); rarely are fathers thought of in this situation. Feeding help is generally given to the mother; how often does a nurse help a father with feeding? The nurse may assume that a mother will instinctively know how to feed her infant. Community health nursing

and nursing in clinics have also largely focused on the mother as the primary caregiver because contacts have been made during the day, when many fathers are working.

What about the parents who ask about maternal employment after childbearing? From what perspective can nurses answer if they view this behavior as "deviant"?

In some hospitals, support persons other than husbands are not allowed in the labor/delivery areas. Again, the assumption seems to be that any relationship other than the nuclear family relationship represents deviance.

Aside from clinical implications, functionalism is not a particularly useful theory for the researcher. If roles and functions are fixed, the researcher is limited as to the measurement of adjustment/deviance. In a society in which the behavior of men and women within the family is changing markedly for many individuals, a researcher's commitment to fixed roles and functions is not only nonproductive for research but potentially destructive for families influenced by the results of such research.

Symbolic Interaction

Symbolic interaction might better be termed a theoretical orientation or perspective than a theory per se in that it is more a body of insights than a systematic theory. By definition, a theory requires concepts that are connected in order to explain and predict and that are tested and refined through the gathering of data. Symbolic interaction encompasses a number of perspectives including reference group theory, perceptual theory, role theory, and self theory. However, the various subtheories have not been integrated with one another nor have they been tested. Nevertheless, insights from symbolic interaction theory are important conceptual frameworks for nurses.

Role is a basic concept in symbolic interaction. Although role for the functionalist is a prescribed norm or script and thus static, for at least some symbolic interactionists role is a more dynamic concept in which "there is usually considerable room for individual differences in roles, and there is no clear-cut normative script for much of what persons do in a role" (Burr et al. 1979). Turner (1962) uses the term *role making* to describe the way in which individuals improvise, explore, and judge what is appropriate in a particular situation rather than act on the basis of previously learned scripts or expectations. Burr and associates (1979) write, "It is indefensible to argue that roles are a static aspect of structure, because roles are dynamic and processual. . . . Even those parts of roles that are the most clearly and precisely defined by social expectations are ongoing, dynamic processes rather than static events."

Role theory is a major concept in maternity nursing. Reeder and colleagues (1976) described roles in the tradition of George Herbert Mead as "defined, created, stabilized or modified as a consequence of interaction between the self and others," a concept that "allows for innovative, individualistic designing of a person's role performance." Moore (1978) writes of "the period of preparation for childbearing as an ideal time for helping individuals and couples think about the way in which they view the roles of mother and father." Ziegel and Cranley (1978) view roles as negotiable, with the increased participation of fathers in both pregnancy and child care. They suggest that nurses can facilitate role negotiation in their discussion of infant care with the couple.

The *quality of role enactment* (Sarbin and Allen 1964) or *quality of role performance* (Biddle and Thomas 1966) describes how well a person performs a role relative to the expectations for that role. It is a concept that is part of the basic nursing assessment of parents. For example, "alterations in parenting" is one of the accepted nursing diagnoses identified by the National Group for the Classification of Nursing Diagnosis (Gebbie 1976), indicating a role performance that is expected by nurses as professionals. Depending on the basis of nurses' expectations, this diagnosis may or may not be appropriate.

Parents, too, have expectations for themselves, for each other, and for others. These expectations may be discussed between individuals (e.g., mother and father), but frequently they may be understood or thought to be understood but not expressed. For example, a prospective father may expect his baby to breast-feed because that is traditional in his family, or a grandmother may expect the baby's mother to give up her job and remain at home once the baby is born. In a given situation there may be a high level of *consensus or role expectations* or little or no consensus. Some authors use the term *role conflict* to describe a low level of consensus or lack of consensus, but others feel this term is too ambiguous.

The concept of *role strain*, originally developed by Goode (1960), a functionalist, is defined as "felt difficulty in fulfilling role obligations." Role strain can be thought of as a continuous variable that can range from absence to a very high level. As role strain increases along the continuum, i.e., as individuals become increasingly uncomfortable in complying with the expectations of a role, anxiety, stress, and loss of self-esteem may occur. Labeling this concept as "role strain" is less valuable than identifying the behaviors that produce stress, but because the term is widely accepted, it is used here.

Utilitarianism

Although symbolic interaction offers a number of useful concepts it does not, as previously noted, really deal with the basic issue of what happens in families in an integrative fashion. Functionalism does, of course, by suggesting that families exist and operate because of societal norms. Nursing practice has drawn upon both perspectives in a somewhat eclectic fashion, fitting concepts with clinical experience and (I believe to some extent) with traditional biases of society (e.g., the idea of nuclear families as the norm).

A contrasting solution is offered by a theory termed *utilitarianism* by Ellis (1971). Exchange theory and conflict theory are utilitarian theories; our focus here will be on exchange theory. The basic assumption of this perspective is that persons (and groups) behave as they do to gain rewards and avoid costs. Whereas some exchange theorists approach rewards and costs from an individualistic perspective (e.g., Nye), others focus on interaction between individuals or groups (e.g., Scanzoni).

Childbearing can certainly be examined in a reward-cost framework. Perceived rewards may include being recognized by the community as an adult member of society, having a sense of personal achievement, achieving survival of family name, and receiving affection (Scanzoni and Scanzoni 1976). Moore (1978) suggests many perceived rewards of childbearing such as a steppingstone into the adult world, a means of saving a relationship or a substitute for a relationship, a way to please others, an escape from an undesirable situation, a replacement for a lost child, a means of affirming masculinity or femininity, and a way to act out rebellion. In a recent survey, Hoffman and Mannis (1979) found that the rewards of childbearing included love and companionship, stimulation and fun, and expansion of self.

Costs receive some attention in maternity texts although not in the reward-cost framework. Jensen, Benson, and Bobak (1977), drawing on Eshleman (1974), write of the "rather profound and negative effect on marital satisfaction, particularly for the mother, who may even feel her basic self-worth is threatened." Moore (1978) notes that "pregnancy and adaptation to a new member of a family can add strain to even a firm, stable union," whereas Ziegel and Cranley comment on the frustrations of parenthood for the mother and the straining of the relationship between parents.

One concept important to exchange theorists is *resources.* Resources may be either tangible (money, job status, education, etc.) or intangible (e.g., self-esteem). The possession of resources is a principal source of *power,* which is defined as the ability to achieve intended effects, although other factors such as preferences, goals, and prevailing social values may influence power (Rodman 1972).

Issues like power and resources have not traditionally been a part of the conceptual framework of maternity nursing, probably because they were not dealt with by the sociologists whose concepts had been utilized. Contemporary sociologists, however, are turning their attention to this facet of childbearing. LaRossa's 1977 volume, *Conflict and Power in Marriage: Expecting the First Child,* draws attention to the issue even in the title. Scanzoni (*Sex Roles, Life-Styles, and Childbearing: Changing Patterns in Marriage and Family,* 1975) and Lamb's chapter in Lerner and Spanier (1978) explore these issues in some detail. The emphasis is on the *processes* that occur in families in the period surrounding childbearing.

What does happen to couples when a child arrives? Let us assume that this is a first child and that the couple is either married or committed to each other over a period without marriage. The changes that childbearing brings will depend on the current pattern of interaction in the relationship.

Three styles of marital interaction, described by Scanzoni (1979), may be thought of as on a continuum from traditional to egalitarian (Fig. 11–1). Some couples interact in the traditional way described by the functionalists. Scanzoni has called this type of marriage "head complement," in that the man, as head of the family, continues to hold greater power than the woman over areas such as family finance. The wife is his complement.

In the senior partner–junior partner relationship, the woman possesses resources that give her increased power in the relationship, although her power is not equal to that of her mate. Her power

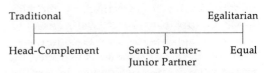

Figure 11–1. Three styles of marital interaction. (Derived from Scanzoni *In* Levinger and Moles: Divorce and Separation. Basic Books, 1979.)

may be derived from a job that gives her increased economic resources, for example.

The equal partner marriage is similar to the dual-career marriage described by Rapoport and Rapoport (1976), in which men and women are coproviders in the economic sphere (possessing resources that are close to being equal) and in which no issues are non-negotiable. There are relatively few marriages at this time that approach this degree of equality, but as women's educational levels and job opportunities increase, it can be expected that equal-partner marriages will also increase.

If we accept the existence of various family patterns, the question becomes, Does childbearing affect each pattern equally? Lamb suggests that as childbirth approaches, the relationship between couples becomes more traditional. He cites as an example the wife's withdrawal from work which "may facilitate a change from the more egalitarian values and role demands of dual-career couples to the more stereotyped role set of traditional nuclear families" (Lamb 1978). Exchange theory suggests that if she does indeed withdraw from work, she will have fewer resources (such as her own source of income) and thus be more dependent, less equal, and less powerful than her husband.

Hoffman (1963) found that agreement with the statement "Some equality in marriage is a good thing, but by and large the husband should have the main say-so" increased with the birth of the first child and never returned to prechild levels. Whether this agreement would be found in the 1980s is questionable.

This change in relationship may be stressful to at least some women, particularly young women in the 1980s who place a high value on equality. This process may explain earlier reports of decreased marital satisfaction following childbirth. For some women, the costs of the altered relationship may be perceived as outweighing the rewards, and the woman may begin to negotiate with her partner for what she perceives as a more equitable solution.

For example, she may negotiate to return to work, which could help to restore the balance of power. Such a move would probably require increased participation of the father in child care and house care.

EXCHANGE THEORY AS A CONCEPTUAL FRAMEWORK FOR NURSING PRACTICE AND RESEARCH IN THE CARE OF CHILDBEARING FAMILIES

Exchange theory provides insights that can be useful at each stage of the nursing process. What is the couple's current style of interaction? Is the relationship traditional, senior partner-junior partner, or egalitarian? Are both partners satisfied with their current style? How do they expect the birth of the baby to change their style? How do they feel about that? What are the rewards of childbearing for them? What costs do they perceive?

Such questions might be raised on individual assessment, but they could also be raised in a childbirth education group discussion or in a class for new parents after delivery. These and similar questions could also be the basis of research into the needs of childbearing couples.

A better understanding of an individual couple's needs enables the nurse to plan teaching and support to meet those needs. If the father is to have a major responsibility for child care, how can the nurse help him, as well as the mother, to gain skill and confidence? If the mother who wants to breast-feed for just a few weeks before she returns to her job asks, "Will that be worthwhile?" what should the nurse tell her? What do the nurse's casual comments and gestures communicate when parents communicate "nontraditional" attitudes or behaviors?

Exchange perspectives can also serve as a conceptual framework for other childbearing clients. Hoffman and Mannis (1979) suggest that if one is dealing with teenage pregnancy, identifying the perceived rewards of parenthood for teenagers (e.g., the desire for adult status) and providing alternate sources of satisfaction may be ameliorating. (An alternate explanation in some instances may be indifference to costs rather than interest in perceived rewards.)

A cost-reward framework could also further understanding of a woman's choice of alternatives when faced with an unwanted pregnancy. Although childbearing may appear a costly choice to some women, for others the alternatives, such as abortion or relinquishment, may appear even more costly.

SEX STEREOTYPING: AN EXAMPLE OF CULTURAL VALUES AND BEHAVIOR TOWARD NEWBORNS

From the moment of birth, when the announcement is made, "It's a boy" or "It's a girl," beliefs about what is appropriate for the socialization of an infant of that gender become important. In a time when gender roles are of concern to many persons, including new parents, knowledge of the research in this area is important for nurses.

Rubin, Provenzano, and Luria (1974) asked 30 pairs of primiparous parents, 15 with sons and 15 with daughters, to describe their baby as they would "to a close friend or relative" and to then rate their baby on 18 11-point, bipolar adjective scales such as firm-soft, relaxed-nervous, noisy-quiet, and hardy-delicate. There were no significant differences in the male and female infants in birth weight or length or in Apgar scores at five and 10 minutes.

Fathers rated their infants almost immediately after delivery; they were not allowed to be present during delivery and had seen their infants only through the nursery window. Mothers rated their infants during the first 24 hours; they had delivered under general anesthesia but had handled and fed their infants.

Both mothers and fathers differentially labeled their infants according to gender. Daughters were rated as softer, finer featured, littler, and more inattentive. When the relationship between the sex of the parent and the sex of the infant was analyzed, fathers were more extreme in their ratings of both sons and daughters than were mothers. On one variable (cuddly — not cuddly), mothers rated the sons as more cuddly, whereas fathers saw their daughters as more cuddly, a finding that appears in slightly different form in the study of Gerwitz and Dodge (1975).

Given the obstetrical situation at the time this study was done (particularly, lack of fathers' participation in labor, delivery, and the first hours of life), it seems reasonable to ask if the results would be different under current conditions of care. Since the mothers, who interacted with the babies, stereotyped their infants less, would the fathers who interacted with their babies also stereotype them less?

Although these babies were alike in specific characteristics such as weight and Apgar scores, it could nevertheless be argued that there were other discernible differences in their appearance or behavior such as state (Chapter 6).

Attempts to disentangle the effects of infant behavior on the attitudes of adults from the effects of the attitudes themselves have focused on experimental situations in which the subjects view or hear the same infant but receive different gender information. Although these studies involve children beyond the newborn period, the effects of cultural beliefs are apparent.

Gerwitz and Dodge (1975) conducted an experiment in which subjects viewed a videotape of interaction between a three-year-old and the experimenter. A cover story disguised the true purpose of the experiment; questions indicated that the subjects believed the cover story. Half the subjects (13 male and 13 female college students) were told the child's name was Christopher Mandel; the other 13 male and 13 female subjects were told the child was named Christine Mandel. On tape the child, who was dressed in shorts and a tee shirt and had a Dutch-boy style haircut, identified himself as Chris (he was actually Christopher Mandel). Behaviors on the videotape, selected because they were considered nonsex-specific, included reading a story from a book *The Very Hungry Caterpillar,* coloring pictures, and putting together a puzzle. Interaction was unrehearsed and the tape was unedited.

After viewing the tape, the subjects were asked to do the following:

1. Rate the child on 26 dichotomized personality items on a seven-point scale (e.g., inhibited-spontaneous; restrained-assertive, not at all self-reliant–self-reliant).
2. Rate the child on five items reflecting ability:
   a. Child has won a puzzle contest; predict his place of finish in a second contest.
   b. Child has won second contest; explain victory on a scale from 1 (good luck) to 7 (ability).
   c. In a third puzzle contest, child finished last; estimate child's ability from 1 (below average) to 7 (above average).
   d. After (c), child complained of stomachache; was this a believable explanation for performance on third puzzle?
   e. Subjects were told child threw puzzle, screamed, etc.: what would they do if the child were theirs?; rank on scale of 1 to 7 according to permissiveness.

The subjects viewed Christopher as somewhat louder, more mischievous, lovable, energetic, and extroverted and having greater potential for intellectual achievement than Christine ($.05 < p < .15$).

Condry and Condry (1976) also utilized a videotape; the stimulus infant was nine months old and was dressed in neutral clothing. Half of the subjects (45 male and 159 female college students) were told that the infant was a girl named Dana; the remainder were told that the infant was a boy named David. During the course of the 10-minute videotape the infant was presented with each of four stimuli for a period of approximately one minute each. The stimuli were a teddy bear, a jack-in-the-box, a doll, and a buzzer. The first three stimuli were presented five times, the buzzer only three times because of the

infant's reaction. After the presentation of each stimulus, the videotape was stopped and the subjects were asked to indicate the intensity of the child's reactions in relation to three emotions (pleasure, anger, fear) on a 10-point scale. If not all emotions were observed, those not observed were rated zero. The subjects were also asked to describe their experience with infants on a five-point scale. Following the videotape, the subjects were asked to describe the infant on a semantic differentiation scale in relation to activity, potency, and evaluation. Condry and Condry report:

1. When an infant is labeled a boy it is seen as showing more pleasure across all situations than when an infant is labeled a girl.
2. Males are more likely to evaluate the male baby as showing pleasure.
3. Experience with children leads to greater sex-label differences in male subjects but slightly less sex-label differences in female subjects.
4. In the jack-in-the-box situation, in which the meaning of the response (crying and screaming) is ambiguous, there was a marked difference in interpretation ($p < .02$), with "anger" attributed to the boy and "fear" attributed to the girl.

On the semantic differentiation scale, the infant labeled as a boy was perceived as more active and more powerful ($p < .05$); there was no difference in the evaluative measures (good-bad, ugly-pretty, and friendly-unfriendly).

Seavey, Katz and Zalk (1975) asked 42 nonparent volunteers (half male, half female from academic, business, and secretarial populations) to participate in a study involving infant response to strangers. Subjects interacted with a three-month-old infant; three toys were available to them: a small rubber football, a Raggedy Ann doll, and a flexible plastic ring. One group of subjects were told they were to play with a three-month-old *girl,* one group a *boy,* and a third group a *baby* with no mention of sex or name. When queried after the experiment, 57 per cent of the male subjects and 70 per cent of the female subjects of the third group thought the infant was a boy.

Both toy choice and physical handling varied with the sex of the infant and the sex of the subject. The only straightforward effect was increased doll play when the infant was believed to be a girl. The fact that a football was the male stereotype toy may have been a confound, since toy footballs are not usually a toy for infants of this age.

Of those subjects who attributed sex to the neutral baby, those who believed the baby to be a boy noted lack of hair and strength of grasp, whereas those who believed the baby to be a girl mentioned the baby's roundness, softness, and fragility.

Sidorowicz and Lunney (1980) replicated the Seavey, Katz, and Zalk study, but three infants were utilized (two male and one female). All infants were dressed only in shirt and diaper; assigned gender varied from actual gender. This variation was in response to the concern that varying the gender label of a male infant would produce different results from when a female infant was used.

Gender label was more important in this study than in the previous study. When the infant was designated male, 50 per cent of the male subjects and 75 per cent of the female subjects chose to give the baby the football. When the infant was designated female, 72.7 per cent of the female subjects and 88.8 per cent of the male subjects chose to give her a doll. No male gave an infant designated female the football, whereas 28 per cent of the females did. As in the previous study, the subjects asked or tried to guess gender, and following debriefing, attributed stereotyped characteristics to the baby. For example, one male subject said the infant was a girl because "she is friendly and female infants smile more" (the baby was actually male).

CULTURAL BELIEFS OF FAMILIES

There are three reasons why nurses cannot overlook the importance of cultural beliefs:

1. If a belief is accepted by a mother or father whether or not a nurse feels the belief has any scientific validity, it will be valid in the parents' eyes and will affect their baby both before and after birth. Many of these beliefs are not based on reason but have strong religious overtones. For example, if a mother feels she must eat certain foods or perform certain acts during pregnancy to ensure her baby's well-being, telling her that this is not so is not likely to make very much of an impression. "Who are they to question the wisdom of my people?" she thinks.

2. Reexamination of some traditionally held beliefs show that not all of them are completely valueless. If nurses can work with some beliefs and see them as being neutral, causing no special good but causing no harm either, they may be in a better position to deal with those beliefs that do have a potential for harming the infant.

3. Often cultural beliefs fulfill a very special need of the people who hold them.

The Possible Validity of Cultural Beliefs

For at least 30 centuries in India, a drug known today as *pegal-kesawa*, the insanity herb, has been sold at village fairs and has been used by the people of that land. Holy men have chewed it during meditation; mothers have given it to fretful babies; and people in general have used it for vomiting, fever, certain eye problems, and a variety of other symptoms. The claims made for the drug were so extravagant that Western scientists ignored it for hundreds of years. It was not until 1947 that Western researchers began to consider seriously the properties of this drug, known as rauwolfia, although Indian physicians and chemists had begun to take a scientific interest in its properties in the late 1920s and early 1930s (Kreig 1964).

Rauwolfia has also been known in Africa for a number of centuries. Dr. Raymond Prince, a psychiatrist from McGill University who has spent considerable time in the western bush country of Nigeria studying the methods of witch doctors in the treatment of mental illness, found that their therapy included, along with "talking things over," the use of a yellow liquid medication. Analysis revealed that it chemically resembled reserpine, widely used by contemporary Western psychiatrists as a tranquilizer (Kreig, 1964).

Should we tend to overlook the possible merits of these traditional beliefs, it seems worth remembering that Western medicine "discovered" the concept of psychosomatic medicine approximately 40 years ago; traditional people have known for generations that body and mind are not separate entities and that no treatment can be completely effective if it does not cope with psychological as well as physiological needs.

Willow bark tea, taken by the Chinese for centuries as a remedy for stiff joints and rheumatic pains, is chemically related to the salicylates used for similar purposes today (Kreig 1964).

Ross and Van Warmelo (1965), in reporting on the Bantu approach to skin disease, comment, "It is not generally recognized how advanced the ideas of some native tribes are on the identification, causation, and treatment of skin diseases. At times their knowledge is surprising. . . . There is always a theory behind their viewpoint, and a meaning attached to many of the names for the conditions they recognize."

There is no suggestion here that every cultural belief, whether about pregnancy, newborn, medical treatment, or whatever, is valid. For each jewel hidden in the rubble of cultural belief there are thousands of ideas representing beliefs that do neither harm nor good and some that can actually cause harm. One such practice in this last category is geophagy — the eating of clay — which can harm an unborn baby. Whereas a practice such as this is harmful in itself, other beliefs can have a more subtle effect by keeping the mother away from the medical care that she or her baby needs (although cultural traditions are not the only reason mothers fail to seek medical help).

Cultural Beliefs That May Meet Special Needs

It is interesting to consider the possibility that some cultural beliefs can prove valid, but it is even more important to realize that these beliefs often fulfill some special need for the women who hold them. In this regard we might consider a very widely held traditional belief, even among middle-class Americans, that certain foods are craved during pregnancy. Tradition suggests that if a woman does not get the food she craves, her baby will be marked, often in the shape of the food desired.

Obeyesekere (1963), in dealing with the customs of the Sinhalese of Ceylon, discussed a possible function of such cravings in that country, where the term *dola duka* refers both to food cravings and to certain other "minor complications" of pregnancy, specifically nausea, vomiting, and weakness. Although recognizing physiological and individual psychological components in *dola duka*, Obeyesekere sees it chiefly as an opportunity for the pregnant woman to express pressing needs in a socially approved manner.

A Sinhalese girl marries shortly after puberty. In a brief period of time she must make a rapid change in role from carefree girl to wife and mother. In addition she often must leave her own village to live in the village of her husband. The young wife is very likely to have an ambivalent feeling toward pregnancy or toward having a child, for children are associated with the social roles of wife and mother, roles that determine a woman's inferior status in Sinhalese society. Moreover, the continual birth of babies virtually destroys any freedom a woman might have and ties her down to a life of domesticity.

Dola duka is a defense provided by the culture — an opportunity for expressing some important needs in a way that society sees as appropriate. Its most conspicuous aspect is a craving, not equated with hunger, that has to be satisfied. The woman will not be satisfied with a larger quantity of food but only with the consumption of a specific kind of food. To deny a woman what she craves may seriously damage one's chances of rebirth. More immediately it is believed that the ears of the fetus will rot if the cravings are not satisfied.

And so for the woman who takes on an adult role at an early age *dola duka* offers the opportunity to escape from that role into an emotionally gratifying phase of childhood. For the woman who is ambivalent toward her pregnancy, again there is a certain amount of gratification. From another standpoint *dola duka* might be considered a culturally approved way of expressing male envy. Whereas normally Sinhalese women are expected to obey and serve their husbands, *dola duka* inverts the roles and the husband is compelled by custom to serve his wife.

For another example of the possible function of traditional belief, consider the following ways in which the sex of a coming child is supposedly foretold: If a woman is larger in front during pregnancy, the child will be male. If a father wears his boots while his offspring is being born, the child will be male. If your first-born is a girl and you want a boy, turn your bed around. A child born on a shrinking moon will be a boy (White 1961). If a woman carried a baby high, it's a girl; low, it's a boy. If a baby first moves on its left side, it's a boy; and vice-versa (Clark 1966).

Could these beliefs not reflect a certain amount of anxiety over the sex of the coming child and thus afford a way to deal with that anxiety through what can seem like a never-ending wait? Once the child is born, that anxiety will disappear. One will rarely look back to validate prior assumptions, particularly if one has been incorrect. And at any rate, any prediction has a 50 per cent chance of being right — far better odds than are necessary to keep traditions in active circulation.

Cultural Beliefs About Health Care That Affect Newborns

It is not possible here, nor is it our purpose, to catalogue the wide variety of beliefs that are held about childbearing and infants. The examples that follow are meant to serve as illustrations. Each nurse, whether she works in a hospital or a clinic or with mothers at home, has to understand the varying life-styles, ideas, and beliefs of the people she is serving. The available literature, particularly that of medical sociology and medical anthropology, can be helpful.

SPANISH-SPEAKING PEOPLES

There are Spanish-Americans in many areas of the United States today — the Southwest, the Northeast, and the Southeast. Some are descendants of families that came to the United States many years ago; others are recent immigrants. Because of language barriers, low social status, poverty, fear of discrimination or insult by Anglos (a fear that for many is based on experience), and a desire to avoid the conflict caused by introducing new ways of doing things, many Spanish-speaking Americans have retained their own cultural heritage rather than accepting the beliefs and practices of twentieth century America.

Among these beliefs and practices are some very specific ideas about the cause, prevention, and cure of illness, about how an individual must act in the face of illness, and about the way in which the curer — doctor, nurse, or curandera — should behave. Baca (1969) feels that many Spanish-speaking people are unable to seek care from someone who does not understand their beliefs.

As previously mentioned, many Spanish-speaking people believe in *el mal ojo*, the evil eye; it describes symptoms of restlessness and unusual crying, which are believed to be caused by the admiration or coveting of the baby. The intention of the admirer need not be malicious; usually he is not accused of wishing the baby ill. But in spite of himself he brings sickness to the infant. As a result, "Hispanos" do not admire or praise babies as many American mothers do. Or if they do they follow any praise with a mild slap.

Consider the consternation, then, that a nurse could cause in a clinic waiting room filled with Spanish-speaking mothers if she should go from one baby to the next commenting on how pretty or how good each seemed to be.

When a baby falls ill and *el mal ojo* is believed to be the cause, the parents can resort to several types of folk cures. It is generally considered useless to consult an Anglo doctor, who may deny the existence of the evil eye and thus prove himself or herself either a liar or a fool. Clark (1959) quotes a resident of Sal si Puedes, California: "How can a doctor cure something he doesn't even know about?"

Another Spanish belief concerns a condition called "fallen fontanel" *(mollera caida)* and illustrates the difference that may exist between traditional ways of thinking and medical beliefs regarding what is cause and what is effect. One common symptom of dehydration in infancy is a depressed fontanel; rugae of the soft palate are also often exaggerated. Since severe diarrhea and vomiting produce dehydration rather quickly in a small baby, a depressed fontanel and elevated rugae are often associated with vomiting and diarrhea. But in Spanish traditional belief the symptoms are seen not as the end result of dehydration but as the cause. A *bolita* (elevated rugae) on the hard palate is thought to cause the baby to nurse poorly, with the gastrointestinal symptoms as sequelae. Traditional treatment is directed toward elevating the fontanel — by suspending the child upside down over a pan of tepid water, by slapping the soles of his feet while he is held inverted, and so on. In view of this belief about cause, the treatment seems logical.

Since gastrointestinal disorders are the major cause of infant morbidity and mortality in most of the countries from which Spanish-Americans come, depressed fontanels and elevated rugae are hardly uncommon conditions. But the belief concerning this condition is not limited to the poor and uneducated, or even to Spanish areas. A graduate student from British Honduras revealed an identical belief among his people (where the *mollera* is

simply called "the mole") in asking about the size of his own new infant's fontanel.

Air *(aire, mal aire)* is seen as another source of illness. Air and particularly night air is thought to enter the body through any of its cavities. In the newborn, the cord stump is seen as a portal of entry for the air, and a surprised nurse may find a raisin placed over the umbilicus as a preventive measure (Baca 1969).

To people who hold a belief in air as a cause of illness, the fear of surgery takes on an added dimension, for any incision increases the avenues through which air may enter the body. Thus the intestinal distention that frequently accompanies abdominal surgery only serves to support this traditional belief.

Sometimes the reactions of a Spanish-American mother to treatment recommended for her sick infant may confuse the nurse or physician involved. But it should be remembered that culture plays a major role in determining how a mother will act when she learns that she or a member of her family is ill. For example, if a middle-class American mother is told by her doctor that her infant has pyloric stenosis and requires immediate hospitalization and surgery, she would most likely accept the diagnosis and carry out the physician's directions. Undoubtedly either she or her doctor would call her husband to tell him what was taking place, but the diagnosis of the illness would lie in the physician's hands and would be accepted by the parents.

This is not as likely to be true if the family is Spanish-American. There may be a discussion between family members, relatives, and neighbors as to the proper course of action. All of this talk may seem to be a waste of valuable time to the medical team, and there is no question that the time involved can be a real problem in some instances. The delay, however, is not due to a lack of concern over the baby's welfare; actually it is a sign of truly conscientious parents. The opinions of nurses and doctors are not accepted as final; it is the family group that has the ultimate authority to make the decision. In the eyes of the Spanish community, the role of the curer is to advise, not to dictate. Authoritarianism is likely to drive patients away. The parents will rarely be openly defiant; they will smile and answer, "Si." But unless family consensus confirms medical opinion, medical advice may be ignored: medicine is not given, a return appointment is not kept, and the medical team wonders why the mother is so unfeeling and uncaring (from their point of view).

Culture, then, decrees the way in which the doctor or nurse is expected to behave. Clark (1959) describes the behavior of Paula, a curandera in California, who typifies the role. "Paula's manner is as warm and friendly as her kitchen-dispensary. She observes the requisite social amenities and always behaves in a manner which her clients regard as courteous. For example, she is always careful to wait for an invitation to enter the house before she goes in. She knows that she is expected to sit down with the family, drink a cup of coffee, and make small talk before getting down to the business at hand. . . . After a decent interval, the illness can be mentioned and the patient seen."

AMERICAN INDIANS

American Indians also have a distinct cultural heritage. In fact, many Indians have never been assimilated into what we call American culture. Most are isolated both geographically and culturally from other Americans; the majority are poor, and many are limited in their comprehension of English. Because of poverty and isolation, health care for Indian people has also been limited. Even when care has been available, the lack of understanding of Indian culture on the part of many of the doctors and nurses has complicated Indian acceptance of new health measures.

Although ideas and beliefs vary from tribe to tribe, a majority of American Indians, like traditional people in many parts of the world, tend to see health and illness as intimately connected with religious life. Yet changes and innovations

can be made. Just as ways of curing have been borrowed by one tribe from another (e.g., the Navaho have borrowed hand trembling from the Apache and masks and fetishes from the Pueblo), certain aspects of Western medicine have been integrated into Indian culture when shown to be truly helpful. Today most medicine men, as well as their patients, recognize that there are conditions — appendicitis, for example — that Western medicine can treat far better than Indian medicine. Other conditions, however, are virtually unknown to Western medicine; only the medicine man is able to help people with these illnesses. In still other instances both physician or nurse and medicine man are called upon. The medicine man may begin to care for a baby, feel that the baby needs additional help, send him to a clinic for treatment, and then complete his rites when the baby returns, even if the interim has been several weeks.

Farris (1978) describes a number of tribal customs surrounding childbearing. Pregnancy is considered a natural process among the tribes discussed, which include the Seminole of Florida, the Crow of Montana, the Navajo, and the Laguna Pueblo, but special precautions may be prescribed. For example, the pregnant Laguna Pueblo woman may drink an herb tea and is expected to walk slowly.

Breast-feeding was traditionally practiced by Indian women but is reported to be decreasing. Sevcovic (1977) reports that many Navajo women at Shiprock, Arizona, still follow the traditional practice of not placing the baby to breast until the milk comes in. Nurses have been able to encourage mothers to initiate breast-feeding at delivery.

Many Navajo babies share their parents' bed after they return home, and rooming-in mothers may sleep with their babies in the hospital. Sevcovic reported that in three years of rooming-in in Shiprock, no infant has smothered or fallen out of bed.

A cradle board (Fig. 11–2) is used by a number of tribes; although designs vary from simple to elaborate, the use of the cradle board to move the infant about

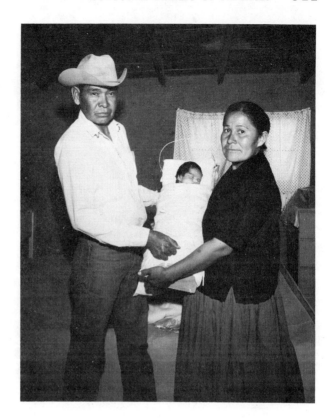

Figure 11–2. A Navajo family living in Arizona. Note the traditional cradle board. (Courtesy of U.S. Public Health Service: Indian Health Service.)

easily while providing security is similar from one tribe to another (Farris 1978).

For many Indian families, hunger, malnutrition, and poor health are constant facts of life (Fig. 11–3). Even water, so taken for granted by most of us, must be hauled many miles on some reservations. Although neonatal mortality (death within the first 28 days of life) has declined, infant mortality (death within the first year) remains higher on reservations than for the United States as a whole. Maternal mortality is also higher.

Health care for Indians who live on reservations, other than the traditional care of the medicine man, is provided through the Division of Indian Health of the United States Public Health Service. Because of a shortage of personnel, it is largely crisis-oriented and overcrowded. An Indian may travel 90 miles to a clinic to find 200 to 300 persons ahead of him, with no hope of even being seen.

Transportation presents a major barrier to health care. Many families live miles from the nearest improved road. The *New York Times* (February 19, 1969) tells of a Navajo woman who carried her sick baby 30 miles from her hogan to the nearest travelled road. The *Times* noted that in the previous year 20 infants from the Pine Ridge Reservation in South Dakota were dead on arrival at medical stations. Eighteen of the deaths were attributed to delay in reaching medical aid.

Although most nurses may never give direct care to Indian families, I believe that anyone interested in people and their care should become aware of the problems Indian peoples face in order to serve, whenever possible, as an advocate for better opportunites for them.

ASIAN AND MIDDLE EASTERN SOCIETIES

Many families living in the United States are from Asia — from China, Japan, India, Korea, Vietnam, the Pacific Islands, and many other Far and Middle Eastern nations. Some of these families have lived in the United States for several generations;

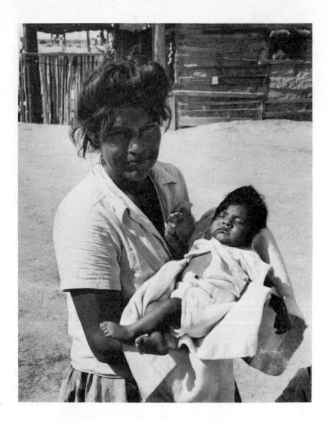

Figure 11–3. A Papago Indian mother and her baby. Because of isolation and poverty, perinatal and infant mortality is high in many Indian societies. (Courtesy of U.S. Public Health Service: Indian Health Service.)

others have only recently immigrated. Although families from Middle and Far Eastern cultures are not homogeneous, many share certain characteristics that are important for nurses to recognize if they are to help these families cope with and grow during childbearing.

The importance of family support   When many of us think of family support during pregnancy, we think first of a nuclear family and the support that comes from the husband. For many Middle and Far Eastern women, however, the traditional support during pregnancy comes from women in the extended family — mothers, aunts, and sisters.

The male role   The traditional Asian husband sees pregnancy as "women's business"; his cultural values often tell him that it is not proper for him to be actively involved with his wife's pregnancy, labor, or delivery. To judge his degree of participation by our Anglo standards and thereby label him as uninterested is, at the very least, unfair. Fathers of Asian descent,

however, who have been in the United States for a number of years may attend childbirth classes and participate in the birth. Thus the wishes of the individual family must be assessed.

Because males are traditionally not expected to care for women, many Asian and Near Eastern women prefer a woman physician or midwife and are very uncomfortable with a male physician. If they live in a community where there is no woman available for total obstetrical care, a nurse can help to some extent by protecting the mother's modesty with particular care and by reminding colleagues of this special concern.

Traditional practices   Traditional practices associated with childbearing vary with the society and with the individual family (see Cultural Assessment). A prolonged convalescence is customary for many societies, with special proscriptions about diet, bathing, and avoiding the "outside" or "unclean" world. Although these customs may seem unusual to us, from the viewpoint of ancient societies such practices probably served the new mother well by protecting her and her baby from infection when there was no way to treat it.

Similarly, prohibiting the father from entering the room of the new mother and baby, which is common to many traditional societies, may have served to protect the new mother from intercourse and possible pregnancy too soon after birth during century after century when abstinence was the only sure means of contraception.

Circumcision is not acceptable in some Asian cultures. Stringfellow (1978) reports that many Vietnamese women who deliver in American hospitals are unaware when they consent to such a procedure for their sons. Chinese also believe circumcision is unnecessary. On the other hand, circumcision is a part of the religious beliefs of Moslem and Jewish families.

APPALACHIAN MOUNTAIN PEOPLE

More than 24 million people live in Appalachia (Fig. 11–4); another 3½ million Appalachians live in urban areas including Cleveland, Detroit, and Pittsburgh, where they have migrated in search of employment, in many instances with minimal success. The poor and working class people of Appalachia tend to share values that may be misinterpreted by health care professionals with middle-class values. A few examples are cited below.

Time orientation Middle-class Americans are largely *future oriented;* they plan today for events that are going to happen at some future time. Appalachians, like many of the world's peoples, are commonly *present oriented.* Prenatal care, which involves seeking medical care *now* to pre-

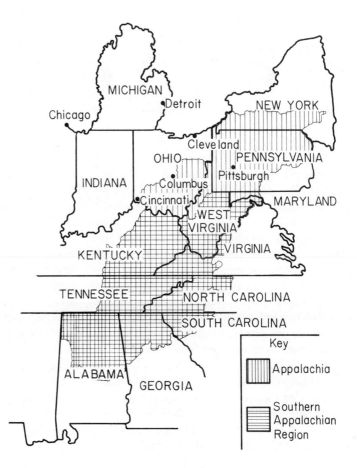

Figure 11–4. Location of the Appalachian and Southern Appalachian regions. (From Nurs Clin North Am 12(1):43, 1977.)

pare for a *future* event, may have low priority. Another aspect of time orientation — a flexible attitude toward schedules — may lead to broken appointments. An appointment at 8 AM today may be kept "sometime today" or "sometime this week."

Relationship of man and nature Whereas middle-class Americans tend to believe that man controls his own destiny to a large extent, Appalachians (again like many of the world's peoples) believe that man has very limited control, if any, over the forces of nature. If one has no control over events — if "What will be will be" — then preventive health care such as prenatal and well-baby care makes very little sense.

Importance of the extended family The most important group influencing the Appalachian woman is her kinspeople, the members of her extended family. Their advice, especially about age-old matters like pregnancy and birth, will often take precedence over the advice of professional strangers.

THE COUNTERCULTURE: ALTERNATIVE LIFE-STYLES

"Any family, any commune, is like a Rorschach test. What you see when you come here says more about who you are than what it is. Visitors . . . completely miss what's really going on because they don't see what these things mean to us" (Melville 1972, quoting a member of an Oregon commune).

Knowledge of the counterculture, those young men and women who have chosen to live in a style different from that considered to be "mainstream American," is important not only so that nurses may give care to these young people but also because some facets of their alternative life-styles may be signals of changes that will later become part of the society as a whole. This is already evident in matters such as hair style and dress, and I think

we are seeing examples in facets of childbearing as well.

The decision to live apart from the mainstream of life is hardly unique to the twentieth century. The Old Testament Jews saw themselves as a people set apart; so did the early Christians. Convents and monasteries offered medieval women and men the opportunity for communal living. Nineteenth century America saw both successful communities (e.g., Shakers, Oneida, The Harmony Society) and many brief, less successful attempts at communal life (Brook Farm, Oberlin, Utopia, and a long list of others). Nathaniel Hawthorne lived at Brook Farm for a time. Bronson Alcott, the father of author Louisa May Alcott, was one of the founders of a small, short-lived group called Fruitlands.

Many of the expressed values of the counterculture concerning childbearing and childrearing are not very different from the ideals expressed in this and other nursing texts. For example, there is emphasis on the role of the father during pregnancy, at delivery, and in childrearing. "Natural" childbirth is common, although many nurses would find it difficult to accept delivery within the community with others serving as midwives. Breastfeeding is almost universal within the countercultures, as is intimate contact between mother and baby during infancy. In some groups the child is rarely left with anyone but his parents, whereas in others childrearing tasks may be shared, even to the point of exchanging breast-feeding infants among several lactating mothers.

There is considerable interest in nutrition, particularly in organic foods and herbs. One potential problem during pregnancy is that protein intake may be low. Diets with adequate protein can be planned within the framework of the dietary desires of most mothers, but some education and care in menu planning are necessary. For some mothers, the expense may be prohibitive.

The emphasis on naturalness and intimacy may put couples in conflict with the traditional medical world of hospitals and clinics — a world in which from their point of view, technology and bureaucracy often seem to be more important than people and relationships.

Bell (1975) talks of this conflict and his reaction to it in describing the birth of Stephen Benson.* At the time he wrote his book, Bell was a pediatric house officer in an intensive care unit of a medical center — practicing medicine in a way as foreign to life in the commune as the bloodletting of the eighteenth century is to the use of cardiac pacemakers. Stephen's parents, Kristin and Peter, lived on a farm with 13 other people. Kristin had received prenatal care from an obstetrician who was unwilling to participate in a home delivery. She said of him, "I don't think he likes us very much," and added, "We want to do everything possible for our baby. We don't want it to be unsafe, but we feel that it would be better for the child to be born at home." The couple agreed that should complications arise, they would go immediately to the hospital, a 15-minute drive.

Bell was asked to witness the delivery. In describing the labor he comments, "We were witnessing something we had never seen in a hospital, a child being born in an atmosphere of love and caring. I wondered if the baby would somehow recognize this and, as Kristin and Peter believed, be a better, happier person because of it." A friend sang quiet songs during the long hours of labor. Kristin ate ice chips and drank sips of tea. At the time of Stephen's delivery Bell records,

> Finally, the vagina had stretched enough, and with a push the infant's head came out. Peter held the head and slowly guided out the shoulders and body of his son. The wet, warm, slippery body began to move, and after a cough, he began to cry. . . . Peter and Kristin began crying, sobbing with joy as their son moved about, flexing his arms, opening his eyes, looking around for the first time. . . . The door opened and the

other house members came in, everyone laughing, crying, hugging each other, rejoicing, and welcoming the new child. . . . Still overcome with joy, he [Peter] dried the baby, handing him carefully to Kristin, and they cried together for the joy of the new life they had produced. Their son was not crying but moving about, carefully studying this strange new world in the arms of his loving parents (Bell 1975).

What kind of people will Stephen and his contemporaries, the children of the counterculture, be as adults? Melville (1972) quotes a father in Taos Pueblo: "The test of this whole thing . . . will be the next generation . . . the kids who grow up here, they're going to be really high people, absolutely out of sight." Veysey (1973), in looking at the children of earlier generations who sought alternative life-styles, found that most of their children "slipped back into more conventional beliefs and styles of living" and at least some "were soon enthusiastically playing baseball." He comments, "In America it seems little easier for radicals to hold on to their children than it is for any other parents."

PICA

Cultural differences are by no means limited to people who espouse a radically different life-style or who speak a different language. Practices that affect newborns can occur right in our own communities. Yet many medical professionals, both physicians and nurses, are either totally ignorant of them or are so vaguely aware of their existence as to consider them insignificant in scope. One such example is pica, including the eating of dirt or clay (geophagy), and the related practices of starch and flour eating (Fig. 11–5).

Clay eating, an ancient practice recorded from the time of Pliny in the first century A.D. and undoubtedly dating to much earlier times, is very much a factor in the United States today. The practice in this country apparently originated in the South, but it exists as well in many north-

---

*Dr. Bell's book, *A Time to Be Born*, highly recommended to all nurses who care for mothers and babies, describes in very readable fashion the first days of four infants: Stephen Benson and three sick babies born in a medical center hospital.

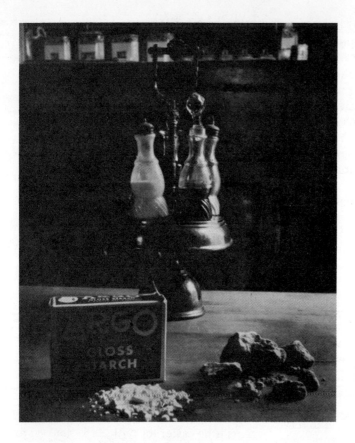

Figure 11–5. The eating of clay and starch, particularly during pregnancy, is a cultural practice that affects the newborn. (From Moore: The clay eaters. RN Aug. 1970. Photographed by Ray Solowinski. Courtesy of RN magazine.)

ern cities to which southerners have migrated.

There seems little doubt that clay eating can have an adverse effect on the newborn. But is it really prevalent enough to be of major concern? Only a limited number of studies, as to both incidence and specific effects on the fetus and newborn, have been conducted to date, but more extensive investigations are being undertaken. One survey of 49 pregnant teenagers in one southern community revealed that 46 of them, all black, were familiar with clay and starch eating (Li and White 1970). Forty-five admitted that they had eaten starch at one time or other. Twelve of these women had also eaten clay or dirt as well as starch but expressed a distinct preference for clay, which is the more deleterious from the standpoint of the fetus' health.

In a small sample of 13 women in another community, one-fourth reported eating clay, half favored starch, and the remaining fourth preferred raw flour (Hochstein 1968).

Lackey (1978) studied pica in East Tennesseee and found that substances consumed included clay, dirt, cornstarch, laundry starch, coke magnesia, soot, charcoal, slate rock, flour, raw coffee and coffee grounds, cigarette ashes, chalk, coal oil, and coal.

Various reasons have been offered to explain the phenomenon of pica. They include spasms due to hunger, the relief of menstrual cramps or uterine sensations that occur during pregnancy, and the belief that the clay may contain substances essential to the well-being of the mother or child. Hochstein points out that just as the physician may recommend soda crackers to the middle-class mother who is nauseated during early pregnancy, neighbors and relatives of the poorer mother may guide her to clay or starch for the same purpose.

Regardless of the historically reported reasons for pica, Li and White found that women in their study ate clay because it was "good," "gummy," "crunchy," or "bitter." Their descriptions of starch included "good," "smooth," "sweet," "bitter," and "thick." In short, they enjoyed eating the clay or starch, just as the woman who smokes cigarettes or chews gum enjoys that particular habit. In no way did the women in the study attribute any special food value to either starch or clay. The habit seemed so natural to them that there was no reluctance to discuss it; it was no different from expressing a preference for a candy bar. The findings of other researchers support this matter-of-fact attitude.

Many observers feel that the ingestion of clay and related substances by pregnant women is not merely a curiosity but of concern because of a possible association with iron deficiency anemia. Some studies support this association whereas others find no association (Lackey 1978). Some researchers postulate iron deficiency anemia as a cause of pica; others suggest anemia to be a result of pica.

THE CULTURE OF POVERTY

The practice of eating clay or starch is but one aspect of the culture of poverty, in this particular instance for the black poor. There are many differences between the culture of the very poor and that of the middle-class. Lower-class behavior may be just as difficult for nurses to understand as is the behavior of a Spanish or Indian mother.

Families living in poverty, whether they live in crumbling tenements or rural shacks, often have inadequate sanitary facilities and suffer all degrees of malnutrition and disease. Many poor mothers have no prenatal care; the incidence of prenatal care is actually decreasing in some areas. One reason is economic: In some clinics a mother must pay before she can be examined, even though the charge is somewhat lower than what she would pay a private physician. But if she appears at the emergency room in labor it is more difficult to turn her away, even though she has no money. So she just waits until this moment.

Long delays in clinics, poor facilities, seeing a different doctor on each visit, the attitude of many clinic personnel, and a tendency to face today's problems rather than plan for tomorrow's (i.e., to be oriented to the present rather than to the future) are other factors limiting prenatal care among the poor.

What is the very poor mother like? She may be very young or the mother of many children. Her education is likely to be limited, and perhaps because school and formal learning may have been an unpleasant experience for her, she may be hostile to people in authority (including nurses). She may have difficulty in making herself understood, and she may have just as much difficulty understanding others.

Barriers to communication can include differences in the pronunciation of words, differences in the meanings attached to the same words, and different words used by the nurse and mother to refer to the same object or behavior. In addition, many words the nurse may feel are rather commonplace may be totally unfamiliar to the patient.

The limited education of the low-income mother has special significance for nurses interested in mother-baby health, for there is so much to teach the mother about caring for her baby. One test of mothers who came into the pediatric emergency room of Los Angeles County Hospital revealed that 15 per cent read at the fourth grade level or below, 30 per cent at the sixth grade level, and 55 per cent at the eighth grade level or above. (The test consisted of four paragraphs about pediatric health problems which the mother was asked to read, followed by four multiple choice questions which the mother answered on the basis of what she had just read.) Reading level correlated with the number of years of education; those who had the highest levels of education tended to have the highest scores. But only 60 per cent of those mothers who had attended high school were able to read at the eighth grade level (Wingert, Grubbs, and Friedman, 1969).

It seems that most of the printed material nurses give to mothers from low-income neighborhoods is beyond their comprehension and thus of little value. Wingert and colleagues suggest that reading material should be written at no higher than a sixth grade level for it to be understood by approximately 85 per cent of all mothers. In addition, printed material of this type should be extensively illustrated to catch the attention of the nonreading mother, and it should certainly be discussed thoroughly with all mothers and not just handed to them.

Husband-wife relationships in the lowest socioeconomic class frequently differ from those in middle-class families. Men and women tend to operate in separate spheres for both work and play. This has real significance when a baby is born. In most lower class families the father, if he is present at all, is going to feel uncomfortable about performing tasks such as changing diapers and feeding or even holding the baby; this is "women's work." He probably feels uncomfortable about visiting his wife in the hospital and might not want to stay with her in the labor or delivery room (nor might she be comfortable having him there). The worlds of men and women of this culture are too far apart for this kind of sharing.

It is easy for nurses with a middle-class bias to interpret this behavior as an indication of lack of affection. All the family pictures in our textbooks and the articles in popular magazines reinforce our beliefs of family togetherness, which are generally accurate for middle-class patients like ourselves. But here again both our attitudes and our teaching must be modified to fit the life-styles of the people for whom we care.

Assessment of Cultural Practices

Individual differences within cultures have been emphasized as well as differences between persons from various cultures. For the nurse to be most helpful to an individual family, a cultural assessment is essential. Rose (1978) suggests an assessment of Chinese Americans, which I have modified to provide a basis for a sociocultural assessment of any childbearing family (Table 11–1).

Working Within the Framework of the Parents' Beliefs

Perinatal and infant mortality and morbidity rates in the United States are, in general, higher in those groups whose cultural heritage differs from that of middle-class America. It does not necessarily follow that these increased rates are merely the result of different beliefs. Both the increased incidence of death and illness and the maintenance of traditional values and ideas are related to the isolation of groups of people — because of poverty, color, differences in language, and a multitude of related factors. To introduce better health measures into these communities, nurses and their fellow health workers must overcome these barriers.

Aichlmayr (1969) has described what can happen when nurses have some understanding of, and appreciation for, cultural beliefs and values different from their own. The project began when six students in a community nursing class observed a government speaker addressing a group of Indians in a highly condescending manner. The purpose of the meeting has been to explore the health and welfare needs of the Indians, yet it seemed that the speaker ignored both the expressed needs of the Indians and their contributions. He appeared to typify a very common attitude: that the Indians were "lazy, unappreciative, and unreachable" — a sentiment resulting from the Indians' failure to cooperate with health programs that the white community had prescribed without first consulting them.

It was only with difficulty that Aichlmayr and her students were able to arrange a meeting with health aides in the Indian community, not because the Indians were reluctant to meet but because the local director of the Office of Economic Opportunity (OEO) felt that as a result of previous bad experiences with whites the Indians would be unwilling to accept the

Table 11–1   Cultural Assessment*

Area Assessed	Significance
Family	
Birthplace of parents-to-be	Younger generation may have different ideas of family tradition and culture, particularly if older generation was born in "home" country and younger generation was born in United States
Birthplace of grandparents-to-be (maternal and paternal)	
Residence in culturally identifiable neighborhood (e.g., Indian reservation, Chinatown)	Residents of identifiable neighborhood may have more traditional values
Nuclear or extended family	It is essential to understand family influence on young parents when teaching and counseling
Grandparents living in home	
Role of grandparents in decision making	
Family support	In some societies a male labor coach is unusual; males may not expect to help in infant care
Companion or coach during labor	
Assistance during postpartal period at home	
Diet: Traditional foods	Nutritional counseling must utilize foods acceptable to individual clients; appropriate foods must be provided to the mother during hospitalization
General	
During and following pregnancy	
For infant	Understanding cultural beliefs about infant diet (e.g., delayed breast-feeding) must precede infant care and teaching
Pica	Pica is frequently deleterious
Traditional health care practices	Understanding traditional values of health and child care must precede both care and teaching
Use of herbs	In assessing drug use (Chapter 3), traditional herbs must not be overlooked
Herbs used	
Western medicines used	
Beliefs about value of herbs	
Ritual practices	
Beliefs related to health and illness (e.g., *el mal ojo*)	
Utilization of traditional healers (e.g., faith healer, curandero, medicine man)	When advice is being received from other healers, knowledge of that advice is essential (Scott 1974)
Child care practices	Understanding traditional values of health and child care must precede both care and teaching
Feeding	
Circumcision	
Bathing, dressing, sleeping, etc. (e.g., is a belly band believed to be necessary; does baby sleep alone or with parents?)	
Special protection for infant	
Rituals or customs (e.g., cradle boards)	

*Adapted from Rose *In* Clark, A. (ed.): Culture, Childbearing, Health Professionals. F. A. Davis, 1978.

students and their instructor on their reservation. Nevertheless, a meeting was arranged. When the Indian aides were told that the students wanted to get to know the Indian people and that it was up to the Indians to decide what information they wanted to obtain from the students, the aides began to discuss among themselves topics such as their high rate of infant mortality and the paucity of medical facilities for their people.

In a subsequent meeting on the reservation, one Indian woman said, "We are so tired of having people come to the reservation with their prescribed programs and telling us what our needs are and how we should live." One example cited was the manner in which whites from large cities admonished the Indians to bathe daily, without ever considering the availability of bathing facilities or the supply of water, which is tremendously scarce on many reservations.

Aichlmayr and her students came to be accepted by the Indian women as the Indians discovered that the students truly did want to help in the way in which the Indians desired. At the same time the nurses learned things about the Indians; they found that the Indians valued sharing more than saving, cooperation more than competition, anonymity rather than individuality — all in direct contrast to the values of most middle-class whites. They learned that even such a seemingly simple act as asking a woman a direct question about herself violated valued anonymity.

Perhaps most important of all was the fact that they did learn. By going to the reservation with neither fixed ideas nor a set program they were able to win friends and offer specific help in a number of health areas. It may be another generation before all the results of such a program can be evaluated; cultural change is usually a long, slow process that can't be hurried. But it would seem that the right beginning has been made in this instance.

PROJECT IN A BLACK GHETTO

As has already been mentioned, we do not have to go to an Indian reservation to enter a world with ways that seem foreign to us. But we can learn from the experience of Aichlmayr and her students. The same principles of listening first to the mothers so they can tell us of their needs and then planning with them, rather than for them, are equally applicable in an urban ghetto or a rural southern county.

"The Mom and Tots Neighborhood Center" is an example of an attempt to meet the needs of poor, black, urban mothers in one of the "most deprived and alienated" areas of the city of Detroit (Milio 1967). Even the name of the center came from the women of the community; Milio had planned to call it the "Maternity Satellite Center" but was told by the women that no one would understand such a title.

The center was envisioned by the Visiting Nurse Association of Detroit, but it actually began only after Milio, the only full-time professional person on the project staff, talked with neighborhood mothers in their block clubs and at their church meetings. The mothers pointed out that they were often unable to go to prenatal and birth control clinics because they had neither transportation nor baby sitters; that they often had to spend long hours waiting if they did go; and that no one had time to answer their questions. They were concerned about keeping their children away from the streets and keeping the rats away from their babies. Some mothers wanted the project to be staffed only by local blacks. Many wanted full-time day care for the children of working mothers. A great many of the ideas were incorporated, in whole or in part, into the plans for the center. An empty neighborhood store was found, local men and women renovated and decorated it, and operations began.

In Milio's description of the prenatal clinic the planning that went into meeting specific community desires is obvious. "Cribs, playpens, and a baby-sitter are available for the children while their mothers wait to see the doctor. Coffee is served by our clinic aide, Tommie, who lives two blocks away. Tommie brings her own year-old daughter, so that she can work an eight-hour day. While waiting, the women may be shown a pertinent sound filmstrip or color slides made by the center staff. They may discuss with Tommie and the public health nurse the pictures, diets, or sample intrauterine contraceptive devices displayed on the walls. They may go to the kitchen to observe a bath demonstration using one of the center babies. Group discussion is encouraged and enjoyed. Increasingly, we are filtering more health information through Tommie, who is a most effective intermediary."

PROJECTS IN OTHER COUNTRIES

Understanding what a particular group of mothers value and what motivates them can solve specific problems as well as long-range ones. Although both of the examples that follow are drawn from experiences outside the United States, the situations are similar to those many nurses have met or will meet.

Prenatal care in Mexican health centers In Mexico City's prenatal programs, the major goals were to (1) persuade women to come to the health centers at the first sign of pregnancy and to return at regular intervals until delivery, and (2) to promote hospital delivery rather than home delivery.

One hospital in the city, the Maternidad Isidro Espinosa de los Reyes, is considered the most prestigious of the government hospitals because of its location in an elegant section of the city. If a woman comes to the health center early in pregnancy and keeps all of her appointments, she receives a card entitling her to delivery at this hospital. Women who delay their prenatal care or who are less regular in attendance are admitted to hospitals that offer competent medical care but are located in less affluent neighborhoods. In a study of the factors influencing mothers to use government maternity services, Garcia found that many mothers carefully followed the rule of the health center for the status they gained by having their infants born at the prestigious hospital (Foster 1969).

The distribution of powdered milk in a Venezuelan health clinic Powdered milk has been distributed in many areas of the world as well as in the United States in an attempt to improve nutrition at relatively low cost. In Venezuela powdered milk was distributed at maternal-child health clinics for nutritional purposes and as an incentive and a reward for faithful attendance. Clinic attendance did indeed improve, but there was little evidence of change in nutritional status. Investigation revealed that rather than drinking the milk, mothers were exchanging it for adult food and liquor. Several factors were found to be responsible.

1. Giving powdered milk implied that the mother's breast milk was inadequate and threatened her role as a mother.

2. The mothers were never shown how to mix the milk or how to incorporate it into other foods.

3. Some mothers felt that by exhanging the milk for other food, the whole family, not just the mother and baby, would share in the benefits of a government program.

Clinic nurses then began to spend more time teaching the mothers how to mix and use the milk powder; they awarded prizes for ingenious ideas from the mothers themselves; and they began to open cans of milk before giving them to the mothers, so that it was more difficult to exchange them. As a result of these steps milk consumption seemed to increase (Foster 1969).

Summary

Cultural beliefs determine to a large extent the way in which all of us view every aspect of our lives. The term *ethnocentrism* describes the fact that all people believe that the ways of their group are better than those of any other group. Nurses in the United States are the products of a particular cultural point of view. From this cultural heritage, they have derived certain ideas about infant care (as well as other aspects of life) that are seen as "right" or "best." It is very important for nurses to recognize their cultural "biases."

On the other hand, some of the mothers for whom nurses care have grown up with cultural beliefs that are very different from their own. They in turn are likely to feel that their ways are correct and the ways of the nurse are strange, or that the nurse does not understand their beliefs. The clash of beliefs between nurses and mothers can be a real barrier to health care for infants.

At times the beliefs of other cultural groups, like our own, are helpful; at other times they are detrimental. When we see people practicing beliefs that we feel are detrimental we want to change both belief and action. But ignoring or ridiculing the ideas of other groups is rarely successful in bringing about change. Such an approach may very likely break down communication. The mother may simply take her baby home and fail to return. Other barriers between mother and nurse include a lack of knowledge of the ideas of other groups, differences in language, and differences in level of education.

Nurses can help lower the barriers to good health for newborns in a number of ways.

1. Nurses can treat every mother with dignity and as a person rather than a case, regardless of how poor she seems to be, of how inadequately she speaks English, and of any other factor that makes her seem "different."

2. They can talk to each mother so that she can understand. This may mean understanding a different language, such as Spanish, or understanding the idiomatic use of the English language. The latter is equally as important as the former. Conversing with a mother who talks of cooking her "salat" with fat-back and serving it with the "pot licker" can be as difficult as conversing in a foreign tongue.

3. They can understand the social organization of the families with whom they work so that they will see why in some families the mother must defer decisions about the baby to the father and in others to the family group.

4. They can recognize the importance of "traditional" cultural beliefs in people's lives and realize that ridiculing or ignoring them not only serves no useful purpose but injures the pride of the mother. There are times when these beliefs can be incorporated into the health practices nurses wish to encourage. For example, suppose nurses feel that all the water given to a particular baby should be boiled, perhaps because they know that the water supply used by the family comes from a questionable source. But the mother has been lax in boiling the water, and the baby may even have diarrhea. If the mother follows a tradition of giving an herb tea for illness, she can be encouraged to boil the water, to which she can add the tiniest bit of herb, giving the baby only this boiled water. Thus the medical goal has been achieved within the framework of the cultural tradition.

5. By responding to needs felt and expressed first by the mothers, nurses can begin to bring about practices they feel are important. Both Aichlmayr's work with the reservation Indians and Milio's project in the Detroit ghetto illustrate this well.

6. They can try to understand the role expected of them by mothers of different cultural heritages and work within these expectations insofar as possible. This may mean, for example, that nurses slow the pace of activity — admittedly a very difficult thing for many nurses to do — so that they can observe the necessary social amenities essential to rapport. To the mother for whom "el tiempo ando" (time walks), the nurse's attitude of "time flies" can seem brusque at the very least. But in the long run, such an approach may prove more economical in terms of time, because if the mother has accepted the health suggestions made and is raising a healthy baby, she will not have to seek the nurse's help as frequently.

7. When a cultural change seems important for health and safety reasons, focusing on concrete behavior patterns and specific practices has been found more effective (Harrison, Tymrak, and Friedman 1978). If individuals can make a public commitment (such as the raising of hands in a class) to a proposed change, the acceptance of that change has been shown to be increased (Lewin, 1958).

Working with parents and babies from a diversity of cultural backgrounds adds richness and depth to nursing careers. However, if we underestimate the role played by culture in the lives of all people, we will never be able to adequately care for infants and their parents in the fullest sense. When cultural values differ extensively from our own, we may not even be able to establish basic communication. And if we cannot do this, all of us — family, baby, and nurse — will be losers.

Bibliography

Adair, J., Euschle, K.: The People's Health: Medicine and Anthropology in a Navajo Community. New York: Appleton-Century-Crofts, 1970.
Aichlmayr, R. H.: Cultural understanding: a key to acceptance. Nurs Outlook 17:20, 1969.

Baca, J. E.: Some health beliefs of the Spanish-speaking. Am J Nurs 69:2172, 1969.

Bartlett, F.: Infants and Children: Their Feeding and Growth. New York: Farrar & Rinehart, 1932.

Bell, D.: A Time to Be Born. New York: William Morrow, 1975.

Biddle, B., Thomas, E.: Role Theory: Concepts and Research. New York: John Wiley & Sons, 1966.

Burr, W., Leigh, G., Day, R., Constantine, J.: Symbolic interaction and the family. In Contemporary Theories About the Family. Vol. 2, W. Burr, R. Hill, F. I. Nye, and I. L. Reiss (eds.). New York: Free Press, 1979.

Cahill, I.: The Mother from the Slum Neighborhood. Columbus, Ohio: Ross Laboratories Conference on Maternal and Child Nursing, 1964.

Christensen, H. (ed.): Handbook of Marriage and the Family. Chicago: Rand McNally, 1964.

Clark, A., Affonso, D.: Childbearing: A Nursing Perspective. 2nd Edition. Philadelphia: F. A. Davis, 1979.

Clark, J.: North Carolina superstitions. N C Folklore XIV, I:3, 1966.

Clark, M.: Health in the Mexican-American Culture. Berkeley: University of California Press, 1959.

Condry, J., Condry, G.: Sex differences: a study of the eye of the beholder. Child Devel 47:812–819, 1976.

Cunningham, M. P., Weatherly, P.: We went to Mississippi. Am J Nurs 67:801, 1967.

Ellis, D.: The Hobbesian problem of order: a critical appraisal of the normative solution. Am Soc Rev 36:692–703, 1971.

England, N. C., Daugherty, M. C.: Prenatal care in North Florida Negro dialect. Unpublished, 1970.

Eshelman, J.: The Family: An Introduction. Boston: Allyn & Bacon, 1974.

Farris, L.: The American Indian. In Culture, Childbearing, Health Professionals, A. Clark, (ed.). Philadelphia: F. A. Davis, 1978.

Foster, G. M.: Applied Anthropology. Boston: Little, Brown, 1969.

Gebbie, K. (ed.): Classification of Nursing Diagnoses. Summary of the Second National Conference. St. Louis: Clearinghouse, National Group for Classification of Nursing Diagnoses, 1976.

Gerwitz, S., Dodge, K.: Adults' evaluations of a child as a function of sex of adult and sex of child. J Pers Soc Psychol 32:822–828, 1975.

Goode, W.: A theory of role strain. Am Sociol Rev 25:488–496, 1960.

Harrison, G., Tymrak, M., Friedman, G.: The Riverside school heart project: a laboratory in applied medical anthropology. In The Anthropology of Health, E. Bouwens, (ed.). St. Louis: C. V. Mosby, 1978.

Hochstein, G.: Pica: a study in medical and anthropological explanation. In Essays on Medical Anthropology, T. Weaver, (ed.). Athens: University of Georgia Press, 1968.

Hoffman, L.: Parental power relations and the division of household tasks. In The Employed Mother in America, F. Nye and L. Hoffman (eds.). Chicago: Rand McNally, 1963.

Hoffman, L., Manis, J.: The value of children in the United States: a new approach to the study of fertility. J Marriage Fam 41:583–596, 1979.

Jacobson, P.: The Y Family. Am J Nurs 69:1951, 1969.

Jensen, M., Benson, R., Bobak, J.: Maternity Care: The Nurse and the Family. St. Louis: C. V. Mosby, 1977.

Kay, M.: The Mexican-American. In Culture, Childbearing, Health Professionals, A. Clark, (ed.). Philadelphia: F. A. Davis, 1978.

Kreig, M.: Green Medicine. New York: Rand McNally, 1964.

Lackey, C.: Pica — a nutritional anthropology concern. In The Anthropology of Health, E. Bauwens (ed.). St. Louis: C. V. Mosby, 1978.

Lamb, M.: Influence of the child on marital quality and family interaction during the prenatal, perinatal and infancy period. In Child Influences on Marital and Family Interaction: A Life-Span Perspective, R. Lerner and G. Spanier (eds.). New York: Academic Press, 1978.

LaRossa, R.: Conflict and Power in Marriage: Expecting the First Child. Beverly Hills: Sage, 1977.

Lerner, R., Spanier, G. (eds.): Child Influences on Marital and Family Interaction: A Life-Span Perspective. New York: Academic Press, 1978.

Lewin, K.: Group decision and social change. In Readings in Social Psychology, E. Maccoby, T. Newcomb, and E. Hartley (eds.). New York: Holt, Rinehart and Winston, 1958.

Li, S., White, R.: The Presence of Geophagy in North Carolina. Unpublished, 1970.

Marquez, M. N., and Pacheco, C.: Midwifery lore in New Mexico. Am J Nurs 64:81, 1964.

Melville, K.: Communes in the Counter Culture: Origins, Theories, Styles of Life. New York: William Morrow, 1972.

Milio, N.: Project in a Negro ghetto. Am J Nurs 67:1007, 1967.

Moore, M. L.: Realities in Childbearing. Philadelphia: W. B. Saunders, 1978.

Nye, F., Hoffman, L.: (eds.): The Employed Mother in America. Chicago: Rand McNally, 1963.

Obeyesekere, G.: Pregnancy cravings (Dola-Duka) in relation to social structure and personality in a Sinhalese village. Am Anthropol 65:323, 1963.

Parsons, T. The Social System. New York: Free Press, 1951.

Pitts, J.: The structural-functional approach. In Handbook of Marriage and the Family, H. Christensen (ed.). Chicago: Rand McNally, 1964.

Prugh, P. H.: A yearning for clay by pregnant women alarms some doctors. Wall St J, Dec. 10, 1969.

Rapoport, R., Rapoport, R.: Dual-Career Families Re-examined. New York: Harper & Row, 1976.

Reeder, S., Mastroianni, L., Martin, L., Fitzpatrick, E.: Maternity Nursing. 13th Edition. Philadelphia: J. B. Lippincott, 1976.

Rodman, H.: Marital power and the theory of resources in cultural context. J Comp Fam Stud 3:50–67, 1972.

Rose, P.: The Chinese American. In Culture, Childbearing, Health Professionals, A. Clark, (ed.). Philadelphia: F. A. Davis, 1978.

Ross, C. M., Van Warmelo, N. J.: Bantu concepts of skin disease: dermatological fact and fiction amongst the Venda. Arch Dermatol 91:640, 1965.

Rubin, J., Provenzano, F., Luria, Z.: The eye of the beholder: parents' views on sex of newborns. Am J Orthopsychiatry 44:512–519, 1974.

Sarbin, R., & Allen, V.: Role enactment, audience feedback, and attitude change. Sociometry 27:183–193, 1964.

Saunders, L., Hewes, G.: Folk medicine and medical practice. J Med Educ 28:43, 1953.

Scanzoni, J.: A historical perspective on husband-wife bargaining power and marital dissolution. *In* Divorce and Separation, G. Levinger and D. Moles, (eds.). New York: Basic Books, 1979.

Scanzoni, J.: Sex Roles, Life-Styles, and Childbearing: Changing Patterns in Marriage and Family. New York, Free Press, 1975.

Scanzoni, L., Scanzoni, J.: Men, Women and Change: A Sociology of Marriage and the Family. New York: McGraw-Hill, 1976.

Scott, C.: Health and healing practices among five ethnic groups in Miami, Florida. Public Health Rep. 89:524, 1974.

Seavey, C., Katz, P., and Zalk, S.: Baby X: the effect of gender labels on adult responses to infants. Sex Roles 1:103–109, 1975.

Seham, M.: Poverty, illness and the Negro child. Pediatrics 46:305, 1970.

Sevcovic, L.: Traditions of pregnancy which influence maternity care of the Navajo people. *In* Transcultural Nursing Care of Infants and Children, M. Leininger (ed.). Salt Lake City: University of Utah College of Nursing, 1977.

Sidorowicz, L., & Lunney, G.: Baby X revisited. Sex Roles 6:67–73, 1980.

Spiegel, J. The resolution of role conflict within the family. *In* The Patient and the Mental Hospital, M. Greenblatt, D. Levinson, and R. Williams. (eds.). New York: Free Press, 1957.

Starch and clay as food. Sci News 95:35, 1969.

Stringfellow, L.: The Vietnamese. *In* Culture, Childbearing, Health Professionals, Clark, A. (ed.). Philadelphia: F. A. Davis, 1978.

Turner, R.: Role-taking; process versus conformity. *In* Human Behavior and Social Processes, Rose, A., (ed.). Boston: Houghton Mifflin, 1962.

Veysey, L.: The Communal Experience: Anarchist and Mystical Counter-Cultures in America. New York: Harper & Row, 1973.

Watts, W.: Social class, ethnic background, and patient care. Nurs Forum VI:155, 1967.

White, I.: The Frank C. Brown Collection of North Carolina Folklore, Vol. 6. Durham: Duke University Press, 1961.

Wingert, W., Grubbs, J., Friedman, D.: Why Johnny's parents don't read. Clin Pediatr 8:655, 1969.

Wolfenstein, M.: Trends in infant care. Am J Orthopsychiatry 33:120, 1953.

Ziegel, E., Cranley, W.: Obstetric Nursing 7th Edition. New York: Macmillan, 1978.

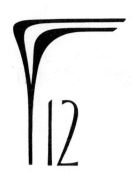

PERINATAL NURSING — YESTERDAY, TODAY, AND TOMORROW

by
*Karen G. Galloway, R.N., M.S.N.**

Technology

The field of perinatology resembles the aerospace industry in one respect — the changes that have occurred in both fields in the last 15 years are mind boggling! Today, most of us do not give a second thought to satellites, manned space flights, or even daily weather maps of the entire country — photographed by the ever-present satellite.

Similarly, rarely do we realize that just about 15 years ago a new medical field was born. Neonatal intensive care units and maternal monitoring during labor were new concepts at the time. Prepared childbirth classes were not yet accepted in many hospitals, and a husband in the delivery room was unthinkable. The world of obstetrics and the new field of neonatology were closed, enigmatic, and profession oriented.

These developments, however, marked the beginning of a totally new approach to

*Karen G. Galloway was formerly an Assistant Professor in the Graduate Program at the University of Arkansas for Medical Sciences College of Nursing in Little Rock, Arkansas. Her previous experience included working for two years as Maternal-Fetal Clinical Nurse Specialist at the Wisconsin Perinatal Center, South Central Region, in Madison, Wisconsin; and teaching maternity nursing in the baccalaureate programs at the University of Missouri-Columbia, Michigan State University, and the University of Wisconsin-Madison.

care during childbearing. During the last 15 years, new knowledge and attitudes have made it possible for the discipline of perinatology to emerge.

In the 1970s, research was conducted on the relationships between fetal and neonatal risk and the medical complications of pregnancy. Maternal intensive care programs were established, emphasizing careful supervision during the prenatal and intrapartum periods.

Knowledge concerning maternal high risk criteria increased, as did the technology for detecting fetal distress. Fetal monitoring, while questioned by patients seeking natural birth, became invaluable for the pregnant woman in danger of losing her fetus; such monitoring aids not only in fetal assessment but in reassuring the mother by allowing her to hear her baby's heartbeat.

The use of the fetal monitor to assess placental function is now a common practice. As described in Chapter 3, the nonstress and oxytocin challenge tests are major advances in fetal assessment. Another test of placental function is the determination of the serum or urinary estriol level. Major advances in ultrasonography that enable professionals to assess gestational age, breathing movements, and other fetal characteristics, including sex, are also described in Chapter 3.

In addition to advances in perinatal knowledge and technology, progress in other fields has greatly contributed to the care of the pregnant woman with specific medical complications. An excellent example is the care of the pregnant woman with diabetes. Currently, clinical research is being done utilizing assessment of hemoglobin A_1 to provide data on the patient's blood glucose levels for the preceding six to eight weeks, not just the usual single check. Portable insulin infusion pumps that administer insulin over a two-month period are being tested, and an artificial pancreas is being investigated for use in labor. The intravenous infusion system continuously measures the blood glucose level and delivers insulin or glucose on the basis of the patient's need (Pfeiffer, Kerner, and Beischer 1979).

Neonatal technology has also progressed rapidly during this 15-year period. Major advances and current clinical research are described in Chapter 8.

The late 1960s and the 1970s were indeed filled with space-age advancements in technology. Yet there was another movement occurring simultaneously: a growing interest in consumer knowledge and increasing pressure for consumer participation.

Consumer Power

As women assumed more responsibilities outside the home, their mates began to share the childrearing and homemaking tasks (although behind closed doors in the beginning). Parents wanted more knowledge about childrearing. They asked the reasons for old-fashioned methods, and if dissatisfied they tried new approaches.

Similarly, couples sought to increase their knowledge of childbearing, from the beginning of pregnancy through labor and delivery. Childbirth preparation classes based on the theories of Lamaze and others were organized and taught to interested parents-to-be. Emphasis was placed on education and relaxation to prepare for labor and delivery. Fathers became "coaches," and were pleased—if

slightly trepidatious—at the reprieve from the "Vice President of Pregnancy" position: at long last, they had a role in more than the conception in this childbearing process!

The classes were a success. Suddenly physicians and hospitals were being asked by pregnant patients, "Can my husband/partner be with me in the labor room? In the delivery room?" If the answer was "No," the couple sought another physician and hospital. Physicians and hospitals put up a battle but, in the end, when few cases of "fainting fathers" actually materialized, the policy book was rewritten. Family-centered care was born.

In an effort to help parents get to know and be able to care for their baby prior to discharge, rooming-in programs were established. The father of the baby was permitted — and then encouraged — to hold, feed, and learn to take care of his child. Visiting hours were relaxed for fathers and eventually opened to siblings in many hospitals. In certain perinatal centers, even parents of a high risk neonate may now spend a couple of days rooming-in with their infant prior to discharge.

In addition, new concepts of increasing the natural and family-oriented attitudes toward birth have arisen. Labor and postpartum units are now designed to look more natural and homelike. In some hospitals, siblings and other family members and friends participate in the birth. Many hospitals have combination labor and delivery rooms, called "birthing rooms."

In some birthing centers, parents are admitted for the labor and delivery and then discharged within 12 hours postpartum if both mother and infant are normal. Other areas of the country have a large number of home deliveries attended by lay or nurse midwives.

Consumer activities and enthusiastic participation in educational groups and family-centered care are not limited to natural births. Couples who had prepared themselves for a normal labor and delivery but instead required cesarean section recognized a need for support and education following such a birth. They organized groups to allow parents to express their feelings about their experiences with cesarean births, and the groups often utilize professional resources to help educate members about how and why cesareans are done and the implications for future pregnancies. Many childbirth preparation classes also include information about the possibility of a cesarean birth.

Consumers alone, of course, did not achieve all these changes in the care of families expecting a child. Although many physicians, hospitals, and (although I hate to admit it) nurses opposed these changes in the beginning, some professionals recognized that with preparation and support, there were behavioral differences in the mother during pregnancy and delivery. These professionals became leaders and client advocates in the prepared childbirth and family-centered care movements.

The extent of this commitment to the pregnant woman and her child was exemplified by the development of a document proclaiming the rights of the pregnant patient. The "Pregnant Patient's Bill of Rights" describes the rights of the pregnant woman to information, participation in decision making, support in labor and birth, care of her infant, and access to her own medical records (American Hospital Association, 1977).

Regionalization

With advancing technology, some hospitals — often university medical centers — were able to acquire the latest equipment and techniques for caring for high risk neonates. Accordingly, when infants with problems were born in nearby hospitals, they were sent to the medical centers. These neonatal intensive care units were frequently developed without the forethought or knowledge that this would be the beginning of a regional perinatal plan.

As mortality rates were studied and referral problems multiplied, it became obvious that equipment and skilled professionals in one center were not sufficient

to supply all aspects of high risk care. In Wisconsin, as in some other states, special studies were done to determine the current status of care in the state, mortality rates, professional resources, and causes of perinatal mortality that might be prevented (Callon 1975). Following this study, the concept of a perinatal center that would meet the needs of the state was developed.

The Perinatal Center in the Wisconsin plan is the unit which assumes responsibility for educating health care professionals in the region in the area of antepartum, intrapartum, postpartum and neonatal care. It assumes responsibility for the complete and comprehensive health care of high-risk or seriously ill mothers or neonates throughout the hospital stay. This includes not only the health care of the baby, but the education of the parents and any other personnel who may be involved with the infant following discharge from the hospital.

The center also works with the primary physician, local public health personnel and hospitals for the follow-up of the high risk mothers and newborns. Thus, the center is not a repository in which sick patients are placed, but rather an institution in which education, current and comprehensive medical and nursing care and ongoing study and evaluation of all facets of perinatal health care are coordinated and carried out with a responsibility for an entire region within the state (Callon, 1975, p. 267).

On the basis of this concept, perinatal teams went out to the community hospitals in the state and presented educational programs and conferences regarding care of the neonate in the first few hours of life, emphasizing early identification of risk factors, thermoregulation, early referral, and preparation and care en route. Neonatal transport units were developed to provide skilled professionals who would care for the neonate in transit to the intensive care unit. Private physicians in the community were enlisted as associates and were recognized as the "first line" in prevention/detection of problems.

Attention was also focused on the high risk mother. High risk criteria were identified, and more community education programs were instituted, emphasizing early identification and referral of the woman with a high risk pregnancy. Maternal intensive care programs were established, including prenatal clinics. Whenever it was appropriate, the local referring physician would continue to provide part of the prenatal care, with intermittent checks at the maternal intensive care clinic. For more severe high risk conditions, such as diabetes, the mother received all her prenatal care at the regional center, with reports sent to her referring physician.

The planners of this regional perinatal center also developed a highly specialized perinatal team. In addition to the neonatologists, obstetricians, and perinatologists who provided the medical expertise, there was recognition of the need for specialized nursing, dietary, and social work support. Accordingly, a dietitian and social worker were placed on the team caring for high risk mothers and neonates.

Neonatal and maternal/fetal clinical nurse specialists were added to the nursing staff. In addition, a nurse clinician program was developed and funded to prepare neonatal and obstetrical nurses for high risk care (Aure and Schneider 1975; Schneider, Ziegel, and Patteson 1975). The clinical nurse specialists and nurse clinicians would become the nursing team that now help provide continuity, individuality, and advocacy in caring for the high risk pregnant woman and her family. Their roles include direct patient care, patient education, staff education, and active teaching in workshops and educational programs within the region.

The Maternal Intensive Care Program in Madison, Wisconsin, at the South Central Regional Perinatal Center provides the opportunity for families to receive genetic counseling and amniocentesis for possible defects; carefully monitored care throughout the prenatal period; diagnosis of fetal maturity via history, physical assessment, ultrasound study, and amniotic fluid analysis; carefully monitored labor (or treatment for premature labor); and follow-up care.

One of the reasons this program is so effective is its communication system. The maternal/fetal specialized team meets for weekly conferences after the maternal intensive care clinic and discusses each patient seen within the past week; the team discusses present status, recent changes, proposed treatment, and long-term plans. These discussions are documented on the patient's chart so that no matter when the patient is admitted or which member of the team is caring for her there is no doubt about the plan of care for her. Whenever possible, members of the neonatology team also attend the conferences, to give opinions on the effects of a woman's present problems on the fetus or to report on the current status of infants in the neonatal intensive care unit.

This permanent perinatal team is augmented by other auxiliary professionals when necessary — endocrinologists, cardiologists, ophthalmologists, etc. Their recommendations are also documented on the patient's record and discussed in the weekly conferences.

In addition to the initial community education efforts, the center employed an outreach nurse, who continuously visited the outlying hospitals with a physician who was designated as having outreach responsibilities. This team assessed problems or educational needs and planned outreach programs addressing both maternal and neonatal topics.

Wisconsin's system has been very effective in decreasing the perinatal mortality rate in that state and is well known for the successful outcomes for both mothers and infants at high risk. Each state may set up a very different system and utilize other approaches in an attempt to decrease mortality rates and provide high quality care to women at risk. Some states are just beginning the regionalization of perinatal care and have not yet developed their basic concepts.

Perinatal care, and even the process of regionalization, continues to be plagued by some very persistent problems, which thus far have withstood all efforts at solution. Addressing these problems will become our goal for the next decade.

Persistent Problems

The most urgent, frustrating, and difficult problem remains an unreversed high perinatal mortality rate. Mortality and morbidity rates continue to decrease in the United States and other nations; however, the United States is still lagging far behind advanced countries (Fig. 12–1; Tables 12–1, 12–2).

Why, with all of our resources and technology, can we not show more significant progress in reducing perinatal morbidity and mortality? One reason is the divergence of economic resources in various regions of the country. Those states with low standards of living have higher mortality rates; those states with higher standards of living and well-developed perinatal systems have lower mortality rates.

In addition to the problems of poverty and inadequate living conditions, many people in those states with high mortality rates have never been educated in health care or health maintenance. Since they have to pay for health care, they may delay seeking prenatal care until late in the pregnancy. Thus, patients with significant high risk factors may not receive prenatal care until near term or even until labor begins. Still others deliver at home with lay help or no help at all. Clients who are seen in high risk clinics often have a history of previous stillbirths at home. The actual perinatal mortality rate may be even higher than statistics demonstrate, since some of the births, stillbirths, and deaths may go unreported.

These families may have no means of transportation, so that even if they sought medical attention, they would have difficulty reaching the facilities. For many rural communities, there is no public transportation — no taxis, bus service, trains, etc. The only way to travel is by car *if* the family can afford the gas, or perhaps they may be able to persuade a neighbor or friend to drive over tortuous roads to a hospital that will accept them — often a distance of 200 miles.

Maternal malnutrition during pregnancy is also a problem in states with much poverty. Protein intake may be almost nonexistent. If a partner is present in the home, diet may consist of whatever fish or game he can catch when weather permits and whatever vegetables they can grow. One mother who came to a high risk clinic had been eating soup and cereal for the past two weeks because she had no money for other food. It is not hard to imagine such a client delivering a high risk infant.

As if these problems were not enough to increase perinatal risk, they are compounded by the steadily rising adolescent pregnancy rate in the same states with high mortality rates. It is not uncommon to see pregnancies occuring at age 12 — second or third pregnancies by ages 14 or 15. In addition to the high risk nature of these pregnancies, this pattern obviously perpetuates the poverty cycle.

These factors simplistically indicate some of the problems of pregnant women that increase their perinatal risk and prevent the current perinatal morbidity and mortality rates from decreasing more rapidly. As yet, we have no solutions for these socioeconomic problems.

Another aspect that must be mentioned as a problem in the successful reduction of perinatal mortality in poverty-ridden rural states is the problem of the quantity and quality of professionals available to provide health care services. There is little financial enticement in these areas, so it is difficult to recruit leaders or specialists in the health professions. Health care may be several years or a decade behind accepted standards of practice in more progressive states. The educational institutions in these areas may also be far behind, so even recent professional graduates may not have the knowledge to provide significantly improved health care — and so again, the vicious circle continues.

An attempt is being made by some states to increase the availability of health services. The regional perinatal programs being developed by these states include "satellite" clinics — physicians and nurses who reside in or travel to various communities and provide prenatal health care at reduced or little cost to consumers. This plan allows prenatal assessment for

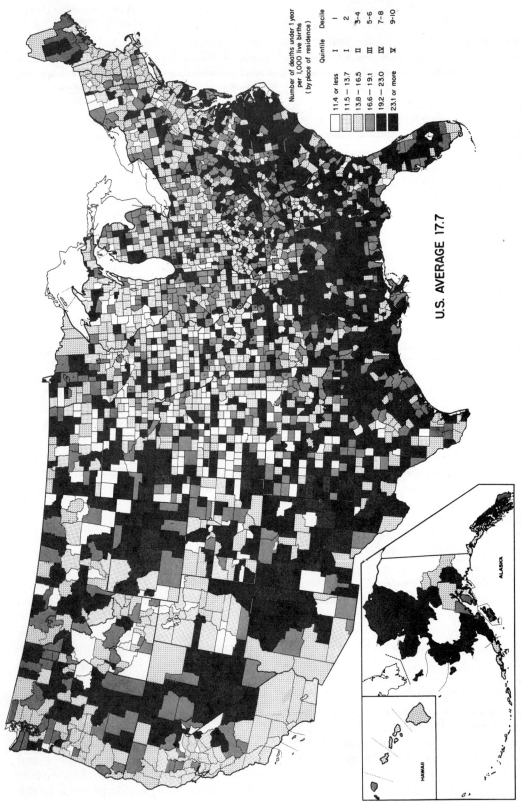

Figure 12–1. Infant mortality rates. United States and each county, average annual rate, 1971–1975. (From Infant and Perinatal Mortality Rates by Age and Race, 1966–1970, 1971–1975, prepared by Maternal and Child Health Studies Project, ISRI, Washington, D.C.)

U.S. AVERAGE 17.7

Number of deaths under 1 year
per 1,000 live births
(by place of residence)

	Quintile	Decile
11.4 or less	I	1
11.5 — 13.7	I	2
13.8 — 16.5	II	3–4
16.6 — 19.1	III	5–6
19.2 — 23.0	IV	7–8
23.1 or more	V	9–10

ALASKA

HAWAII

Table 12–1   Infant Death Rates — United States: 1960–1977*†

State	1960 White	1960 Black and Other	1970 White	1970 Black and Other	1977 White	1977 Black and Other
United States	**22.9**	**43.2**	**17.8**	**30.9**	**12.3**	**21.7**
New England	**21.7**	**35.2**	**16.8**	**30.3**	**11.3**	**19.1**
Maine·	25.7	12.9‡	21.0	25.0‡	9.6	4.1‡
New Hampshire	23.7	10.6‡	18.0	20.5‡	10.2	6.2‡
Vermont	24.2	—	17.6	19.2‡	10.0	—
Massachusetts	21.2	34.4	16.0	31.4	11.6	16.7
Rhode Island	22.4	44.4	19.3	27.7	11.2	24.0
Connecticut	20.0	36.9	15.5	30.4	12.2	22.2
Middle Atlantic	**22.0**	**41.4**	**17.3**	**31.7**	**12.3**	**22.4**
New York	21.5	41.6	16.9	30.2	12.3	21.7
New Jersey	21.9	41.7	16.9	33.0	11.8	24.0
Pennsylvania	22.6	40.6	18.2	34.2	12.6	22.9
Eastern North Central	**22.1**	**39.4**	**17.8**	**31.0**	**12.5**	**23.4**
Ohio	22.2	39.4	17.2	28.7	12.7	21.0
Indiana	22.6	37.7	18.5	27.8	13.3	21.6
Illinois	22.2	39.6	18.3	33.6	13.0	26.1
Michigan	22.1	40.4	18.6	30.4	12.2	23.1
Wisconsin	21.2	35.3	16.0	29.8	10.8	17.8
Western North Central	**21.7**	**42.5**	**17.3**	**31.4**	**12.2**	**21.6**
Minnesota	21.6	22.6	17.3	24.0	10.8	17.0
Iowa	21.7	35.2	18.3	31.4	12.2	18.0
Missouri	21.4	45.4	17.0	33.4	12.4	23.6
North Dakota	24.1	43.3	14.3	14.3‡	12.6	27.3
South Dakota	24.2	76.0	16.7	37.3	14.8	26.4
Nebraska	21.3	34.3	18.5	34.6	12.6	14.2
Kansas	21.3	33.4	16.7	27.5	12.8	19.4
Southern Atlantic	**23.6**	**47.2**	**18.0**	**32.6**	**12.6**	**23.0**
Delaware	17.8	50.6	16.3	31.6	11.4	20.8
Maryland	22.3	44.6	16.4	29.0	11.5	20.6
District of Columbia	29.4	39.6	26.3	29.5	15.0	29.7
Virginia	24.6	45.5	17.0	33.3	13.3	23.4
West Virginia	24.8	37.7	22.8	27.7	14.3	20.9
North Carolina	22.3	52.4	19.3	36.1	12.2	23.3
South Carolina	23.9	48.5	18.2	31.1·	13.1	24.2
Georgia	24.6	48.1	17.2	32.9	12.5	20.4
Florida	23.6	46.1	17.8	33.2	12.2	24.0
Eastern South Central	**25.6**	**48.4**	**18.7**	**35.2**	**13.3**	**23.5**
Kentucky	26.0	48.3	18.8	27.8	13.7	21.0
Tennessee	25.3	43.5	18.8	30.6	13.3	22.6
Alabama	24.9	45.0	18.6	36.0	13.4	23.6
Mississippi	26.6	54.3	18.7	39.2	12.1	24.6
Western South Central	**24.9**	**44.3**	**19.6**	**31.4**	**13.1**	**23.2**
Arkansas	22.5	38.7	18.3	31.1	12.3	24.4
Louisiana	22.6	46.9	19.8	32.3	12.4	26.2
Oklahoma	22.7	42.8	20.3	26.3	12.7	17.7
Texas	26.3	43.9	19.6	31.8	13.4	21.7
Mountain	**25.7**	**51.7**	**18.1**	**27.0**	**11.9**	**17.1**
Montana	24.2	34.5	21.2	24.7	13.6	14.7
Idaho	22.7	33.3‡	17.3	11.6‡	11.3	10.9‡
Wyoming	27.5	48.6‡	19.6	27.6‡	13.9	13.1‡
Colorado	26.9	44.0	19.7	23.5	11.9	14.3
New Mexico	30.9	52.8	19.5	28.9	12.9	18.7
Arizona	26.6	60.8	16.0	28.0	12.4	19.3
Utah	18.8	54.0	14.9	17.5‡	9.9	14.6‡
Nevada	29.6	33.9	22.2	37.0	13.5	16.4
Pacific	**22.6**	**30.5**	**16.7**	**21.9**	**11.6**	**14.4**
Washington	22.7	36.7	18.1	26.4	11.9	14.1
Oregon	23.0	29.2	16.0	14.1	12.0	14.7
California	22.5	29.7	16.5	22.1	11.4	15.0
Alaska	27.9	68.2	20.3	29.0	14.7	16.3
Hawaii	21.5	24.0	17.8	18.9	10.5	11.8

*Deaths per 1000 live births by place or residence. Represents deaths under 1 year old, exclusive of fetal deaths. Beginning with 1970, excludes deaths of nonresidents of the United States.
†From Statistical Abstracts of the United States, 1979, p. 75. U.S. Department of Commerce, Bureau of the Census.
‡Based on a frequency of less than 20 deaths.

Table 12–2 Infant Mortality Rates* by health service area,† 1971–1975‡

State						Health Service Area								
	1	2	3	4	5	6	7	8	9	10	11	12	13	14
Alabama	19.6	21.1	19.0	23.1	25.6	21.5	22.2							
Alaska	17.5	17.4	19.3											
Arizona	15.7	14.1	22.4	22.9	14.6									
Arkansas	16.8	19.1	18.7	20.2										
California	14.6	14.4	14.7	13.5	14.8	14.5	13.2	14.1	16.9	13.7	15.0	15.9	13.7	14.9
Colorado	15.2	18.9	17.8											
Connecticut	15.7	15.7	15.9	15.7	15.0									
Delaware	16.4													
District of Columbia	27.4													
Florida	20.0	18.9	18.6	17.9	18.2	21.5	21.7	17.8	16.3					
Georgia	19.5	20.0	17.5	18.5	22.2	20.7	20.8							
Hawaii	14.9													
Idaho	15.8													
Illinois	17.5	17.9	17.1	19.3	17.7	25.4	15.0	16.4	18.8	17.9	18.7			
Indiana	18.8	16.5	16.9											
Iowa	15.6	17.3	17.9											
Kansas	16.9	14.6	18.5	16.3										
Kentucky	16.7	18.4	15.5											
Louisiana	21.1	19.5	20.6											
Maine	16.5													
Maryland	17.5	12.4	16.4	17.0	19.1									
Massachusetts	15.1	15.1	14.1	15.6	14.0	14.2								
Michigan	19.0	16.3	17.9	16.3	19.1	17.1	15.2	14.8						
Minnesota	16.7	16.4	15.5	15.3	15.2	16.2	15.9							
Mississippi	24.9													
Missouri	16.3	17.6	18.7	17.6	20.0									
Montana	18.7													
Nebraska	16.6	12.6	17.3	15.6										
Nevada	19.9	18.7												
New Hampshire	15.7													
New Jersey	14.7	17.9	19.6	15.2	17.8									
New Mexico	18.6	22.9												
New York	18.0	14.9	16.6	16.0	15.4	15.0	19.1	13.7						
North Carolina	22.0	19.4	20.0	19.4	22.0	22.5								
North Dakota	16.1	16.7	15.5											
Ohio	15.5	17.2	18.6	17.8	16.9	17.2	17.0	16.2	18.2	17.6				
Oklahoma	17.5													
Oregon	16.0	15.5	17.9											
Pennsylvania	19.1	14.9	17.5	14.4	18.1	16.7	17.4	16.0	18.3					
Rhode Island	17.4													
South Carolina	20.1	21.5	26.8	18.8	18.5									
South Dakota	18.5													
Tennessee	18.1	18.4	19.5	17.6	20.8	21.1								
Texas	20.4	23.9	16.5	21.4	18.7	18.5	22.4	17.6	17.4	20.9	18.2	20.8		
Utah	13.0	22.9												
Vermont	14.4													
Virginia	18.2	15.0	19.9	19.4	20.5	18.1								
Washington	15.9	16.2	17.8	18.8										
West Virginia	19.3													
Wisconsin	14.0	14.7	13.4	15.0	14.8	13.4	16.4							
Wyoming	20.2													

*Rates per 1,000 live births.
†Health service areas that cross state boundaries are shown in each state; rates are for entire interstate health service area
‡From Infant and Perinatal Mortality Rates by Age and Race, 1966–1970, 1971–1975, p. xiv. Maternal and Child Health Studies Project, ISRI, Washington, D.C., 1978.

risk factors and, if high risk factors are discovered, the patient may be referred to a perinatal center.

Other states are utilizing nurse-midwives to provide prenatal care, risk assessment, and delivery for patients. England and other countries have utilized this system successfully for many years. In the United States, the Frontier Nursing Service in Kentucky is well known for its midwives, who provide maternal-child care to the families who live in this region.

In addition to the persistent problems involved in providing prenatal and intrapartum care to these high risk families in high risk environments, we are now much more cognizant of what occurs *after* this child is born. The reality of child abuse, neglect, and failure to thrive of certain infants has been known for some time. Recently, studies have begun to identify those populations that are at risk for parenting problems. More research needs to be done on the success of preventive interventions or very early intervention after maladaptive behaviors are noted. (Interventions to facilitate parent-infant interaction in families at risk are discussed later in this chapter.)

Finally, politics cannot be ignored when considering persistent problems in perinatal care. Politics play an important part in all aspects of health care in our society. Both federal and state governments control which health services will receive funding for personnel, programs, and research. They can choose whether or not a state will have programs in respiratory disease, family planning, well child clinics, and prenatal care.

Regionalization plans and programs have become political prizes, and many mistakes have been made in our efforts to initiate perinatal centers and regionalization programs. *Where* the perinatal center is to be located, *how many* centers will be developed, and sources of financial support are now issues to be argued, lobbied, and bargained for. The perinatal pie has often been divided as "potential financial assets" among various hospitals without consideration of what might be optimal care for families. So, we have the mother in the maternal perinatal center, the infant in the neonatal perinatal center, and often very little coordination of care, continuity, or even cooperation to provide total family care.

Another problem which has been experienced with regionalization programs is duplication of services — for instance, several hospitals establish perinatal centers independently in one community. This angers referring physicians and official planning authorities, who see this as an effort to create financial rivalry and competition between centers for the greatest number of patients. Lack of feedback, communication, and any positive reinforcement for efforts have been stated as reasons that local physicians in outlying hospitals stop referring their patients to these centers.

Besides political issues, other persistent problems remain. Racial biases are still with us and are still a problem. Minority patients or poverty patients may be provided minimal health service programs. Private physicians may refuse to see patients who are on medical assistance, so pregnant patients may be forced to wait hours to be seen in a clinic — even with an appointment. Only the physical needs may be assessed by the health care professional. Total care, even for high risk patients, may be provided by residents and interns, with no staff physician present or even consulted.

These are a few of the monumental problems and conditions in our country contributing to our lack of success in further decreasing perinatal morbidity and mortality rates. Realistically, we have significantly reduced the rates for the country overall in the past 15 to 20 years. However, our knowledge and technology indicate that we *could* reduce them even more significantly if we could overcome some of the problems in our socioeconomic and health care delivery systems.

ROLE OF THE PERINATAL NURSE

Assessment

Our lives are often complex patterns of interaction. We can no longer pretend that life is simple or that the pregnant woman exists in a vacuum. Therefore, nursing care in the perinatal period must include assessment of and intervention with other aspects of the client's life that may affect the pregnancy, the fetus, or the new family unit.

Nursing care is especially critical for the high risk or at risk parent. Mercer (1977) defines parents at risk as "parents who, because of a stressful incident occurring around the time of the birth of their infant, experience interruptions in their early parent-infant contact and interactions. As a result of these early interruptions, their acquaintance, claiming, and attachment processes, as well as their cueing-in to their infant's unique needs, are likewise interrupted."

It is difficult to imagine an area in which nursing care has more impact on a family than assessment, planning, intervention, and evaluation with the family at risk in the perinatal period. Nursing care during this period involves advocacy for this family, provision of continuity of care, and realistic problem solving with the family.

Medical efforts may well keep the pregnant diabetic patient's blood sugar at a level of less than 100, even if this means long-term hospitalization. But the physical well-being of her infant will mean little if this mother totally rejects her pregnancy and her newborn. Medical success in pulling a 14-year-old mother through severe eclampsia will likewise not help her to be a good parent. Nurses are the professionals who pick up on cues that indicate unrealistic expectations of newborns and possible future child neglect or abuse.

Because of the many and varied areas in which nursing can help the family solve problems during the childbearing cycle, it is necessary to look at nursing in a broad context during the perinatal period. How can the nurse provide the most effective care for the family expecting a child?

In many settings, it is possible for the same nurse to follow a family throughout the pregancy. This has the obvious advantages of building a trust relationship and allowing more in-depth assessment without repetition.

It is ideal if a primary nurse can be assigned at the family's first prenatal visit. This is especially important in high risk pregnant women. If at all possible, the pregnant woman and the father of the baby should be encouraged to attend the clinic together the first time. Again, ideally, the initial interview with the couple by a physician and nurse should take place in an environment that is comfortable and conducive to conversation (versus the patient disrobed in a sterile-appearing cubicle). The former approach gives the nurse an idea of the client as a person and the relationship and support between the couple.

Wherever and whenever the nurse-family interview is made, assessment should include factors with potential risk to the family's psychosocial or physical well-being.

CRISIS

Crisis at birth, especially the birth of a sick infant, has been discussed in Chapter 10. Assessment of crises — or potential crises — is also part of prenatal nursing care. Are any family members undergoing maturational crises (Hessick and Aguilera 1979), i.e., is the pregnant woman a teenager entering the world of adulthood? Is the pregnant woman an "elderly primigravida" preparing to enter middlescence? Are the developmental tasks of the particular maturational stage being achieved successfully? Are maladaptive behaviors noted? Are other members of the family entering a new stage of maturational development? One of the most difficult situations for family members may be a pregnant middle-aged mother with a daughter who is going through either adolescence or a pregnancy.

Are there situational crises present within the family concurrent with the pregnancy (Hessick and Aguilera 1979)? This may affect the way the family is able to view the pregnancy. The addition of other situational crises may also make this pregnancy a crisis. Families who are experiencing loss of an income, illness of a family member, family problems, death of a loved one — any of these could, with the addition of a pregnancy, place the family in crisis.

Along with the identification of crisis or potential crisis situations, an assessment is made of the developmental level of this family and the coping patterns utilized in crises. Does the family have a "firm handle on things" and the ability to think through and evaluate possible actions? Do the individual members act independently or interdependently? Or is this family still at the level of total engrossment with meeting basic needs, turning to dependence on parents or others in times of crisis?

There may be a need to assess the family's knowledge of and ability to utilize resources in preventing or dealing with crises. Some families are unaware of avenues for support; others are unwilling to seek help; and still others fear the social stigma they feel is attached to helping agencies, personnel, or programs. Before crisis intervention can be addressed, the family's attitudes toward resources and professionals need to be identified.

STRESS

There may be many life events occurring within the family that are not seen by them as crises but nevertheless require a great deal of energy for adaptation. These "life stress events" have been described by Holmes and Rahe (1967), who also developed and tested a social readjustment rating scale. The magnitude of the life stress event, as well as the cumulative number of life stress events currently being experienced, may have implications for the health of the pregnant woman or a family member (Holmes and Masuda 1971). Certainly if nurses judge that the family is experiencing an inordinate amount of stress, they should delve more deeply into the family's adaptive and coping mechanisms and the need for additional resources.

The course of the pregnancy itself may produce additional stresses for the family. A "normal" pregnancy requires both physical and psychosocial adaptations on the part of the pregnant woman. A high risk pregnancy compounds the potential adaptation problems.

A woman who is diagnosed as having a high risk pregnancy may have difficulty in adapting to the assault on her body image; she is required to attend a special clinic designated as "high risk" or "medical complications clinic." She may have an "insulting" diagnosis, such as "elderly primigravida," "incompetent cervix," or "habitual aborter." The clinic or center where she receives care may be some distance away, requiring transportation arrangements. She may feel like a stranger in this new place, with no support from nearby friends. She may fear for the health of herself and her infant. And this medical problem may require additional tests, treatments, visits, and/or even hospitalizations — all of which add to the emotional, physical, and financial strains on the woman and her family (Galloway 1976). Thus, the high risk family may need much guidance in how to adapt to these, at times, overwhelming stressors.

ROLES

An in-depth initial assessment should also include roles within the family. In addition to the commonly assessed roles of mother, father, wife, and husband, who is the bread winner, the financial planner, the disciplinarian? What are the *demands* of the current roles? Are any of the roles requiring excessive amounts of energy at this time? Is the mother just completing her high school or college education? Are other roles demanding time, energy, commitment? One pregnant woman related that her husband had just been diagnosed as having cardiac disease and would require open heart surgery. She felt that her major role at this time was that of "wife" and "supporter" for her husband, and all other roles took on secondary significance.

When one role demands maximal time and energy, this has major implications for the family member in his or her ability to accept or adapt to new roles. The adaptation to the pregnancy and to mothering or fathering roles may be delayed, ignored, or rejected.

The reciprocity of roles within the family is also an area that commonly needs assessment. Although the pregnant woman may see her role as "mate and mother," the father of the baby may not identify with his role of "mate and/or father." At times it is very helpful for the pregnant woman and the father of the baby to explore their expectations of themselves and each other in terms of roles. If this can be accomplished during the pregnancy and they can have open discussion about the approaching roles as parents, some problems may be prevented.

Role conflict may occur during the pregnancy or postpartum. Especially after the birth of a sick infant or an infant with a defect, the woman may assume the major role of "mother," spending almost all her time with her child. The father may both be hurt by and resentful of this change, feeling a need for her major role to be "mate." This kind of role conflict can have serious significance for the future of this family.

COMMUNICATION/SUPPORT

Another area of assessment is the parents' ability to communicate effectively with each other and with their other children. Both verbal and nonverbal cues can be utilized to identify problems or potential problems in communication.

During the initial interview session, do the couple appear comfortable with each other? Is one partner the spokesperson, the other the listener? Does the conversation shift back and forth easily, or is every point argued between them? Does one partner frequently place blame on the other?

Do the couple sit close to each other; do their eyes meet for reassurance, confirmation, or permission? Does one lend physical reassurance to the other with a pat on the arm or an arm around the shoulders or by holding hands?

If the family is observed with their other children, what kind of interaction occurs between the parents and the children? On what level do they interact? Do the parents attempt to communicate, explain to the children —or is all verbal interaction "instructions" or "admonitions"? Does the family express and explore their feelings, needs, fears, and concerns with one another? Is one member the primary support person? Is one member always blamed for everything?

The family may or may not be the woman's main support system, so nurses also need to assess other resources. Besides her mate, to whom would she turn if she needed help, had an emergency, or just needed to talk? There may be a variety of resources she would utilize, depending on the need. She might feel most comfortable calling on her parents for help in an emergency in case of hospitalization; a neighbor for fast transport in labor; a friend if she needed someone to listen. On the other hand, she may have great difficulty communicating her needs to anyone or asking for help. She may feel extremely alone, isolated, and helpless.

CULTURE

The cultural context of the family may dictate whether our health care efforts are successful or not. Cultural background, beliefs, and environment play a large part in our lives, though we often do not fully realize the impact. Though it may sound ridiculously simplistic and repetitious, one of the fundamental rules is to assess cultural practices *prior to* planning or implementing interventions. Although this is a simple rule, it is violated many times a day. For example, how often have you heard a nurse or nutritionist "teaching" a client with a low hematocrit about the importance of foods high in iron *before* taking a diet history? Talking about the importance of meat will be wasting time if the client cannot afford or does not believe in eating meat. This energy and time could be much better used in discussing alternative iron sources.

Those clients who believe that everything in their lives should be *natural* may present even more complex problems. In addition to assessing adequate protein intake in a vegetarian diet, the entire health care system approach to this client may need to be evaluated. The client may seek home delivery without aid and may refuse laboratory tests, ultrasonography, amniocentesis, or stress tests during pregnancy. This client seeks care to try to assure a healthy newborn but will only accept those aspects of care that do not violate her or his family's philosophy. To provide care for a high risk client with these limitations is a critical challenge to perinatal professionals.

The nursing approach to assessing a

client's cultural practices is important. The first step is to realize our own cultural biases and to try to be objective in learning about beliefs that differ from our own. When a client sees a look of disbelief or disapproval on a nurse's face, the sharing and trust end. The client truly believes in the cultural heritage that has been practiced for generations and is sincere in these beliefs. Therefore these beliefs are not to be dismissed lightly.

An example of this can be seen in a portion of the black culture in the South; people of this culture still believe in and practice voodoo. Clients who have had a voodoo curse placed on them may seek medical help to try to remove or relieve the effects of this curse. The culture attempts to blend the old and the new. The birth of a premature or ill newborn or an infant with a defect may also be seen by the client as the sign of a curse. When a woman truly believes in this curse, or any other cultural taboo, belief, or ritual, she is likely to be preoccupied with dealing with this and may be resistive to treatment or care.

Nursing assessment, then, must include not only what the client believes but also how the client wishes the situation to be handled. Nurses have to make special efforts to keep communication open and to consider new and perhaps unorthodox ways of providing nursing care. If the client believes that a certain person or thing can remove the curse causing an illness, then that option should be given objective consideration and the potential harm versus benefit weighed. The consideration must always be, What will provide this client optimal opportunity to achieve health?

Religious beliefs are also entwined with culture. A client recently came to our clinic with a history of several previous cesarean births. She related to the staff her belief that God wanted her to have this baby naturally. She was apprised of the medical risks involved, and her answer was that she knew God would take care of her.

This made the staff extremely uncomfortable. A release was signed by the patient stating that she knew the risks involved and that she excused the hospital and staff from responsibility for her decision. The nursing staff continued to work with her and discuss her decision. They did not question her right to make this decision but wished to be sure that she had the knowledge to make it wisely. Although their philosophy differed from hers, the staff felt a commitment to provide this client with the best possible care to try to avoid or prevent the complications that could occur as a result of her beliefs. (She subsequently delivered a healthy newborn with no complications.)

Assessment of the family's cultural practices and attempts to learn and understand these traditions or beliefs communicates to the family the nurse's interest and desire to help. Through this understanding, the nurse can work with the family to select appropriate and acceptable approaches for problem solving.

24 HOURS IN A DAY

It may seem a bit overwhelming when one considers what an in-depth perinatal nursing assessment should include (in addition, of course, to basic medical and nursing history and physical assessment). However, this assessment takes place over time. As the relationship develops, new questions and new areas of discussion arise. During assessment of knowledge about pregnancy or premature infants, nurses also learn of the parents' beliefs and practices. During problem solving, they learn the developmental levels of the parents.

Probably not all areas will be covered with every client. As in all things, nurses must use judgment and set priorities. Often they gather cues in some other areas of assessment that tell them that these areas are not priorities, not problems. Because they may not formally think of this intuitive sorting of cues as assessment and they have not formally recorded these cues, nurses may not realize that these cues are, nonetheless, part of the data base. And it is this data base, both formal and informal, that leads nurses to prioritize problems and begin planning interventions.

Interventions

Once the initial assessment has identified priorities for care, these priorities must be shared and validated with the client/family. Does the client agree with the assessment? Does this assessment reflect the client's greatest concerns and needs? Is the client ready to commit herself to a contract to work on this area at this time?

PROBLEM SOLVING

When this formal or informal contract is made, the exploration of problem-solving interventions can be initiated. The client and the nurse identify whether similar problems have been experienced by the family, how these or the current problem has been handled, and whether the approach was deemed effective.

The nurse may be able to identify strengths this family demonstrates on the basis of her assessment and observations or on the client's description of past experiences. At times it is hard for families to see the positives when everything seems to be "crashing in." Identification and sharing of family strengths may help the family members see themselves and the problem more objectively so that these strengths can be maximized.

One client with cardiac disease, Mrs. A, was beginning her third trimester of pregnancy when her husband presented her with divorce papers. She was devastated and cried continuously. She could not keep food down and lost seven pounds. After one week, she came to the clinic seeking help. In talking with the nurse, Mrs. A. acknowledged that she and her husband had never been close and she was sure that he had had a number of affairs. However, she felt overwhelmed by his leaving at what she considered to be the most crucial time in the pregnancy. She felt she could not make it alone.

After the initial grieving reaction, Mrs. A. reviewed the course of her six-year marriage with the nurse. They had moved four times in that period, as the husband frequently changed jobs. Mrs. A, a secretary, had worked throughout their marriage to help make ends meet. When their first child was born three years before, the husband had disappeared for four months after the birth. This pregnancy was unplanned.

As she explored her past experiences, the client realized that she had always been the strength in the family and had always managed throughout their crises. She depended on her family for her main support and positive reinforcement. This realization did not diminish her grief at losing the person she loved, but it did help her place her life in focus. She knew she could survive this crisis as she had survived others. Her support system was mobilized, and she began utilizing coping mechanisms that would help rebuild her self-esteem. Her family helped her plan for the birth of this child, and for her postpartum life as mother of two with little financial support until she could return to work.

Identification and realization of her own strengths and support systems helped Mrs. A. to utilize these strengths in planning alternatives when faced with the crisis. Some clients, however, are not so fortunate as to have family support systems or "back-up" experiences of being strong in previous crises. These clients may need more help in identifying potential alternatives and outcomes, progressing through the decision-making process, and implementing decisions and plans.

The pregnant diabetic is a good example of a client who needs both long- and short-term help in problem solving. It is ideal if the woman with diabetes seeks medical care prior to conception and can discuss what such a pregnancy will mean. However, this is the exception rather than the rule. At the first visit, whenever that is, her family needs to learn the care involved in a diabetic pregnancy and needs to receive support in planning for potential problems. The diet changes, lab tests, insulin therapy, and possible hospitalizations are realities that need to be considered. Other factors such as distance, lack of transportation, work schedules, and financial limitations will require planning for emergencies. The support and communication patterns in the family may need to be strengthened.

As the nurse helps this family to think through these potential problems, she also helps them identify possible alternatives. To save time, travel, and money, is there a laboratory in their home town that could perform blood glucose tests? Can the husband be taught to administer glucagon at home in an emergency? Can the pregnant woman's coworkers be taught to recognize her characteristic signs of approaching hypoglycemia? What stresses would hospitalization impose, and how could these be handled?

The potential situations are endless. The emphasis is on identification of potential problems and development of realistic plans and alternatives to resolve, or at least decrease the stress of, such problems. The decisions are, of course, to be made by the family. The nurse's responsibility is to see that the family has the appropriate knowledge and support to be able to make intelligent decisions and to realize the outcome of those decisions. Once the decisions are made, the nurse may help implement those plans — such as teaching the husband to recognize hypoglycemia and administer glucagon.

CRISIS

In discussing problem solving, we have already mentioned one client in crisis. Mrs. A. had a readily definable source of her crisis, and therefore interventions were fairly easy to identify.

For a client experiencing a crisis or multiple crises the nurse may need to help the client identify the exact source of the crisis prior to attempts at resolution. Mrs. T., for example, had experienced several crises during her pregnancy. In her second trimester, her father suffered a severe myocardial infarction. Returning from a visit to him in the hospital, she and her husband were involved in a freeway accident, that left her husband with a broken back. He was still in the hospital when she delivered an infant with major cardiac anomalies. The neonatologists informed her that the infant would need immediate surgery. Mrs. T. could not make the decision about the surgery.

When the nurse and physician talked with her, this mother stated that she had been strong for so long and had carried most of her family's burdens that she just could not go through one more battle. She felt unable to decide anything and was still in shock from learning of her infant's diagnosis of cardiac anomalies. She agreed that a decision had to be made, but she could not bring herself to make it. She spoke with her husband on the phone, and he felt it was her decision to make. She notified the physician that she could not decide what was best for the baby and asked that the decision be taken from her hands.

The physicians sought and received a court order authorizing the surgery. The mother was extremely relieved and said that she felt that an "unbearably heavy burden" had been lifted from her shoulders.

The surgery was successful, and Mrs. T. did accept and attach to her infant. The removal of sole responsibility for her infant's surgery was necessary for her to cope with the infant's possible death. In later therapy, it was learned that she felt responsible for her husband's accident and hospitalization and feared both his death and the death of her father. She thus could not withstand the guilt attached to yet another decision that could mean life or death for someone she loved.

This client's crises during and following her pregnancy were exceptionally dramatic, yet crises do occur. Unless nurses take the time to explore the family's *reasons* for their responses — the cause of their crisis — they are likely to "label" the parents and make incorrect assumptions about their parenting attitudes or abilities.

STRESS

Similarly, nurses may need to explore more deeply how some clients adapt to stress in their lives and to utilize and teach stress management techniques that are appropriate and acceptable to each client. As nurses identify clients who are experiencing life stress events, they can ask "How do you handle stress?" or "What do you do to reduce tension?" Often clients come to the clinic describing classic symptoms of stress or tension without realizing the cause.

For any client, relaxation and stress management techniques may be very helpful, but this is especially applicable to clients with medical problems in which stress could be detrimental to their health. A pregnant woman with hypertension, for example, may need to identify those situations that cause her the greatest stress and then learn coping mechanisms that will be effective in reducing that stress.

One client, Mrs. Q., who had multiple high risk factors, including hypertension, recurrent pyelonephritis, and an anatomic defect in the uterus, had to be hospitalized at 28 weeks gestation for the remainder of her pregnancy. Initially, she was concerned about her three children at home and cried frequently, talking about how much she missed them.

Mrs. Q. was a very outgoing patient, and since she could have some limited activity, she soon made up her mind to be the friend of every patient on the unit. She greeted new arrivals, said goodbye to all those being discharged, helped pass out water and juices, and so on.

After a month, her interest in those around her seemed to decline and she began having frequent headaches. She would stay in bed for two days at a time. Her blood pressure began to creep slowly but surely higher. She was having difficulty sleeping.

Her primary nurse from the clinic visited daily, and they discussed her change in behavior and mood and her symptoms of increasing tension. She asked Mrs. Q. if she could identify the cause of the problem or if she knew when it began. She could not identify any specific cause.

The nurse taught Mrs. Q. stress management techniques appropriate for limited activity patients — breathing concentration, relaxation exercises, and imagery. As the nurse left each day, Mrs. Q. would be practicing her stress management techniques.

These techniques did seem to help, and Mrs. Q. began to take more interest in things and to be a bit more active. She still seemed to be withdrawn, however, and so a psychiatric clinical nurse specialist was consulted with the permission of the patient. The clinical specialist was able to help this client work through her feelings about herself and her family, which were the cause of her stress. She continued the stress management exercises and expanded on them with new techniques. Mrs. Q. even began helping other long-term patients practice relaxation and breathing techniques. Her blood pressure stabilized, and the rest of her hospitalization was uneventful.

Unfortunately, there are also times when teaching strategies are *too* effective. One client with hypertension, Miss V., was a member of a commune. Miss V. believed that everything about her pregnancy should be natural. She ate a well-balanced vegetarian diet and looked to be the picture of health. She refused most laboratory procedures and stress and non-stress tests. She did agree to have a serial ultrasound scan performed at 26 weeks.

This client was taught stress management techniques, and she was able to relax very well using these methods. She sought instruction in other methods, such as meditation and yoga, on her own. She continued, however, to have a very high blood pressure reading at each visit, despite all treatments. At 28 weeks, it was becoming dangerous.

Miss V. maintained that her blood pressure was lower at home and rose only on clinic days. An effort was made to decrease the stress of her clinic visits. She was scheduled first, so she would not have to wait. She saw the same nurse and physician each visit and received positive reinforcement from them on weight gain and other signs of progress. Still, her blood pressure was too high. Finally, a public health nurse arranged to stop by her commune several times for "spot" blood pressure checks. To the clinic staff's surprise, the client was correct: her blood pressure *was* significantly lower at home over a two-week period.

Thereafter, this client canceled all clinic visits and never returned. A nurse made a home visit and advised Miss V. again of the staff's interest in her and their concern about the risk of intrauterine growth retardation and the need for medical supervision. She stated she had no problem except when she tried to conform to the "establishment."

Miss V. notified the clinic when, at 41 weeks gestation, she delivered a nine-pound baby girl at home, unassisted. One imagines that she must have managed her stress very well.

PRENATAL ATTACHMENT

Postpartum attachment to a newborn and interventions for follow-up nursing care are discussed in Chapter 10. Often we do not think, however, of enhancing or encouraging attachment in the prenatal period. Since high risk families are "at risk" for parenting problems, perhaps nurses should focus more on this aspect of prenatal care.

It has already been mentioned that the high risk pregnant woman is made to feel very "different" by attending a special clinic, being identified by her diagnosis, and being very cognizant of any threats to her health or that of her fetus. In addition, this client may be placed in the "sick role" as health care personnel focus on the medical complication and its management. Much of the medical attention this client receives is related to her disease, its treatment, and its effect on the fetus. Limitations, rules, regulations and medications prescribed for this client are justified by the words, "It's for the good of the baby." Even though she may want this baby very much, might a mother not begin to resent the imposition this fetus is placing on her life? People are paying more attention to the fetus than to her feelings and needs.

To foster attachment, nurses need to focus on the pregnant woman as a person, not as a vessel with a disease. She may not be ready to deal with this fetus yet. First, nurses need to explore her knowledge and feelings about her medical complication and what care this will entail during the pregnancy. Second, nurses need to deal with other stress or crisis factors in the woman's life at this time (as described earlier in Interventions). She cannot relate to the fetus if she is grieving for a loved one, her husband has just lost his job, or her oldest child just suffered third degree burns in an accident.

When the parents are ready, nurses can begin planning interventions to facilitate adaptation. One of the most important strategies in perinatal nursing care of the high risk family is: Do not forget the *normal* aspects of pregnancy. Nurses need to help this family work through the developmental tasks of pregnancy, especially focusing on recognition of the fact that the woman is carrying a fetus, a separate individual; she will have a *baby*. She is not just a "high risk pregnancy."

Nurses can encourage her to listen to the fetal heartbeat — even with a fetoscope if a doptone is not available. (Using a fetoscope requires some contortions but can usually be accomplished except by the very obese.) This simple intervention is probably one of the most effective ways to begin bonding — and one of the most rewarding. Every mother's face goes through a transformation as she hears her child's heartbeat for the first time.

This is also a good way to begin a discussion of the fetus. Nurses should let parents know that it is normal to think, fantasize, and dream about their baby, and they should encourage the parents to talk about how they think and dream about this infant. What does this baby look like in their dreams? Is it a boy or a girl? Do the parents have a nickname for the baby? If so, this can be noted on the chart and used on successive visits, emphasizing the individuality of this fetus. Nurses also need to assure parents that it is normal to have some fears, bad dreams, and nightmares, and they should encourage them to also share these experiences and feelings.

Throughout the pregnancy with a high risk client, nurses need to remember to explain the normal changes of pregnancy and normal fetal growth and development. Parents love to hear (or better, see pictures) of what their fetus looks like during development.

Parents are encouraged to attend prenatal classes to increase their knowledge and confidence about pregnancy, labor, and delivery. Usually, no one in the class needs to know theirs is a high risk pregnancy, and so they are treated like everyone else and can share experiences and feelings with other couples (the instructor may be informed confidentially about the medical complication).

At the same time that nurses are directing care to meeting the needs of the pregnant woman as a person, they may also gear some interventions toward the specific needs of the baby. They can discuss the mother's basic nutritional needs *and* the need to feed the baby in utero just as she would feed it if it were already born.

One creative nurse, recalled the "Eggbert" cartoons (depicting a remarkably mature fetus in utero talking to his mother), made a large "uterus" and put an Eggbert-like fetus inside it. She asked a pregnant woman to describe what her baby would say about her diet yesterday, and the nurse gave her several examples like, "Mom, you gotta lay off the pizza, I'm getting heartburn!" or "If you eat one more carrot, I'm gonna have x-ray vision!" This helps the mother begin to imagine what her fetus might be thinking or saying if he could talk, making him more like a person; it also focuses on the fact that a pregnant woman's dietary intake affects the fetus; and it is fun for the mother to have permission to fantasize about her fetus!

Thus, nursing interventions have a dual focus — to assess and meet the needs of the pregnant *person* (not the pregnancy), and to help the mother recognize her fetus as an individual (not just the cause for her treatment regimen) so that she may begin the attachment process while the baby is still in utero.

There are families, however, in which these prenatal interventions to foster attachment are not appropriate. In families who have experienced repeated losses, nurses often find a deep fear of being hurt again. These families are afraid to hope. They may experience anticipatory grief before the baby is born. They make no preparations for the baby, demonstrate no nesting behaviors, and are unable to talk about the baby — almost as if they are afraid of "jinxing" their chances if they dare to think positively. With these families, nurses need to accept their behavior and go only at their pace. Their attachment will proceed rapidly when they do have a live infant.

ANTICIPATORY GUIDANCE

The preparation and planning for the new family's transition to parenthood and discharge is almost solely a nursing responsibility. Especially for new parents, this preparation can mean the difference between confidence and total panic when a crisis situation arises in the home setting.

Parents need to be prepared for the additional stresses that will arise with a new infant. Planning during the pregnancy often may be idealistic in terms of what effect a new baby will have on the couple's lives. One hears them saying confidently, "We plan to just take the baby with us wherever we go, so nothing will really change."

Nurses can help families to anticipate how a child *will* affect their lives. If the couple will be going from two incomes to one, for example, they may need to discuss financial planning necessary for a simultaneous decrease in income and increase in expenses.

Although mobility is certainly still possible and encouraged, it will take more planning and preparation time. Also, babies have been known not to cooperate with plans. How would they handle a situation in which the parents and infant are all ready to leave the house on an outing with another family when the baby suddenly starts screaming at the top of his lungs, soils every stitch of clothing he has on, or begins to act as if he is ill? How will the parents deal with such problems and frustrations?

Especially in the postpartum period, it is important to foster confidence in each partner's role as parent of *this* infant. How well does this parent *know* this infant?

Nursing intervention can help the parents to really individualize their child — not just what he *looks* like, but *who* he is. What kind of personality does this infant have? Does he quiet easily? Does he frighten easily? Is he easily awakened by sudden sounds?

Brazelton and Berry (1979) and Affonso (1979) describe ways to help parents understand the unique characteristics of their own child. Knowing these characteristics, parents can understand their infant's responses and plan an environment and care that complements these responses. For example, an infant who startles and awakens easily would not sleep very well if his crib were placed next to a television that was always on. An infant who consoles easily when a parent is visualized might be put in a playpen in a room that is the center of activity, like a kitchen or a family room.

Nurses can help parents realize that there is no right way to parent every child — that because each child is unique, they should determine what will be most effective with *this* infant. The parents need the reassurance that they will soon know their infant and his needs and responses better than anyone.

This confidence in their new role of parent of *this* infant will also help them to deal with role conflicts that may be stressful. Grandparents of the new infant — and sometimes other relatives or friends — may feel a need to instruct the new parent on how to best care for the child. If their well-meaning advice is in agreement with the parents' beliefs, all goes well. However, if there is disagreement, family arguments or strained family relationships may begin.

If a parent is confident in the role of knowing and being able to care for this infant, it is much easier to be patient and objective rather than defensive. Parents can listen to advice and simply reply something like, "Thank you, I'll take your advice into consideration as I make my decisions on what is best for Tommy."

Thinking through some of these potential crisis situations can help parents prevent or deal with problems more effectively. Another potential role conflict to discuss with the couple is the possible conflict *between* parents. Not only just disagreements about what to do in any given situation but also conflicting feelings. What if the father feels left out, jealous of the mother-infant pair, anxious to return to "what it was like before." Could he express his feelings? What if the mother begins to feel closed in, resentful of a world of diapers and formula, tired, and in need of adult intellectual stimulation? How would she handle it? What parts of the childrearing will be shared, and what parts will *not* be shared between parents?

Sibling rivalry can also be a shock unless parents are expecting it. Although the three-year-old may very well be excited about the new baby, new babies get tiresome for three-year-olds faster than broken toys at Christmas. Parents need to understand that some feelings of jealousy are normal, as are some regressive behaviors. They need to consider how they will handle these situations *before* they are caught unprepared and react without thinking.

On the positive side, parents need to think through ways to make the older siblings still feel very special. Parents have shared with me these ideas for dealing with sibling rivalry:

> Having the father carry the new baby into the house so mother is free to greet older children with hugs and kisses, and "introduce them" to the new baby. Dad's been there all week, anyway, so the children aren't as likely to be jealous of him holding the new baby. This also prevents Mom's first words from being: "Watch out! Be careful! Don't hurt the baby!!"

> Bring the older children some kind of memento to show them "Mommy's been thinking about you and missing you." It

could be as simple as little paper medicine cups or, well planned before delivery, a prebought toy or book.

Plan some time each day that is just for the older child, and he or she can choose the activity to do during that time.

Put a sign on the door to remind friends to "say 'Hi' to Sally first before rushing directly to the new baby." If the child is old enough, he or she may enjoy having the job of "taking everyone to see" the new baby brother or sister.

Include older children in the care of the infant and/or provide a doll so they can pretend.

Make baby feeding time also "story time." This makes it special and anticipated by the older children too, rather than the time solely devoted to the baby. The newborn will have the voice stimulation he needs as well.

There are many other ideas, but these suggestions from experienced mothers are among my favorites. So, when exploring the parents' plans for handling sibling rivalry, nurses should discuss these ideas and others. In a four-bed room in a hospital, the suggestions, anecdotes, and questions are soon flying.

In addition to anticipatory guidance about potential stresses and role conflicts, parents also need education about health maintenance — for the mother, the newborn, and the marriage. The mother should be taught proper care of herself postpartum including nutrition and contraception. Any restrictions of her activity should be discussed and the rationale explained — e.g., many post-cesarean mothers could not understand why their physicians told them not to drive a car. When they understood that postoperative patients guard against pain — not making any fast or jerky movement — and that this increased response time could cause an accident, they were much more willing to comply with the physician's orders.

The mother should also know what is normal and abnormal behavior in her infant and what signs indicate that she should call her physician. Similarly (in addition to "normal" newborn care), she

should be taught signs of infant illness and basic skills in emergencies: how to take the infant's temperature, how to help him if he is choking or regurgitating, etc. The parents can demonstrate these skills prior to discharge on a "practice run" to increase their confidence in case they have further questions.

Couples are very conscious of their new role as parents, and most partners have a sincere desire — sometimes ranging to obsession — to be a "good parent." Parenting consumes most of their time, energy, and attention. Parents need to know that their marriage relationship needs and deserves some time, energy, and attention also. They still need to be able to communicate with one another as husband and wife (or significant others). They need some time alone, away from the house and their child.

Some physicians include on their postpartum instruction sheets orders for the parents to "go out without the baby for an evening alone together within four weeks after delivery," and some add, "and at least once per month following." The physicians emphasize this verbally to both parents prior to discharge.

Parents may say, "But we can't afford a baby sitter." Again, they may need help in problem solving to find a relative, neighbor, friend, or another couple with a child with whom they could take turns going out and sitting for each other.

In addition to taking time out to keep their marriage healthy, parents also need to know about keeping their sanity. Some days they will wonder why they ever decided to have a baby. One mother reported reading an article in a woman's magazine suggesting an idea that she immediately adopted: two women, both parents of three children, arranged with each other for what they called "panic days." When one of them had absolutely *had it* with motherhood and the walls were closing in, she would give the other a call, take her children to her friend's house, and take a "mental health day." She would do something just for herself that afternoon. Her friend (the one keeping the kids), would also prepare a casserole for supper. At the end of the afternoon, the revitalized mother would pick up her children and her casserole supper and return home. And, of course, she would be prepared to do the same thing when she received the call for help.

The mother who described this system to me said, "You know, we don't even use it that often — but it just helps your whole attitude to know you *could* take today off if you wanted to. That way, you save it up and just kind of bask in the knowledge that it's there until you really need it!"

Thus, there are a lot of creative ways to help parents care for themselves as persons and as partners. Nurses need to emphasize to couples as never before the vital part that *communication* plays in both their parenting and their continuing partnership as a couple. This is caring for the *family*.

EDUCATION FOR PERINATAL AND NEONATAL NURSING

The rapid changes that have occurred in perinatal and neonatal nursing require nurses to continually update their knowledge and skills. Some nurses choose self-study and participation in continuing education programs; others may elect graduate education leading to a master's degree with a major in perinatal or neonatal nursing.

Continuing education includes not only seminars and lectures but also short courses that offer participants opportunities for guided clinical practice, library research, and classroom discussion. The North Carolina Perinatal Nursing Education Program is an example of this type of continuing education. Two modules were offered in 1979: a two-week course in ambulatory prenatal care for nurses in high risk clinics throughout the state of North Carolina and a three-week course in neonatal nursing care for nurses from community hospitals. The course was offered at Bowman Gray School of Medicine; funding was provided by the Department of Human Resources for salaries,

educational materials, and stipends to help defray the participants' costs. Only four to five nurses are accepted into the program at one time to allow the instructor to individualize the program to best meet the needs of each nurse in her own practice setting. All participants identify those areas of their practice that they would like to change and plan strategies for both change and the continuing education of colleagues in their home agencies. Follow-up evaluation indicates that changes do occur.

Other types of programs have been developed in which a nurse consultant is available to community hospitals and health agencies to provide clinical and classroom instruction. In addition, a wide variety of study guides and audiovisual resources have been developed throughout the nation to supplement continuing education.

SUMMARY

Perinatal nursing is one of the most exciting specialties today. It encompasses prenatal, intrapartum, postpartum, and neonatal fields. The challenges in working with families throughout the childbearing cycle offer opportunities for the nurse to promote positive adaptation to pregnancy, birth, and new roles in the family unit.

To provide effective perinatal care, the nurse must conduct a thorough assessment, validate her findings, and plan interventions with the help of clients and families. Evaluating that care and devising new and creative alternative approaches are essential.

The role of the perinatal nurse involves *advocacy* for clients and their families. This is necessary to individualize and personalize the health care delivery system to meet the needs of each client. It also means that this advocacy will attempt to assure that the expectations of the client/family are realistic.

Perinatal nursing requires *collaboration* with many other professionals and services. The perinatal nurse must interact with those other health care delivery components to assure the client quality care. This collaboration involves effective communication with the other members of the health care team. The client's written record needs to have clear documentation of plans, interventions, progress, consultation, etc.

Also, perinatal nursing requires thoughtful and collaborative planning for *continuity of care*. As mentioned before, the client does not exist in a vacuum. Therefore, nurses need to communicate with local health care providers — physician, office nurse, public health nurse — whoever referred the client or whomever the client is being referred to. Nurses need to share assessments, approaches, current needs, and long-term plans.

Although the regionalization plans and programs have had their share of problems, they have also had phenomenal successes. Perinatal nurses continue to play an important role in seeking and providing educational offerings in regional programs, being patient advocates in regionalization planning, and providing the link between the referring care setting and the tertiary care setting.

Finally, perinatal nursing is beginning to realize the vast potential of research to determine causes of infant morbidity and mortality and to test preventive interventions. Nurses could test, for example, whether or not maternal nutrition, weight gain and health maintenance could be significantly altered to affect fetal/neonatal outcome. Nursing needs to focus on research to help plan effective care for the future.

Just as perinatology is a new and developing field, perinatal nursing is just beginning to be recognized as the new and innovative specialty area in nursing — the *bridge* between maternal and child nursing. Perhaps it is the "bridge over troubled water," which makes the path less difficult.

Bibliography

Affonso, D. D.: Psychosocial concepts. *In* Childbearing: A Nursing Perspective, 2nd Edition. A. L. Clark and D. D. Affonso with T. R. Harris (eds.). Philadelphia: F. A. Davis, 1979, pp. 640–654.

American Hospital Association: The pregnant patient's bill of rights. MCN March/April:137–138, 1977.

Aure, B., Schneider, J. M.: Transforming a community hospital nursing service into a regional center. Nurs Clin. North Am 10(2):275–284, 1975.

Brazelton, T. B.: Behavioral assessment of the neonate. *In* Childbearing: A Nursing Perspective, 2nd Edition. A. L. Clark and D. D. Affonso with T. R. Harris (eds.). Philadelphia: F. A. Davis, 1979, pp. 633–640.

Callon, H. F.: Regionalizing perinatal care in Wisconsin. Nurs Clin North Am 10(2):263–274, 1975.

Galloway, K. G.: The uncertainty and stress of high risk pregnancy. MCN 1(5): 294–299, 1976.

Holmes, T. H., Masuda, M.: Psychosomatic syndrome. Psychol Today 5(11):71–106, 1971.

Holmes, T. H., Rahe, R. H.: The social readjustment rating scale. J Psychosom Res 11:213–218, 1967.

Mercer, R. T.: Nursing Care for Parents at Risk. Thorofare, N.J.: Charles B. Slack, 1977, pp. 4–5.

Messick, J. M., Aguilera, D. C.: Crisis. *In* Childbearing: A Nursing Perspective, 2nd Edition. A. L. Clark and D. D. Affonso with T. R. Harris (eds.). Philadelphia: F. A. Davis, 1979, pp. 89–93.

Pfeiffer, E. F., Kerner, W., Beischer, W.: Substitution of islet cell function by mechanical device: extracorporeal artificial pancreas. Adv Exper Med Biol 119:501–508, 1979.

Schneider, J. M., Ziegel, E., Patteson, D. M.: Education of the perinatal nurse clinician. Nurs Clin North Am 10(2):285–291, 1975.

INDEX

Note: Page numbers in *italics* represent illustrations; page numbers followed by t represent tables.

347

Birth (*Continued*)
  multiple gestation and problem(s) in, 92
  mylenization after, 166
  need for warmth after, 94–95
  physiological changes at, 109–114
Birth crisis, attachment and, 287–288
  parental reaction in, 289–290, 291t
  preventive intervention for, 288
  secondary intervention for, 288–291
Birth day, 19
Birth injury, diabetes mellitus and, 50
Birth weight, maternal smoking and, 49–50
Blastocyst, 2, *3*
Bleeding, intestinal, 142t, 143–144
Blindness, from ophthalmia neonatorum, 96–97
Blood, changes in, at birth, 113
  development of retinal supply of, 187–188, *187*
  fetal, production of, 16–17
    in bone marrow, 113
    sampling of, by fetoscopy, 66
    from scalp, 85–86, *86*
    sampling of, in oxygenation assessment, 180–181
Blood clotting factor(s), synthesis in liver of, 112
Blood culture, as sign of infection, 202t, 203
Blood group incompatibility, 52–55
Blood perfusion, in high risk newborn, 196–198, 197t
Blood pressure(s), mean, 197, 197t
Blood volume, problem(s) of, 196–198, 197t
Body measurement(s), relation to gestational age of, 101–102, *102*
Bone marrow, blood production in, 113
Boric acid, as environmental hazard, 154
Bottle caries, *257*, 258, *258*
Bottle-feeding, anatomy of, 249, *250*
  caries from, *257*, 258, *258*
  maternal characteristics in, 242–243, 242t
  schedule(s) for, 257
  support for mother in, 255–257
Bottle mouth, *257*, 258, *258*
Bowel sound(s), 140, 140t
  in thoracic cavity, 125
Brachial plexus, injuries to, from forceps delivery, 92
Bradycardia, fetal, 80, 80t, *81*
Brazelton neonatal assessment scale, and infant stimulation, 226
Breakage, chromosomal, 34
Breast(s), engorgement of, during breast-feeding, 251–252, *251*
  in newborn, 139–140, 139t
  sore nipple(s) and, 251, *251*
  lactating, 246, *247*
  massage of, 255
Breast-feeding, 240, 240t, 241t, 242–243
  anatomy of, 246–247, *247*, *249*, *250*
  and drainage of colostrum, 248, 249
  and excretion of drug(s), 252t, 253t, 254

Breast-feeding (*Continued*)
  and hypernatremic dehydration, 253–254
  and mastitis, 252–253
  breast engorgement during, 251–252, *251*
  first feeding in, 248–249
  hand expression and, 255
  incidence of, 240–241t
  induced lactation for, 263–264
  jaundice and, 131–132
  maternal characteristics in, 242–243, 242t
  preterm infant(s) and, 261–264
  problem(s) of, 250–254, *251*, 252t, 253t
  procedure in, 248–250, *249*, *250*
  schedule(s) for, 257
  sore nipple(s) during, 250–251
  support for mother in, 254–255
Breast nodule, gestational age and, 99
Breast pump, 261–263
Breath sound(s), in newborn, 124–125, 124t
Breathing, assisted, in resuscitation, 106, *106*
Breech position, 90–92, *91*
Bronchopulmonary dysplasia (BPD), from oxygen therapy, 187, 188
Broussard, E., and Neonatal Perception Inventory, 283, *284–185*
Brown fat, 17
  in newborn, 173
Brushfield's spot(s), 134, 134t
Bulbis cordis, 10, *11*

Calcium metabolism, at birth, 114
Caloric requirement(s), of newborn, 240
Calories, supplementation of, during pregnancy, 48–49, 48t
Caput succedaneum, 132t, 133, *133*
Carbohydrate(s), in commercial formula(s), 236–237t
  in human vs. cow's milk, 243
  requirement(s) of, 235, 236–237t, 238
Carcinoma, maternal, 52
Cardiac catheterization, 208–209
Cardiomegaly, 123–124, 123t
Cardiovascular system. See *Circulation.*
Carditis, rheumatic, maternal, and breast-feeding, 252
Care, of newborn, 151–162
  immediately after birth, 93–102
  Leboyer approach to, 93
  meeting physical need(s), 151–153
  parent education in, 156–163
  preoperative, 210–211, *212*
  protection from environmental hazard(s), 153–155
  recognition of illness in, 155–156
Caries, bottle, *257*, 258, *258*
Cartilage, of ear, gestational age and, 99
Casein, in human vs. cow's milk, 236–237t, 243
Cataract, congenital, 135, *135*
Catheterization, cardiac, 208–209
  umbilical artery, for fluid therapy, 234–235

Middle Eastern people(s), cultural
belief(s) of, 311–313
Milia, 126, 126t
Milk, environmental contamination of,
273–274
  human, composition of, 236–237t
    excretion of drug(s) in, 252t, 253t,
    254
    for preterm infant(s), 259–260, 260t,
    261
    hand expression of, 255
      and contamination, 260–261
    immunological factors in, 244, 245t,
    246
    induced lactation of, 263–264
    storage of, 263
    vs. cow's, 243–244, 246
      casein in, 236–237t, 243
      lactalbumin in, 236–237t, 243
Mineral(s), in human vs. cow's milk,
244
  requirement(s) of, 239–240, 239
Miscarriage, general anesthesia and, 44,
45t
  risk of, in amniocentesis, 64–65
Mitosis, 23–24, 24–26
Molding, of newborn's head, 132, 132t
Mongolian spot(s), 126, 126t
Monitoring, fetal. See Fetal monitoring.
  of fetal heart rate. See Fetal heart rate,
  monitoring of.
  of uterine contraction(s), 84–85, 85
Moro reflex, 145, 145, 146t
Morphine, use of, during labor, 89
Mortality, Apgar score and, 94
Mortality rate(s), infant, 329, 330, 331t,
332t
Morula, 2, 3
Mosaicism, chromosomal, 33
Mother, age of, effect on fetus of, 55–56
  anemia in, 60
    clay eating and, 45–46
  assessment of. See Fetal assessment.
  blood group incompatibility in, 52–55
  body of, as fetal environment, 50–56
    See also Development, fetal and
    Teratogen(s).
  bottle-feeding, characteristics of,
  242–243, 242t
    support for, 255–257
  breast-feeding, characteristics of,
  242–243, 242t
    drug(s) and, 252t, 253t, 254
    nephritis in, 252
    rheumatic carditis in, 252
    support for, 254–255
  deprivation by, 273
  diabetes mellitus in. See Diabetes
  mellitus, maternal.
  disease(s) of, effect on fetus of, 50–52
  drug(s) in, effect on fetus of, 42–45
  drug addiction in, effect on fetus of,
  216–217, 217t. See also Drug(s).
  fetal monitoring in, 86–88, 87t, 88t
  hormone(s) in, effect on fetus of,
  42–44
  hyperparathyroidism in, effect on
  neonatal metabolism of, 114
  infant contact and attachment in,
  281–282

Mother (Continued)
  infection in, effect on fetus of, 38–42,
  52
  medical history of, importance of, 152
  neonatal infection and factor(s) in,
  153
  nutrition for. See Nutrition, maternal.
  obstetrical condition(s) in, 56–60
  postpartum attachment, and
  characteristics of, 282–286, 284–285
  smoking in, and birth weight, 49–50
  stress in, as teratogen, 60–61
Mothering, disorder(s) of, 278
Motor maturity, effect of obstetrical
anesthesia on, 90
Mouth, of newborn, 137–138, 137t
Movement, fetal, and abruptio
  placentae, 86
  assessment of, 72–73
  during labor, 86
  to quiet infant, 224
Mucus, excessive, 137t, 138
  in tracheoesophageal fistula, 212
Multiple gestation, birth problem(s) in,
92. See also Twin(s).
Multiple sclerosis, maternal, 52
Multiple stimuli, effect on preterm
infant(s) of, 225–226
Murmur, of heart, with patent ductus
arteriosus, 205
Muscle(s), abdominal, congenital
  absence of, 140t, 141
  fetal development of, 8
  for breast- and bottle-feeding, 249,
  250
  paralysis of, during ventilation, 186
Muscle tone, 121, 121t
  Apgar scoring method of, 94, 94t
  as sign of neuromuscular maturity,
  98, 100
Myelinization, after birth, 166
Myelomeningocele, 141

Naloxone, for drug-related respiratory
depression, 89, 104, 106, 107t
Narcan, for drug-related respiratory
depression, 89, 103
Narcotics. See Drug(s).
Nasal flaring, 124–125, 124t
Nasojejunal feeding, 265, 266t, 267
Natural childbirth, and counterculture,
314–315
  fetal monitoring and, 87
  Leboyer approach to, 93
Neck righting reflex, 146t
Necrotizing enterocolitis (NEC), feeding
in, 244, 270, 270t
Neonatal Perception Inventory, 283,
284–285
Nephritis, maternal, and breast-feeding,
252
Nervous system, fetal development of, 8
Neural tube defect(s) (NTD), 65–66
Neurological impairment, of newborn,
from obstetrical drug(s), 90
Neuromuscular maturity, gestational
age, and, 98–99, 100–101, 100, 101
Neuron(s), myelinization of, after birth,
166

Nevus flammeus, 127, *127*
Nevus vasculosus, 127–128, *128*
Newborn, acidosis in, at birth, 113–114, 114t. See also *Infant.*
  antibiotics toxic to, 204
  auscultation of, 122–125, 123t, 124t
  bathing of, 158–159
  breast engorgement in, 139–140, 139t
  breath sound(s) in, 124–25, 124t
  brown fat in, 173
  care of. See *Care, of newborn.*
  characteristics of, physical, 121–145.
      See also specific area such as
      Eye(s) and *Heart.*
      external, assessment of, 98–100, *99*
      sensory, 145–149, 146–147t
  circulation in, *111*
    persistent fetal, 206
  circumcision of, 142, 160–163
  cleanliness of, 158–159
  clothing for, 159–160
  conjunctivitis in, 136
  cultural belief(s) and, 297, 322. See
    also *Cultural belief(s).*
  development of, effect of Leboyer
      method on, 93
    pattern(s) of, 157, 157t
  during labor and delivery, 77–114
  fluid balance in, 231–235
  high risk. See *High risk newborn.*
  hyperflexibility in, 121
  hypotension in, 196–197, 197t
  hypotonia in, 121
  identification of, after delivery, 95–96, 152
  illness in, recognition of, 154–156
  inclusion conjunctivitis in, 42
  jitteriness in, 122, 122t
  metabolism of, 114, 231
  nutrition of. See *Nutrition, neonatal.*
  obstetrical anesthesia and, 88–90
  passive drug addiction in, 217t
  physical need(s) of, 151–153
  reflex(es) of, 144–145, *145*, 146–147t
  respiratory distress in, 124–125
  resuscitation of, 102–108
  safety for, 158, 158t
  sensory system of, 145, 148–149
  state(s) of, 116–121, 116t
  stimulation of, Brazelton neonatal
      assessment scale and, 226. See also
      Stimulation.
  surgery in, 210–216
  thermoregulation in. See *Heat* and
      Thermoregulation.
Nipple(s), sore, during breast-feeding, 250–251, *251*
Nitrofurantoin, as teratogen, 44
Noise, sudden, newborn's response to, 136t, 137
Nomogram, Siggaard-Andersen, 194, *195*
Nondisjunction, chromosomal, 30, *30*, 34
Nonshivering thermogenesis, 95, 173
Nonstress test (NST), fetal activity and, 82
  for fetal heart rate monitoring, 70–72, 70t, *72*

Nonstress test (NST) (*Continued*)
  preeclampsia and, 60
Norepinephrine, release of, and heat production, 173
Nuchal cord, and deceleration of fetal heart rate, 82, 83t
Nucleotide, 21
Nurse(s), and assessment of cultural belief(s), 318–322, 319t, 336–337
  and crisis intervention, 339
  and family assessment, 333–338
  and intervention(s) for family, 338–345
  and prenatal attachment, 341–345
  and role assessment, 335–336
  anticipatory guidance for family by, 342–345
  consumer power and, 326–327
  education for, 345–346
  grief process in, 293–294, 293t
  intervention(s) for infection and, 203–204, 204t
  problem(s) of, 329–333, *330*, 331t, 332t
  problem solving and, 338–339
Nursery, infection in, prevention of, 153–154
Nursing bottle syndrome, *257, 258, 258*
Nursing care, for apnea of prematurity, 191–192, 191t, 192t
  for high risk newborn, 165–166
  for infant(s) on ventilator, 184–186, 185t
  for preterm infant(s), sensory stimulation and, 226–228
  neonatal state(s) and, 119–120
  regionalization of, 327–328
  technology of, 325–326
Nutrition, adolescent mother and, 55
  for preterm infant(s), 261
  maternal, effect on fetal growth of, 47–49, 47t, 48t, 49t, 102
  neonatal, calorie requirement(s) in, 240
    carbohydrate requirement(s) in, 235, 236–237t, 238
    deprivation of, 272–273
    fat requirement(s) in, 238
    mineral requirement(s) in, 239–240, *239*
    protein requirement(s) in, 235
    vitamin requirement(s) in, 152, 238–239

Obstetrical abnormalities, effect on fetus of, 56–60
Obstetrical anesthesia, effect on newborn of, 88–90
Obstruction, intestinal, 142t, 143, 214–215
Omphalocele, 14, 214
  detection by ultrasound of, 69
Ophthalmia neonatorum, 136
  prevention of, 96–97
Oral contraceptive(s), as teratogen, 43
Organ(s), internal, exposed, during transport, 223t
Organochlorine compound(s), milk and, 274

…

Therapeutic abortion, legal aspect(s) of, 75–76. See also *Pregnancy, termination of*.
  moral aspect(s) of, 75–76
Thermogenesis, nonshivering, 95, 173
Thermoneutral environment, 170–173, 171t
  during resuscitation, 108
  incubator as, 170, 172
  temperature of, by gestational age, 171t
Thermoregulation, during transport of high risk newborn, 219, 220t. See also *Heat* and *Warmth*.
  in preoperative neonatal care, 210–211, *212*
  in preterm infant(s), 170–176
  in SGA infant(s), 177, 177t
Thiazide diuretic(s), as teratogen, 43
Thoracic cavity, bowel sound(s) in, 125
Thrush, 137–138, 137t, *139*
Thyroid disease, maternal, 52
Thyroid dysgenesis, 156
Tissue(s), germ layer origin of, 6–7, 7t
  granulation, 140, 140t
Tocography, external, 85
Tonic neck reflex, 146t
TORCH disease(s), 38–42
Touch, in newborn, 149
Toxemia, in multiple gestation, 92
  maternal, effect on fetal growth of, 102
Toxic erythema, 126t, 127
Toxoplasmosis, maternal, 38–39
Trachea, fetal development of, 8, *8*
Tracheoesophageal fistula, 138, 212–214, *212*
  and distended abdomen, 141
  during transport, 222t
  feeding after repair of, 267
Traction response, 147t
Tranquilizer(s), as teratogen, 43
  use of, during labor, 89
Transcutaneous oxygen electrode, 180, 181–182, *182*
Transcutaneous oxygen monitor, 180, 181–182, *181*
Transfusion, exchange, for hyperbilirubinemia, 200–201
  intrauterine, legal aspects of, 76
Transient hypoxia, early deceleration from, 82
Transient tachypnea, 109, 124t, 125
Transillumination, to detect pneumothorax, 189, *189*
Translocation, chromosomal, 30–32
Transport, of high risk newborn, 217–222, 222t
  equipment for, 219, 220t
  resuscitation for, 218
  stabilization for, 218–219
  thermoregulation for, 219, 220t
  ventilation for, 220t, 221
  vital sign(s) during, 220t
Transposition of great vessel(s), 207, *207*
Transverse crease(s), on sole of foot, gestational age and, 99, *99*
Transverse position, 92, *92*
Trauma, need for resuscitation with, 103
Tremors, 121–122, 121t

Tricuspid atresia, 207
Trimethadione, as teratogen, 42
Trisomy 18, 32–33, *33*
Trisomy 21, 30–32, *31–32*
  age of mother and, 56
  detection of, by amniocentesis, 66
Trophoblast, 2, *3*
Truncus arteriosus, 10, *11*
Tube, chest, for tracheoesophageal fistula, 213
  gastrostomy, feeding infant by, 267
  neural. See *Neural tube*.
Tuberculosis, maternal, 52
  and breast-feeding, 252
Turner's syndrome, 33–34, *34*
Twin(s), 24
Type I alveolar cell(s), 168, 179–180
Type II alveolar cell(s), 168, 179–180

Ultrasonography, amniocentesis and, 64
  Doppler, fetal heart rate monitoring by, 84
  fetal assessment by, 66–70, *67–69*, 69t
  fetoscopy and, 66
  gray scale (B-scan), 66–69, 69t
  real time, 66–69, *67–68*, 69t
  risk(s) of, 69–70
Umbilical artery catheterization, for fluid therapy, 234–235
Umbilical cord, 6, 140, 140t
  compression of, *81*, 82
Umbilical vessel(s), after birth, *110*, *111*, 112t
  number of, 152
Underdevelopment, of heart, 206–207
Undernutrition, 273
Urinary tract infection, maternal, 52
Urine, 142, 142t
  as water loss, 232, 233t
Uteroplacental insufficiency (UPI), late deceleration from, *81*, 82
Uterus, birth contractions of, fetal heart rate and, 80, 82, 83t
  monitoring of, 84–85, *85*
  fertilization in, 1–4, *2–3*
  position of fetus in, abnormal, 90–92, *91*, *92*
  change(s) in, during delivery, *78–79*
Utilitarian theory of family, 301–303, *302*

Vaccine, as teratogen, 43
Vaginal discharge, in newborn, 141, 141t
Valium, as teratogen, 43
  use of, during labor, 89
Variable deceleration pattern, of fetal heart rate, *81*, 82, 83t
Vascular disease, maternal, effect on fetal growth of, 102
Vasoconstriction, and heart retention, 95
Venereal disease, fetal, 39–40, 41
Ventilation, assisted, in resuscitation, 106, *106*
  nursing care during, 184–186, 185t
  CPT during, 186, *186*